Handbook of Laboratory Animal Science

Volume II

Animal Models

Handbook of Laboratory Animal Science

Volume II

Animal Models

Edited by
Per Svendsen and Jann Hau

CRC Press
Boca Raton   Ann Arbor   London   Tokyo

Library of Congress Cataloging-in-Publication Data

Handbook of laboratory animal science / edited by Per Svendsen, Jann
   Hau.
       p. cm.
    Includes bibliographical references and indexes.
    Contents: v. 1. Selection and handling of animals in biomedical
research -- v. 2. Animal models.
    ISBN 0-8493-4378-X (v. 1). -- ISBN 0-8493-4390-9 (v. 2)
    1. Laboratory animals. 2. Animal experimentation. 3. Animal
models in research. I. Svendsen, Per. II. Hau, Jann.
QL55.H36 1994
599′.00724—dc20   93-39121
                                                          CIP

© 1994 by CRC Press, Inc.

No claim to original U.S. Government works
International Standard Book Number 0-8493-4390-9
Library of Congress Card Number 93-39121
Printed in the United States of America   4 5 6 7 8 9 0
Printed on acid-free paper

PREFACE

The *Handbook of Laboratory Animal Science, Volume II: Animal Models* is dedicated to the use of laboratory animals as models for humans. This book explains in great detail the comparative considerations underlying the choice of animal species and strains in different research disciplines. Volume II consists of chapters authored by predominantly Scandinavian experts and covers a wide range of scientific areas. Unlike many other publications, this book is not restricted to laboratory animal models for the study of human disease. It takes a wider approach, which is in accordance with modern interpretation of the animal model concept.

Most of our knowledge of human biology is derived from animal studies and fortunately the conservative nature of animal evolution often renders reliable extrapolation between species the rule rather than the exception. However, we felt that there is a great need for a handbook on the choice of animal species and strains in different areas of biomedical research that are focused on the relevant comparative aspects in the many different contexts in which animals are used.

The authors have, in many instances, included the most recent research information available as well as generally recognized facts to make the book relevant and attractive to other specialists. Reporting from the cutting edge of a scientific discipline involves including some, but obviously not all, of the most recently reported findings. This selection will invariably make some scientists feel that their results have been neglected, and for this we apologize. The editors welcome comments from readers and colleagues that will allow us to keep the text up to date and correct errors.

Both volumes of the *Handbook of Laboratory Animal Science* are, in many ways, very technical books. We hope our readers will find them useful whether they be postgraduate students not familiar with laboratory animal science or experienced scientists looking for an overview and reference text of the large and heterogenous area of laboratory animal science.

Per Svendsen
Biomedical Laboratory
Odense University
Odense, Denmark

Jann Hau
Laboratory Animal Science and Welfare
The Royal Veterinary College
London, United Kindom

THE EDITORS

Per Svendsen is Associate Professor in Laboratory Animal Science and Head of the Biomedical Laboratory of the Medical Faculty, University of Odense, Denmark.

Dr. Svendsen graduated in veterinary medicine from The Royal Veterinary and Agricultural University, Copenhagen, Denmark in 1963. Following research fellowships at the Department of Physiology, New York State Veterinary College at Cornell University, where he completed a Masters degree in physiology and surgery, and at the Department of Surgery at the Royal Veterinary and Agricultural University in Copenhagen, he earned his doctorate in ruminant pathophysiology.

In 1970 he joined the Department of Physiology at the University of Nairobi in Kenya, where he taught physiology to veterinary and agriculture students. In 1974 he joined the newly established medical faculty at the University of Odense in Denmark, where he established the Biomedical Laboratory and the centralized laboratory animal facility. From 1987 to 1989, Dr. Svendsen taught surgery at the Faculty of Veterinary Science at Sokoine University of Agriculture in Morogoro, Tanzania.

Dr. Svendsen has published more than 100 scientific papers and chapters in textbooks. He has published textbooks in animal physiology and ethology and, together with Dr. Hau, he published *Forsøgsdyr og dyreforsøg*, a Danish textbook in laboratory animal science.

Dr. Svendsen's current research interests include digestive physiology, mainly concerning pancreatic and hepatic secretions, and fetal physiology.

Jann Hau, Dr. med., is Professor in Laboratory Animal Science and Welfare at The Royal Veterinary College, University of London, UK.

Dr. Hau is a biologist who specialized in laboratory animal science and did his doctorate at The Medical Faculty, University of Odense, Denmark. Following research fellowships at Odense University he joined the Department of Pathology, The Royal Veterinary and Agricultural University (RVAU) in Copenhagen as Associate Professor and Head of the Laboratory Animal Science Unit in 1983. He was later Head of the Department of Pathology and Dean of the Faculty of Animal Husbandry and Veterinary Science at the RVAU.

In 1991 he joined the Royal Veterinary College in London as Professor in the newly established London University Chair in Laboratory Animal Science and Welfare.

Dr. Hau is responsible for the undergraduate and postgraduate teaching in laboratory animal science and welfare which includes a 1-year Master of Science course specialized in Laboratory Animal Science.

Dr. Hau has organized several international meetings on laboratory animal science. He is the editor-in-chief of Scandinavian Journal of Laboratory Animal Science and editor for the laboratory animals section in the journal Animal Welfare. He is a member of a number of laboratory animal science societies including LASA, ScandLAS, and AALAS.

Dr. Hau has published more than 200 scientific papers and chapters in books and, together with Dr. Svendsen, he wrote the first Danish textbook on laboratory animals and animal experiments published in 1981, 1985, and 1989.

Dr. Hau's current research interests include development of laboratory animal models for studies of biological mechanisms in reproductive physiology, and development of methods to assess long-term stress and welfare state in animals. These studies include ethology as well as studies of physiological and immunological changes associated with changes in the welfare of the animal. Dr. Hau has also concentrated on research projects that are focused on ways to replace, reduce, and refine the use of animals in antibody production.

CONTRIBUTORS

Hans Mogens Kerzel Andersen
Institute of Medical Microbiology
University of Aarhus
Aarhus, Denmark

Karsten Buschard
Bartholin Instituttet
Kommunehospitalet
Copenhagen, Denmark

Anthony M. Carter
Department of Physiology
University of Odense
Odense, Denmark

H. Dieperink
Laboratory of Nephropathology
Odense University Hospital
Odense, Denmark

Harry Donnelly
Laboratory Animal Science and Welfare
Royal Veterinary College
London, England

Ida Hageman
Bartholin Instituttet
Kommunehospitalet
Copenhagen, Denmark

Ernst Hansen
Institute of Toxicology
National Food Agency
Søborg, Denmark

Jann Hau
Department of Pathology and Infectious
  Diseases
Royal Veterinary College
London, England

Kjell Hole
Department of Physiology
University of Bergen
Bergen, Norway

Steinar Hunskaar
Department of Public Health
University of Bergen
Bergen, Norway

Henrik Elvang Jensen
Department of Pharmacology and
  Pathobiology
Royal Veterinary and Agricultural
  University
Frederiksberg, Denmark

E. Kemp
Laboratory of Nephropathology
Odense University Hospital
Odense, Denmark

S.T. Lillevang
Laboratory of Nephropathology
Odense University Hospital
Odense, Denmark

Otto Meyer
Institute of Toxicology
National Food Agency
Søborg, Denmark

Jesper Mogensen
Institute of Neuropsychiatry
University of Copenhagen
Copenhagen, Denmark

Timo Nevalainen
National Laboratory Animal Center
University of Kuopio
Kuopio, Finland

Karl Johan Öbrink
BMC
Uppsala, Sweden

Otto Melchior Poulsen
Department of Chemistry and Biochemistry
National Institute of Occupational Health
Copenhagen, Denmark

Andrew N. Rycroft
Department of Pathology and
   Infectious Diseases
Royal Veterinary College
London, England

Jørgen Rygaard
Bartholin Instituttet
Kommunehospitalet
Copenhagen, Denmark

Jörn C.W. Salén
Department of Pathology and Infectious
   Diseases
Royal Veterinary College
London, England

Ove Svendsen
Scantox A/S
Lille Skensved, Denmark

Arne Tjølsen
Department of Physiology
University of Bergen
Bergen, Norway

TABLE OF CONTENTS

Chapter 1

Animal Models — Principles and Problems

Jörn C. W. Salén

CONTENTS

INTRODUCTION

The large-scale use of animals in research began in the early and middle decades of the last century when, mainly in Germany and France, the rapid advances in physiology were made. Since then, experiments on living animals have developed into an essential part of most biomedical research disciplines, such as microbiology, immunology, surgery, oncology, and pharmacology.

The topic of this chapter is not easy: a general introduction to the following chapters on specific "animal models", an explanation of basic principles for the selection and application of models, the problem of extrapolating results obtained from nonhuman models to humans, and finally some thoughts about the philosophy of the subject. The intention is to take a critical look at laboratory animal models as a counterbalance to the naturally prevailing enthusiasm in which some specialists tend to indulge when they are invited to write about their field of expertise. In a time when the use of laboratory animals is receiving more and more critical attention, we must be self-critical as well. The admittance and highlighting of negative aspects from a researcher may be unusual and will presumably provoke countercriticism, but picking up the arguments of the opposition is the key to the improvement and success of biomediocal research and the undermining of future criticism.

THE HISTORY AND PURPOSE OF USING ANIMAL MODELS

The assumption that *Homo sapiens* are identical to other animals in his/her bodily functions has led to a number of errors in the history of medicine. Galen, the Greek physician and philosopher who lived in the 2nd century A.D. and was to become the leading medical authority for many centuries, is believed to be the founder of experimental physiology in the western world. His anatomical research was based almost entirely on studies of apes and pigs. Unhesitatingly he transferred (i.e., extrapolated) his discoveries directly to humans, thus initiating many errors.[1] The combination of Galen's immense authority and the dogmatic prohibition by the Church of postmortem dissections of the human body conserved these errors well into the late 16th century. Galen was later blamed for using the wrong method.[2] A closer look reveals that his mistake was to draw wrong *conclusions* from the results of these first scientific "animal models" because of uncritical interspecies extrapolation.

In 1865, the famous French physiologist Claude Bernard published a book intended to give physicians rules and principles for the study of experimental medicine: *Introduction to Study of Experimental Medicine*.[3] This work advocated the chemical and physical induction of disease in experimental situations, thus leading the way to the "induced animal models" of today's biomedical research. Bernard also emphasized the applicability of animal experiments to humans. The other authority in France who helped establish and popularize laboratory research as well as the experimental use of animals was Louis Pasteur. He and Robert Koch in Germany introduced the concept of specificity into medicine and the "germ theory of disease". Koch's work on cholera and tuberculosis further promoted the use of "animal models" of infectious diseases and was followed by models for the screening and evaluation of new antibacterial drugs in the 20th century. Today, "animal models" are used in virtually every field of biomedical research as reflected in the respective chapters of this book.

THE CONCEPT OF ANIMAL MODELS

WHAT IS AN ANIMAL?

Ethymologically, the word "animal" derives from the latin *anima*, meaning soul/spirit, thus describing living organisms that are *animated*. Although we certainly see ourselves as the superior animated species, there is a curious linguistic and scientific mistake in the distinction between "animals" and "humans", e.g., in the term "animal models of human disease". To imply that our own species is "non-animal" or that there are such creatures as "subhuman" animal species, is contradictory to our standards in language and our findings in zoological and evolutionary research. It would, of course, mean enormous heuristical difficulties to give up this artificial distinction, so we will have to live with this anthropocentric lack of objectivity. However, we must not forget it, particularly when employing extrapolations.

WHAT IS A MODEL?

A model is an *object of imitation*, something that accurately resembles something else, a person or thing that is the likeness or *image* of another.[4] Prometheus, who is feigned by the poets to have first formed Man, formed the model from water and earth and then stole fire from the sun to *animate* the model.[5] Consequently, combining the two definitions, an "animal model" is an *animated object of imitation*, an "image of Man" (or other species), used to investigate a physio- or pathological circumstance in question.

The U.S. National Research Committee on Animal Models for Research on Aging attempted to define the term "laboratory animal model" as "an animal model in which normative biology or behavior can be studied, or in which a spontaneous or induced pathological process can be investigated, and in which the phenomenon in one or more respects resembles the same phenomenon in humans or other species of animal". Although true in essence, this definition shows two classical mistakes: by trying to cover everything it becomes unpractically long, and by using the term to be defined as part of the wording ("an animal model in which ...") it defines itself superfluous.

What is very often meant by the term "animal model" is *modeling humans*. It is not the image of the used animal that is the focus of research but the analogy of the physiological behavior of this animal to our own (or another) species. It would, thus, be more correct to speak of "human models" in this context. "Laboratory animal science" and "animal experiments" are indeed much more about humans than about any other "animal" species.

THE APPLICATION OF ANIMAL MODELS

TYPES OF ANIMAL MODELS

As 150 years ago, the majority of laboratory animal models are developed and used to study the cause, nature, and cure of human disorders. Usually it is distinguished in the literature between four groups of animal models: induced, spontaneous, negative, and orphan models. The two first categories are by far the most important.

As the name implies, *induced models* are images in which the condition to be investigated is experimentally induced, e.g., the induction of diabetes mellitus with alloxan or partial hepatectomy to study liver regeneration. The induced model is the only category that theoretically allows a free choice of species. Although one might be tempted to presume that extrapolation from a species is better the closer this species resembles humans, phylogenetical closeness (as fulfilled by primate models) is not a guarantee for validity of extrapolation, as the unsuccessful chimpanzee models in AIDS research have demonstrated.[6]

It is just as decisive that the pathology and outcome of an induced disease or disorder in the tested species resembles the respective pathology of the target species. FIV infection in cats may, therefore, be a better model for human AIDS than HIV infection in simians.

A special type of induced disease images that are recently gaining increased popularity are *transgenic* animal models (see Chapter 10). Transgenic animals carry artificially inserted, foreign DNA in their genome. For practical reasons, the preferred species for transgenic models is mice, but other species are now receiving growing interest. The welfare of transgenic animals has to be monitored with extra care as they may develop hitherto unknown disorders or be unable to express signs of distress, conditions that would render their further use in the experiment unethical and interfere with extrapolation.

Spontaneous animal models of human disease utilize naturally occurring genetical variants. Many hundreds of strains/stocks with such inherited diseases, modeling similar conditions in humans, have been characterized and conserved. A famous example of a natural mutant model is the nude mouse, which meant a turning point in the study of heterotransplanted tumors and, e.g., enabled the first description of natural killer cells. The advantages/options of the nude mouse as an athymic animal model were relatively quickly realized by the research community, whereas the nude (athymic) rat was known for almost 20 years before it was allowed into the immunology laboratories.[7]

Almost the opposite of spontaneous and induced images are *negative* models in which a particular disease does *not* develop, e.g., gonococcal infection in rabbits. Negative models also include animals demonstrating a lack of reactivity to a particular stimulus. Their main application is studies on the mechanism of resistance to gain insight into its physiological basis.

The fourth term used to categorize animal models is the *orphan model*. An orphan model disease simply describes a condition that occurs naturally in a nonhuman species but has not yet been described in humans, and which is "adopted" when a similar human disease is later identified. Examples are Marek's disease, Papillomatosis, and bovine spongiform encephalopathy (BSE), the so-called "mad cow disease".

CHOOSING THE RIGHT MODEL

The application of animal models in research is as diverse as the research disciplines themselves. History provides numerous examples that the outcome of scientific experiments is more often unsuccessful than it is successful. Medical research is in no way an exception from this experience, nor are animal experiments, exclusively burdened and justified by the demand of applicability to humans. But often these experiments can only be assessed retrospectively. So, how can the researcher select the most appropriate model to avoid later disappointment — and criticism?

The case of the huge 25-year screening program, undertaken by the prestigious U.S. National Cancer Institute, illustrates the kinds of dilemma possible: in this program 40,000 plant species were tested for anti-tumor activity. Several of the plants proved effective and safe enough in the chosen animal models to justify clinical trials in humans. In the end, none of these drugs was found to be useful for therapy because of too high toxicity or ineffectivity in humans.[8] This means despite 25 years of intensive research and positive results in animal models, not a single antitumor drug emerged from this work. As a consequence, the NCI now uses human cancer cell lines for the screening for cytotoxics.

It is virtually impossible to give specific rules for the choice of the best animal model, because the many considerations that have to be made before an experiment can take place differ with each research project and its objectives. Nevertheless some general rules can be given:

- Is the problem worth investigating/resolving?
- If yes, has the problem already been solved by someone else?
- Could a human model be developed?
- If no, is an animal an appropriate model?
- If yes, is the species to be used an appropriate species for the problem? Has previous unsuccessful research indicated that a particular species might be unsuitable? What helpful conclusions could be drawn from failed research?
- Can genetic and environmental variation be assessed/controlled?
- Can the health status of the animals be controlled over the whole length of the project?
- Can the decision in favor of a particular model be soundly based on scientific arguments or will it largely be overridden by factors such as personal convenience, inadequacy of local facilities, financial, ethical or legal restraints, lack of availability of the species (in contrast, the fact that a species is readily available cannot be considered as a serious criterion for the choice of this species), lack of inter- or innerdepartmental cooperation, and laboratory tradition and convenience (e.g., ease of handling for technicians or experimenters, litter size, breeding success, etc.)?
- Are rates and routes of metabolism of a substance to be tested comparable in the model?

EXTRAPOLATION

PROBLEMS

The prediction of human response is not only one of the most difficult affairs of our daily life, it is also the crucial point that decides success or failure of animal experiments, and is the driving force in numerous scientific and political debates on the overall significance of animal experiments for the health of *Homo sapiens*. Extrapolation of results from experiments on nonhuman species to human beings carries with it enough controversy for decades of research to come.

Uncritical reliance on the results of animal tests can be dangerously misleading and has cost the health and lives of tens of thousands of humans, as in Ciba Geigy's clioquinol scandal, the Opren disaster of Dista Products Ltd., or ICI's Eraldin calamity. Such counteraction in interspecies reactivity is bilateral: what is noxious or ineffective in nonhuman species can be innoxious or effective in humans. For example, penicillin is fatal for guinea pigs but generally well tolerated by human beings; aspirin is teratogenic in cats, dogs, guinea pigs, rats, mice, and monkeys but obviously not in pregnant woman despite frequent consumption.[9] Thalidomide, which crippled 10,000 children, does not cause birth defects in rats[10] or many other species,[11] but does so in primates. The past has repeatedly shown that close phylogenetical relationship or anatomical conformity are not truly reliable features of parallel physiological behavior although this is and may be the case in many instances; however, it is very difficult to predict such conformity.

One of the most commonly used species in toxicology research, the rat, differs substantially from humans: it lacks a gall bladder, is a very effective biliary excretor, displays less efficient plasma binding of drugs, is an obligate nose breather, is nocturnal, and has a different location of the gut flora, different skin characteristics, different hypersensitivity, and different teratogenicity, to name only a few dissimilarities. Rats are consequently considered to be inadequate predicitve models for, e.g., human asthma or bronchitis research,[12] but have nevertheless been extensively used for the experimental study of bronchitis.[13]

The validity of extrapolation is further complicated by the question: to *which humans*? As wishful as it often is to obtain results from a genetically "defined" and "uniform" animal model (inbreds), the humans to whom the results are extrapolated are highly variable outbreds, with striking cultural, dietary, and environmental differences. This may be less important for many disease models but can become significant for pharmacological and toxicological models.

Public views of animal experiments are particularly sensitive to poor quality research including investigators that knowingly or unknowingly care little to select models for their predictive utility to the human condition. Especially quantitative health risk assessments based on animal data from toxicological research are too often performed with the help of biostatistical models that build on the ludicrous assumption that the animal model gives an identical image of the respective human response.[12] To base the extrapolation of results to other species on homology alone cannot be considered appropriate.

SOME GENERAL REQUIREMENTS

So how can the mistakes of the past be avoided and the mentioned difficulties be overcome in the future, if they can be overcome at all? Some vital requirements for verifiable extrapolation are:

- *Taking a plurispecies approach.* Most of the regulating authorities require two species in toxicology screening, one of which has to be non-rodent. This does not necessarily imply that excessive numbers of animals will be used. The uncritical use of one-species models can mean that experimental data retrospectively turn out to be invalid for extrapolation, representing real and complete waste of animals. Using more than one species is of course no guarantee for successful extrapolation, either.

- *Metabolic patterns and speed must match between species.* Drugs and toxins exert their effect on an organism not *per se* but because of the way they are metabolized, the way they and their metabolites are distributed and bound in the body tissues, and how and when they are finally excreted. The metabolism of small rodents is at least several times faster than that of humans. The visceral organs that control and exert metabolism grow slower than body size as a whole. It has been found that metabolism relates to approximately the 2/3 power of total body weight (so-called metabolic body weight, i.e., body weight$^{2/3}$).[14] Experimental doses should consequently generally be calculated according to the metabolic body weight.[15] Russian research has demonstrated that more than 100 highly diverse biological parameters (e.g. creatinine clearance, water intake, hemoglobin weight) are linearly related to body weight, regardless of mammal species.[16]

- *Confounding variables of metabolism must be controlled.* One must be very careful about attributing to a species or strain differences that could be due to, e.g., age, diet, sex, distress, route or time of administration and sampling, dose size, diurnal variation, season of the year, or daily temperature.[12]

- *Experimental design and the life situation of the target species must correspond.* A model cannot be separated from the experimental design itself. If the design inadequately represents the "normal" life conditions of the target species, inaccurate conclusions may be drawn, regardless of the value of the model itself.

CONCLUSION

It is impossible to give reliable general rules for the validity of extrapolation from one species to another. This has to be assessed individually for each experiment and can often only be verified after first trials in the target species. An extensive and useful overview on the problem of predictive antropomorphization, especially in the field of toxicology research, is *Principles of Animal Extrapolation* by Calabrese.[12]

Extrapolation from animal models, like medical art itself, will always remain a matter of hindsight, devoid of guarantees, although we humans usually demand absolutism from the medical profession and the research community. Science is knowledge in flow. And as we drift away towards unknown waters, we discover what is today's state of the art, but tomorrow's fallacy or truth.

REFERENCES

1. Guthrie, D. : *A History of Medicine*. Nelson, London, 1945.
2. Tomkin, O. : *Galenism*. Cornell University Press, Ithaca, NY, 1973.
3. Bernard, C. : *An Introduction to the Study of Experimental Medicine* (1865). Translated by HC Green. Dover, New York, 1957.
4. *The Compact Edition of the Oxford English Dictionary*, Oxford University Press, 1971.
5. De Foe: *Systema Magicum*, 30, 1727, 1849.
6. King, N.W. : Simian models of acquired immunodeficiency syndrome (AIDS): a review. *Vet. Pathol.* 23, 345, 1986.
7. Festing, M.F., May, D., Connors, T.A., Lovell, D., and Sparrow, S. : An athymic nude mutation in the rat. *Nature* 274, 364, 1978.
8. Farnsworth, N.R. and Pezzuto, J.M. : Practical pharmacologic evaluation of plants. *Lord Dowding Fund Bulletin* 21, 26, 1984.
9. Mann, R.D. : *Modern Drug Use. An Enquiry on Historical Principles*. MTP, Lancaster, 1984.
10. Koppanyi, T. and Avery, M.A. : Species differences and the clinical trial of new drugs: a review. *Clin. Pharmacol. Ther.* 7, 250, 1966.
11. Lewis, P. : Animal tests for teratogenicity, their relevance to clinical practice. In Hawkins, D.F. (Ed): *Drugs and Pregnancy: Human Teratogenesis and Related Problems*. Churchill Livingstone, Edinburgh, pp 17-21, 1983.
12. Calabrese, E.J. : *Principles of Animal Extrapolation*. Lewis Publishers, Chelsea, Michigan, 1991.
13. Baskerville, A. : Animal model of human disease: Chronic bronchitis. *Am. J. Pathol.* 82, 237, 1976.
14. Brody, S.: *Bioenergetics and Growth*. Reinhold, NY, 1945.
15. Weiss, M., Sziegoleit, W., and Forster, W. : Dependence of pharmacokinetic parameters on the body weight. *Int. J. Clin. Pharmacol. Ther. Toxicol.* 15, 572, 1977.
16. Krasovskij, G.N. : Extrapolation of experimental data from animals to man. *Environ. Health. Perspect.* 13, 51, 1976.

Chapter 2

Animal Models In Toxicological Research And Toxicity Testing

O. Svendsen

CONTENTS

INTRODUCTION

Synthetic chemicals have contributed substantially to the quality of life and to the economic growth and improved health and hygiene standards. These contributions have derived from the development of products for use in health care, agriculture, industry, nutrition, transport, and the home.

Toxicology is the study of the adverse effects of chemicals on living organisms. The toxicologist is specially trained to examine these adverse effects including their cellular, biochemical, and molecular mechanisms of action. The variety of potential adverse effects and the diversity of chemicals present in our environment make toxicology a very broad science.

The science of toxicology is not only concerned with the safety evaluation of new chemicals. Toxic chemicals naturally present in the environment or in food or produced by human activity can also affect the health of large sections of the community. Toxicology has a role to play in identifying these undesirable chemicals so that appropriate control measures can be instituted. Toxicology is an area of science that has a profound impact on humans and the environment. Decisions made by toxicologists can affect the lives of thousands of people. The consequences of an incorrect decision can be either economic, through unwarranted restrictions on the availability of a useful chemical or medicine, or clinical, when adverse effects on health might result from exposure of consumers or the general public.

The professional activities of toxicologists fall into three main categories: descriptive, mechanistic, and regulatory. The descriptive toxicologist is concerned with toxicity testing, which provides information for safety evaluation and regulatory requirements. The appropriate toxicity tests (as described later in this chapter) in experimental animals are designed to

8

yield information that can be used to evaluate the risk posed to humans by exposure to specific chemicals. This chapter will not describe toxicity tests that are not performed in animal models.

The mechanistic toxicologist is concerned with the mechanisms by which chemicals exert their toxic effects. Results of these studies sometimes contribute to the development of sensitive predictive tests useful in risk assessment. An understanding of the mechanisms of toxic action requires knowledge of basic physiology, pharmacology, cell biology, and biochemistry.

A regulatory toxicologist has the responsibility of deciding on the basis of data provided by the descriptive and mechanistic toxicologist whether a drug or other chemical poses a sufficiently low risk to be marketed for a stated purpose.

LAWS AND REGULATIONS

Stringent regulations have been formulated to control the introduction of new chemicals to the market and to confirm, or otherwise, the safety of chemicals already in use prior to the establishment of current regulations. The nature of these regulations is determined nationally and enforced by national legislation, although in recent years supranational organizations such as the European Community or the Organisation of Economic Cooperation and Development (OECD)[1] have been instrumental in formulating regulatory guidelines. There is considerable agreement about the way in which toxicology studies should be performed and interpreted and this is of great value to international trade.

Most toxicologists believe that regulations, the protocols for studies and, in particular, the interpretation of data should be based firmly upon scientific principles. Toxicology is, in the main, a pragmatic subject built on the science experience of the past rather than a pure science founded upon universal laws. Nevertheless, scientific thought and method play a vital role in the practice of toxicology and in some ways, for example by the application of the principles of Good Laboratory Practice, its execution is more rigorous than many scientific disciplines.

RISK ASSESSMENT

In general terms, the overall purpose of toxicology is to identify and understand toxic hazards and to provide information that will allow the quantitative assessment of risk to exposed populations.

The process of risk assessment can be divided into five steps. The first step is the determination of toxicity for which exist the animal models described below. The next step involves toxicity evaluation, which means extrapolation of experimental toxicological findings to the individual to be exposed to the product. This process is often rather complicated and includes the possibility of either false positive or false negative findings. False positive findings may hamper the development of useful products whereas false negative findings may have disastrous consequences for the exposed individual.

The third step is called hazard assessment, which means identification of the level of the chemical to which humans may be exposed. When this level has been identified, it gives the background for the next step, risk estimation. The final step, risk evaluation, involves considerations as to whether it is acceptable to take the risk. It is obvious that for drugs, a malignant incurable disease justifies a higher risk than a benign trivial disease.

BASIC SCIENCE IN TOXICOLOGY

In most examples involving the assessment of toxic risk, the major uncertainty is the extrapolation from the experimental findings based on animal studies to the assessment of hazard to humans. Where little information is available, it has become the convention to use the most conservative assumptions such as the use of the most sensitive species. Where the issues are more important, studies on the mechanism of toxic action in the experimental animal provide the best scientific approach to the problem.

It is in these types of study that the contribution of basic science to toxicology is most evident. The toxicologist draws not only from the accumulated knowledge in the field, but equally importantly from the theoretical and technical expertise of other scientific disciplines to tackle specialized problems. Very little of the technology of toxicology is unique to the subject. Most is derived from the biological and chemical sciences. It is also to these sciences that the toxicologist turns to develop new methods.

ANIMAL MODELS IN TOXICITY TESTING

Toxicologists base the evaluation and assessment of human risk on laboratory animal studies. An integral factor in any meaningful assessment of risk and safety is the difficulty of extrapolating the data obtained in animal toxicity studies to humans. Before meaningful extrapolations between species can be attempted, a significant amount of information is required on the effects of the chemical in the test species and the similarities and differences in effects between the test species and humans, as far as the similarities or differences are relevant to the toxic effect observed in the test species.

The need to use suitable animal models for extrapolation purposes is evident since human experimentation is largely precluded. The realization of the need to use animal models capable of predicting human response has been apparent for a long time. However, in spite of extensive efforts, relatively little progress has been made in harmonizing the scientific basis on which an appropriate animal species is selected. As a consequence, toxicologists still largely select animal models on the basis of historical precedent or convenience, with little regard to the appropriateness of the selected animal model to man.

In this chapter, animal models for the following types of testing will be presented:

1. acute toxicity
2. skin irritancy
3. eye irritancy
4. allergic contact dermatitis
5. subchronic and chronic toxicity
6. carcinogenicity
7. reproductive and developmental toxicity
8. genetic toxicity

Two main principles underlie all descriptive animal toxicity testing. The first is that the effects produced by the compound in laboratory animals, when properly qualified, are applicable to humans. The second is that exposure of experimental animals to toxic agents in high doses is a necessary and valid method of discovering possible hazards in humans. This principle is based on the dose-response concept that the incidence of an effect in a population becomes greater as the dose or exposure increases. Practical considerations in the design of experimental model systems require that the number of animals used in toxicology experiments will always be small compared to the size of human populations similarly at risk. To obtain statistically valid results from such small groups of animals requires the use of relatively large doses so that the effect will occur frequently enough to be detected.

ACUTE TOXICITY

Acute toxicity is defined as any harmful effect of a chemical or a drug on a target organism. Acute toxicity has been defined by the OECD as "the adverse effects occurring within a short time after (oral) administration of a single dose of a substance or multiple doses given within 24 hours".

Acute toxicity testing began nearly a century ago. In 1927, Trevan[2] introduced the concept of a medium lethal dose (LD_{50}) for the standardization of drugs. High precision of LD_{50} can only be established with a large number of animals. The list of extraneous factors that affect the precision of LD_{50} is long and includes, among others, sex, animal species, strain of animal, husbandry, experimental procedures, route of administration, stress, and dosage formulation (vehicle), as well as intralaboratory and interlaboratory variations.[3] In spite of the many variables affecting LD_{50} determination, most governmental agencies have adopted the LD_{50} as the primary measurement of acute toxicity for classification purposes. However, change in this attitude has emerged, with the development of the fixed-dose procedure for acute toxicity testing.[4] This test has toxic signs and not lethality as end-point.

The objectives of acute toxicity testing are to define the intrinsic toxicity of the chemical, predict hazard to nontarget species or toxicity to target species, determine the most susceptible species, identify target organs, provide information for risk assessment of acute exposure to the chemical, provide information for the design and selection of dose levels of prolonged studies, and, most important and practical of all, provide information for clinicians to predict, diagnose, and prescribe treatment for acute overexposure.

In an acute toxicity test, the test substance is most often given to several groups of animals by gavage. Rats and mice are most commonly chosen for acute toxicity studies. Clinical examination and mortality check are made shortly after dosing at frequent intervals, and at least once daily thereafter. Cage-side observations include any changes in the skin, fur, eyes, mucous membranes, circulatory system, autonomic and central nervous systems, somatomotor activities, behavior, etc. Any pharmacotoxic signs such as tremor, convulsions, salivation, diarrhea, lethargy, sleepiness, morbidity, fasciculation, mydriasis, miosis, droppings, discharges, or hypotonia are recorded.

Necropsies are performed on animals that are moribund, found dead, and killed at the conclusion of the study. All changes in the size, color, or consistency of any organ are recorded. Microscopic examination of a lesion may be essential. Therefore, tissues from such lesions must be preserved in an appropriate fixative.

Dermal exposure is another important route of exposure. The objective of conducting an acute dermal toxicity study is the same as an acute oral toxicity study. Such testing may provide information on the adverse effects resulting from a dermal application of a single dose of a test substance. The general experimental designs and principles of acute dermal toxicity testing are similar to those of acute oral testing. However, there are differences including selection of the animal species, number of animals per dose level, preparation of animals, and dosage and administration of the test substance.

EYE IRRITATION

A test was developed in 1944 by Draize et al.[5] to study eye irritation in rabbits and used to identify human eye irritants. The test is easy to conduct and requires no special instruments. Simplicity is probably the main reason for the popularity of this test. However, the limitation of the test is a factor as well. The Draize test can identify most of the moderate-to-severe human eye irritants, but the test may fail to detect mild or subtle ocular irritation. The result of the Draize test is one of the criteria for classifying and labeling chemicals.

In the original test, 0.1 ml or 0.1 g of test substance is applied to the eye conjunctival sac of albino rabbits. The degree or extent of opacity of the cornea, the redness of the iris, and the chemosis and discharge of the conjunctiva are scored subjectively according to an arbitrary scale at preselected intervals after exposure. Scoring is based on the degree of effects caused by the testing substance. More emphasis is placed on the opacity of the cornea whereas emphasis is less with other effects such as conjunctival changes and iritis. Humane concern about using animals in eye irritation tests has prompted many investigators to turn to alternative methods. The development of alternatives is still in its infancy. Recent research has focused on validation of methods, most of which are *in vitro*. It is generally agreed that *in vitro* techniques will not replace animal testing in the near future, so the immediate concern is to reduce the number of animals used and minimize the pain inflicted on animals during the study. It is the experience of this author that less than 5% of all animals used for this test show any reaction to the treatment.

SKIN IRRITATION

The albino rabbit is the preferred animal species when testing for skin irritation because of its high skin sensitivity and light skin, where usually even slight skin irritant effects of a substance can be detected.

In general, substances or products are tested for skin irritation with a test design first proposed by Draize in 1944.[5] The substance to be tested is applied in a single dose to intact or abraded skin of 3 to 6 rabbits for 4 or 24 hours, whereafter the substance is removed. Each animal serves as its own control. The possible skin reactions of erythema and oedema are described and graded according to a classification system each of the following days. The duration of the study should be sufficient to make a full evaluation of the reversibility of the possible effects observed.

Dermal irritation is the production of reversible changes, whereas dermal corrosion is the production of irreversible changes (scar formation) in the skin.

ALLERGIC CONTACT DERMATITIS

Allergic contact dermatitis (type IV sensitization) is an immunologically mediated reaction. This is in contrast to irritant contact dermatitis, which is a skin reaction caused by a primary and direct effect of the substance on the skin. In humans, the responses to both types of dermatitis are very similar, characterized by pruritis, erythema, oedema, papules, vesicles, bullae or combinations of these. In animals the reactions may differ and only erythema and edema may be seen. Allergic contact dermatitis is a T-cell mediated cutaneous reaction to a substance, characterized by a delayed response (24 to 96 hours) to a patch test with a non-irritating concentration of the substance.

Information about the potential of a chemical to sensitize skin is important in addition to irritation testing for all materials that may repeatedly come into contact with the skin. Numerous procedures have been developed to determine the potential of substances to induce delayed hypersensitivity reaction in humans, including the Draize test, the open epicutaneous test, the Buehler test, Freund's complete adjuvant test, the optimization test, the split adjuvant test, the guinea pig maximization (GPM) test, and the mouse ear swelling test.

The preferred animal species is the albino guinea pig. Mouse models have been developed, but their predictive value has not yet been established. About 15 different guinea pig methods are available in the literature,[6] and all have certain features in common: an induction (sensitization) phase, where the potential allergen is presented to the skin, followed by a rest period of about 2 weeks, and a subsequent challenge phase to prove whether or not sensitization has occurred. Each test employs 20 to 40 animals divided into test groups and a control group.

One of the recognized and most validated assays is the guinea pig maximization (GPM) test described by Magnusson and Kligman in 1970.[7] The method combines the use of Freund's complete adjuvant enhancing the sensitivity of the test and an induction procedure, where both intradermal injections and topical applications are included.

Results from sensitization tests in guinea pigs have to be carefully evaluated. A positive test result in an adjuvant assay may rate the substance as a stronger sensitizer than it appears to be. A negative test result in a sensitive assay ensures a considerable safety margin in the potential risk during human exposure.

SUBCHRONIC AND CHRONIC TOXICITY

Subchronic toxicity studies are designed to examine the adverse effects resulting from repeated exposure over a portion of the average life span of experimental animals. Subchronic toxicity studies give valuable information on the cumulative toxicity of a substance on target organs and on physiological and metabolic tolerance of a compound at low-dose prolonged exposure. By monitoring many different parameters, including histopathological evaluations, a wide variety of adverse effects can be detected. Subchronic studies are also valuable in establishing doses at which no toxicological effects are evident, a critical factor in risk assessment. The results from such studies can provide information that will aid in selecting doses for reproduction and carcinogenicity studies.

In subchronic or chronic toxicity studies, one or two animal species are dosed daily for a period of 3, 6, or 12 months. The rat is the standard animal species of choice. In case of two species, a rodent and a non-rodent species are used. In practice, these two species are represented by the rat and the dog or the mini-pig.

The animals (80 to 160 rats or 24 to 40 dogs or mini-pigs) are divided into four groups. One group serves as control group. The other three groups are given the product in increasing doses. The dose level of the low dose group should be at the level of human exposure. Ideally, the dose level of the high dose group should be toxic. The intermediate dose group is often chosen as the arithmetic mean between the high and low dose in order to establish a no-effect level.

The most common routes of administration employed in subchronic toxicity studies are oral, dermal, intravenous, or inhalation. Subchronic toxicity studies always attempt to expose the animals by the same route as man is most likely to be exposed.

Oral administration of a test substance can be carried out by gavage, in capsules, or in the diet or drinking water. Dietary administration is a very common route of dosing. Basically, the toxic effects of the test substance can be defined by physical examination, daily observations, ophthalmological examination, determination of diet and water consumption, body and organ weights, hematology, clinical chemistry, urinalysis, and pathology studies. In dogs and mini-pigs, electrocardiography may be included. When possible, these parameters are evaluated prior to initiation of the study to obtain baseline information on the animals. Detailed observations of each animal are made at least once and preferably twice daily for the duration of the study. If recovery groups are included in the study, these animals are observed for a period of weeks after withdrawal of treatment. Daily observations include close scrutiny for changes in the fur, skin, eyes, mucous membranes, orifices, the respiratory, circulatory, autonomic and central nervous systems, somatomotor activities, and behavior. Special attention is given to any palpable mass that may be related to tumor incidence. All signs are recorded. If deaths occur during the study, the animals are necropsied within a short period of time and the tissues placed in fixative. Severely moribund animals are killed and necropsied to prevent loss of valuable tissues due to autolysis. At the end of a test period, all animals except those in the recovery groups are killed. The recovery groups are observed during the recovery period and then bled for hematology and clinical chemistry, and killed for pathological studies.

Hematological analysis includes hematocrit, hemoglobin concentration, red blood cell count, white blood cell count (total and differential count), morphology of the red blood cells, and a measure of clotting ability such as prothrombin and thromboplastin time or platelet count. Biochemical measurements comprise electrolyte balance, carbohydrate and protein metabolism, and organ function tests.[8] This information can be important in the establishment of target organ toxicity. The analyses include most if not all of the following parameters: Ca^{2+}, K^+, Na^+, Cl^-, PO_2^{4-}, fasting glucose, serum GOT (ASAT) and GPT (ALAT), alkaline phosphatase, ornithine carbamyltransferase, gamma-glutamyl transpeptidase, blood urea nitrogen, total protein, albumin, globulin, total bilirubin, blood creatinine, cholesterol, acid-base balance, lipids, cholinesterase (plasma, red blood cell, and/or brain), and any other biochemical parameters that may facilitate the definition of adverse effects. The number of biochemical parameters that are examined is based on the class of chemicals and the expected toxicity. For example, cholinesterase activities should be considered if the test substance is an organophosphate or a carbamate, which are expected to be inhibitors of the enzyme.

Urinalysis is generally conducted at the same time as hematology and clinical chemistry. The following parameters are usually determined: specific gravity and/or osmolarity, acidity, protein, glucose, ketones, bilirubin, epithelial cells, urobilinogen and stones.

All animals are subjected to a gross pathology examination. All tissues from the high dose group and control animals and any tissues with lesions in other groups are further examined microscopically. When tissues from animals in the high dose group are detected as having microscopic lesions, those tissues are examined from animals in lower dose groups. Certain regulatory guidelines have provided lists of tissues recommended for histopathological examination.

CARCINOGENICITY

The objective of long term carcinogenicity studies is to observe test animals for a major portion of their life span for the development of neoplastic lesions during or after exposure to various doses of a test substance by an appropriate route of administration. Such an assay requires careful planning and documentation of the experimental design, a high standard of pathology, and unbiased statistical analysis. These requirements are well known and have not undergone any significant changes during the past several years.

In carcinogenicity studies, mice or rats are dosed every day for a period of 18 or 24 months, respectively. The test is normally conducted with oral dosing. The animals are divided into four groups each consisting of 50 males and 50 females. One group serves as a control group. The other three groups are given increasing doses, where the highest dose should ideally cause slight toxicity, e.g., slight reduction in body weight gain.

During the dosing period, the animals are observed for development of clinically detectable tumors. Animals that die or are killed for humane reasons during the dosing period are autopsied and organs and tissues are examined microscopically for tumors. At completion of the dosing period, all surviving animals are killed and autopsied. Organs and tissues from these animals are also examined microscopically for presence of tumors. The tumors are divided into different categories. The incidence of each category of tumours in the dosed groups is compared statistically with the incidence of the same tumor in the control group.

Increased incidence of one or more categories of tumors in the dosed groups suggests that the product tested has the potential of inducing tumors and may be considered as a potential carcinogen.

REPRODUCTIVE AND DEVELOPMENTAL TOXICITY

Reproductive toxicity is broadly defined as including all effects resulting from paternal or maternal exposure that interfere with the conception, development, birth, and maturation to healthy adult life of offspring. The relation between exposure and reproductive dysfunction is highly complex because exposure of the mother, the father, or both may influence reproductive outcome.

There are several protocols that are routinely used to test for toxicity to the reproductive system. The basic types include the single generation reproduction test, and the multigeneration reproduction test. Animal models in reproductive toxicology are described in detail in Chapter 3.

GENETIC TOXICITY

Genetic toxicology involves the identification and analysis of the action of agents whose toxicity is directed towards the hereditary components of living systems. Many agents damage the genetic material at concentrations that produce acute nonspecific cytotoxicity and death. The primary objective of genetic toxicologists, however, is to detect and analyze the hazard potential of agents that interact primarily with DNA, thereby producing alterations in genes at subtoxic concentrations.

Agents that produce alterations in the DNA and associated components at subtoxic exposure levels, resulting in modified hereditary characteristics or DNA inactivation, are classified as genotoxic.

A mutation is a change in the information content of a gene that is propagated through subsequent generations of cells. Genetic toxicology evolved in response to a concern that many chemicals that produce cancer have mutagenic activity and many of the tests that are the basis of genetic toxicology testing are used to investigate chemicals for both mutagenic and possible carcinogenic activity.

Mutations can be classified into two general types: (1) point or gene mutations and (2) chromosomal mutations. Point or gene mutations are changes in nucleotide sequence at one or a few segments within a gene. Chromosomal mutations (aberrations) are recognized as morphological alterations in the gross structure of chromosomes, i.e., they are aberrations of the normal structural organization of the chromosome. Such chromosomal aberrations are usually detected by microscopic examination of cells fixed and stained at the metaphase stage of cell division.

The simplest and most sensitive assays for detecting chemically induced gene mutations are those using bacteria. Gene mutation can also be detected in cultured mammalian cells, as well as in *in vivo* assays such as the mouse spot test, the specific locus test and the dominant lethal test, although these *in vivo* assays are not so widely used.

The simplest and most sensitive assays for investigating chromosomal aberrations are those using cultured mammalian cells. However, two well-established *in vivo* procedures are available. Chromosomal aberrations can be studied in bone marrow cells of rodents dosed with the suspect chemical either by counting micronuclei in maturing erythrocytes (micronucleus test) or by analyzing chromosomes in metaphase cells from various tissues, e.g., bone marrow, gonades, or peripheral lymphocytes. Chromosomal aberrations can also be studied in the heritable translocation test and the dominant lethal test by measuring changes in offspring rats from treated males.

ETHICAL CONSIDERATIONS

Most of the research necessary for the safety evaluation of chemicals requires the use of laboratory animals. Therefore, toxicologists are faced with an ethical conflict between their professional duties and the interests of the animals. Toxicologists are aware of their ethical responsibilities not only for the safety of the human population, but also for the welfare of the animals. They review the classical toxicological procedures critically and require that the maximum amount of relevant information is obtained from the smallest number of laboratory animals. Toxicologists are also aware of the alternative methods that permit the investigation of toxicological responses in unicellular organisms and cell cultures. For further details the reader is referred to a book by Paton[10] and a paper by Zbinden.[11]

REFERENCES

1. *OECD Guidelines for Testing of Chemicals.* OECD, February 24th, 1987.
2. Trevan, J. W.: The error of determination of toxicity. *Proc. R. Soc. Lond. 1.1B, 483, 1927.*
3. Zbinden, G. and Flury-Roversi, M.: Significance of the LD_{50}-test for toxicological substances. *Arch. Toxicol. 47, 77, 1981.*
4. Heuvel, M. J. et al.: The international validation of a fixed-dose procedure as an alternative to the classical LD_{50} test. *Food. Chem. Toxic. 28, 469, 1990.*
5. Draize, J. H. Woodward, G, and Calvery, H. O.: Methods for the study of irritation and toxicity of substances applied topically to the skin and mucous membranes. *J. Pharmacol. Exp. Ther. 82, 377, 1944.*
6. Andersen, K. E. and Maibach, H. I.: Contact allergy predictive tests in guinea pigs. *Current Problems in Dermatology, vol. 14, 1985.*
7. Magnusson, B. and Kligmann, A. M.: The identification of contact allergens by animal assay. The guinea pig maximization test. *J. Invest. Dermatol. 52, 268, 1969.*
8. Loeb, W. F. and Quimby, F. W.: *The Clinical Chemistry of Laboratory Animals.* Pergamon Press, New York, 1989
9. Wilson, J. G. and Warkany. J.: *Teratology: Principles and Techniques,* University of Chicago Press, 1965.
10. Paton, W.: *Man and Mouse. Animals in Medical Research.* Oxford University Press. Oxford, New York, 1984.
11. Zbinden, G.: Ethical considerations in toxicology. *Food Chem. Toxic. 23, 137, 1985.*

RECOMMENDED READING

Amdur, M. O., Duoll, J. and Klaassen, C. D.: *Casarett and Doull's Toxicology. The Basic Sciences of Poisons.* Pergamon Press, New York, 1991.

Grice, H. C. and Ciminera, J. L.: *Carcinogenicity. The Design, Analysis and Interpretation of Long-Term Animal Studies.* Springer-Verlag, New York, 1988.

Haschek, W. M. and Rousseaux, C. G.: *Handbook of Toxicological Pathology.* Academic Press, London, 1991.

Hayes, A. W.: *Principles and Methods of Toxicology,* Raven Press, New York, 1989.

Lu, F. C.: *Basic Toxicology. Fundamentals, Target Organs and Risk Assessment.* Taylor & Francis Group, London 1990.

Marzulli, F. N. and Maibach, H. W.: *Dermal Toxicology.* Taylor & Francis Group, London, 1991.

Taylor, P.: *Practical Teratology.* Academic Press, London, 1986.

Timbrell, J. A.: *Introduction to Toxicology.* Taylor & Francis Group, London, 1989.

Van Roloff, M.: *Human Risk Assessment. The Role of Animal Selection and Extrapolation.* Taylor & Francis Group, London, 1987.

Chapter 3

ANIMAL MODELS IN REPRODUCTIVE TOXICOLOGY

Ernst Hansen and Otto Meyer

CONTENTS

INTRODUCTION

Reproduction is the term used to describe the biological process, which ensures the continuation of the species. Through this process existing genetic material is passed on to the next generation. The reproductive cycle does not consist simply of conception, pregnancy and birth. It actually begins with the formation of the primitive germ cells in the parents at the embryo-fetal stage and does not end until sexual maturity has been reached. A disturbance of the reproductive cycle can, depending on type or timing, prevent or inhibit reproduction or result in developmental defects in the offspring.

Reproductive toxicity testing forms part of the toxicological investigations providing data that are an essential part of the health assessment of exposure to chemicals such as medicines, food additives, pesticides, and industrial and household chemicals. The three main objectives of experimental toxicology are to give information about the spectrum of toxicity, to predict both adverse effects and safe levels of exposure particularly in humans. The spectrum of toxicity covers the detection of adverse effects of chemicals in selected animal species and the description of the dose-effect relationship over a broad range of doses. The animal models in reproductive toxicology must be able to show whether exposure to a substance will cause effects on fertility, prenatal, perinatal, and postnatal development on the ovum, fetus, and progeny, including teratogenic and mutagenic effects, and perinatal and postnatal effects on the mother. The embryo-fetal damage includes spontaneous abortion, interuterine and perinatal

Table 1. *In vivo* tests to determine embryo-fetal toxicity

Test	Type of animal	Dosing	Effect
One, two or multigeneration testing	Rat Mouse	Two or more dose levels administered continously over generations	Fertility in males and females. Prenatal, perinatal and postnatal effects on egg, embryo/ fetus, and progeny; teratogenic and mutagenic effects. Perinatal and postnatal effects on mother
Teratogenicity testing	Rat Mouse Rabbit	Two or more dose levels, usually during organogenesis	Resorption, fetal growth, morphological abnormalities
Perinatal and postnatal studies	Rat Mouse	Usually one dose level during fetogenesis and lactation period	Behavioral changes due to CNS and PNS effects, together with toxic effects on organs
In vivo teratology screen	Mouse	One dose level during days 8–12 of pregnancy	Fetal growth and survival
Combined repeat dose and reproductive/developmental toxicity screening test	Rat	Two or more dose levels. 14 days prior to mating to 4th day after birth	Fertility of male and female, fetus dead or alive, resorptions and toxicity

death, dysmaturity, including inhibited growth, prematurity, morphological malformations, functional disturbances in the child (motor, mental, immunological, and hormonal) and childhood cancer. The fact that chemicals can be teratogenic in mammals was established only in the late 1940s and early 1950s when it was found that trypan blue, adrenocorticosteroids, urethane, and nitrogen mustard were capable of producing congenital malformations in rats and mice. During these years, it was shown that human embryos were susceptible too, as it was reported that aminopterin, used as an abortifacient, was teratogenic.[1] However, it was not until after the thalidomide tragedy in the early 1960s that attention was drawn to the connection between exposure to chemicals and the occurrence of fetal malformations.[2] The years that followed saw increased, active efforts on the part of the authorities in various countries to draw up guidelines for studying the harmful effects of chemical substances on reproduction. Many tests have been standardized and guidelines published by various expert groups.[3-9] The first guidelines for reproductive tests on animals were those of the U.S. Food and Drug Administration, which recommended multigeneration, pre-, peri-, and postgestation studies.[10]

All current data suggest that any potential human teratogen will, in some way, disrupt development in animal tests. However, species differences are common, and there is no *a priori* basis for test species selection.[11] Regulatory toxicology testing generally requires the use of one rodent and one non-rodent species. Data from studies using various animal species exist, but the most commonly used is the rat and to a lesser extent the mouse, representing rodents, and the rabbit as the non-rodent.[12, 13]

The presentation of animal models in reproductive toxicology in this chapter will mainly focus on one, two, and multigeneration studies and the conventional teratology study, and to

a lesser extent the perinatal and postnatal studies, the *in vivo* teratology screen in mice, and the combined repeat dose and reproductive/developmental toxicity screening test. A few other tests will be mentioned (Table 1).

ONE, TWO, AND MULTIGENERATION STUDIES

The purpose of generation studies is to examine successive generations to identify possibly increased sensitivity to a substance, effects on the fertility of male and female animals, pre-, peri-, and postnatal effects on the ovum, fetus, and progeny, including teratogenic and mutagenic effects, and peri- and postnatal effects on the mother.

METHODS

Young virgin animals (generally rats or mice) are used as the parent generation. Growing males are dosed for at least one spermatogenic period (approximately 56 days in the mouse and 70 days in the rat) in order to elicit any adverse effect on spermatogenesis. The parent females are dosed for at least two complete estrus cycles in order to elicit any adverse effect on estrus (approximately 14 days). Dosing continues during pregnancy and until the end of the experiment (for two and multigeneration studies through successive generations).

In the one generation study, the experiment stops at the weaning of the F_1 generation. In the two and multigeneration studies, the dosing continues until the last generation of pups has been weaned.

In reproduction studies it is important to use strains with defined physiological parameters, specifically reproductive parameters, e.g., fecundity. Strains with low fecundity should not be used. It is essential to use healthy animals, and for the multigeneration study SPF animals are recommended to ensure absence of diseases and good survival as these studies can last for several years.

It is important to use a sufficient number of animals in order to obtain at least 20 pregnant females per group for the first generation. For substances that cause sterility, this may not be possible. The objective is to assure a meaningful evaluation of the study.

International guidelines used for safety evaluation of chemicals give a minimal requirement for the number of groups used in the different generation studies. At least three treatment groups and a control group should be used. If a vehicle is used in administering the test substance, the control group should receive the vehicle in the largest volume used. Ideally, unless limited by the physical/chemical nature or biological effect of the test substance, the highest dosed level should induce toxicity but not mortality in the parent generation. Ideally, the intermediate dose(s) should induce minimum toxic effect attributable to the test substance. The lowest dose should not induce any observable adverse effect on the parents or the offspring. The selection of doses should make it possible to establish a dose-response curve.

The animals are observed daily for clinical changes. Body weight is recorded weekly for the parent animals and for offspring normally at birth, on days 4, 7, and 14, at weaning (approximately day 21) and thereafter every week, and weight gains are calculated. Food consumption and occasionally water consumption is measured. The specific parameters of reproduction recorded are: pregnancy rate, duration of pregnancy, number of animals per litter, number of live and dead pups, number of pups with anomalies, and, if necessary, histological examinations of dead or sacrificed animals. The design of generation studies has some limitations as the mother animals tend to eat the malformed pups immediately after birth. As autopsy of the dams is performed on day 21 after delivery, and the estrus cycle is reestablished about 5 days after termination of pregnancy leading to changes in the uterus, embryotoxicity as reflected in an increase in occurrence in resorptions of the embryos and fetuses is not normally detected. However, the use of a specific method using sulphite to stain the small residues of blood at the implantation sites can, to some extent, overcome this problem.[14] The number of live pups on day 4 and at weaning are recorded and the following indices are often calculated:

- Mating index: copulations/estrus cycles required
- Fecundity index: pregnancies/copulations
- Male fertility index: males impregnating females/ males exposed to fertile non-pregnant females
- Female fertility index: females conceiving/females exposed to fertile males
- Incidence of parturition: parturitions/pregnancies
- Live birth index: viable pups born/pups born
- Survival index for 24 hours, 4 days, 12 days, and 21 days

The number of litters per female per generation varies in the different designs from 1 to 2.

Fertility assessment by continuous breeding has been used to study the depletion of oocytes from the mouse ovary in mice exposed to procarbazine. In this study, prenatally treated mice were continuously housed with untreated male mice, and the cumulative number of offspring was measured by removing the female when noticeably pregnant and then returning the female to the male's cage immediately after delivery to establish a pattern of forced repetitive breedings.[15]

For developmental toxicity covering interuterine and perinatal death, dysmaturity, including inhibited growth, prematurity, morphological malformations, functional disturbances, etc. other specific studies are used.

THE CONVENTIONAL TERATOLOGY STUDY

The teratology study is the best developed and most used *in vivo* method for studying embryo-fetal toxicity during pregnancy. Current guidelines, i.e., minimum requirements for carrying out acceptable teratogenicity tests, include those issued by the U.S. Food and Drug Administration,[10] the OECD,[7] and the EEC.[16] There are many textbooks that describe the methodology in detail.[6, 17-19] This paper represents a brief summary focusing on methods using mice, rats, and rabbits.

METHODS
Animals
Young mature virgin females are artificially inseminated or mated with males. The time of mating is established by observation of mating (e.g., rabbits), identification of a plug (mixture of sperm and cellular material from the vagina of rats and mice), vaginal smear (in rats), or by noting the time of insemination (e.g., for pigs and rabbits).

Dose Levels
Normally, three dose levels and a control group (untreated or vehicle control) are used in order to establish a dose-effect relationship.

Dosing Period
The pregnant females are exposed during the period of organogenesis (Figure 1), i.e., between day 6 when implantation occurs and day 15. (The corresponding periods for mice and rabbits are days 6 to 15 and days 6 to 18, respectively). This period has been found to be the most sensitive to the induction of structural, anatomical malformations (the corresponding sensitive period for humans is between the 18th and 60th day of pregnancy).

Days 6 to 15 are the indicated dosing period for pregnant rats. However, this may vary depending on the substance administered or whether the effect on a specific organ is to be

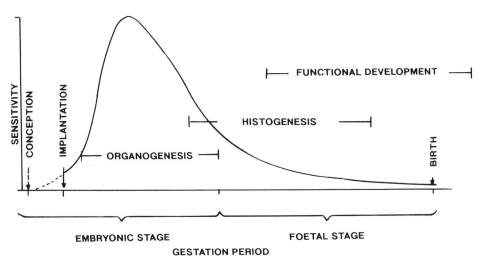

SENSITIVITY

CONCEPTION

IMPLANTATION

ORGANOGENESIS

HISTOGENESIS

FUNCTIONAL DEVELOPMENT

BIRTH

EMBRYONIC STAGE   FOETAL STAGE

GESTATION PERIOD

Wilson 1973

Figure 1. Curve approximating the susceptibility of the human embryo to teratogenesis from fertilization throughout intrauterine development.

studied. A short overview of the most common time periods for the organogenesis of different organs is given in Table 2.

Clinical
Daily observation of the dams is important. Body weight and food consumption are recorded throughout gestation. After cesarian section, an autopsy is carried out to identify any pathological changes. These parameters are important in assessing whether a teratogenic effect is due to a direct effect on the fetus or a toxic effect on the dam. They may also provide information on whether pregnant animals are more sensitive than non-pregnant animals.

Autopsy
Mothers
The fetuses are removed by cesarian section and examined the day before anticipated birth. Where dosing is initiated before or at the time of implantation, the preimplantation loss, i.e., the number of embryos lost prior to implantation is investigated. The total number of implantations, i.e., living embryos, dead embryos, and resorption (embryos that die early and are reassimilated, corresponding to early abortions in humans) are noted. The degree of resorption (i.e., the extent to which the embryo has been resorbed) gives an idea of the time of death of the embryo during pregnancy and may therefore indicate the most sensitive period to study the effect of the substance on the development of the embryo, malformations, etc. Such information may, for example, be of value for follow-up studies.

Fetuses
The fetuses are sexed, weighed, and examined for gross malformations. The main aspects considered are retarded growth and visceral and skeletal development. In larger animals (e.g., rabbits and pigs) organ development is examined at necropsy and histological examination performed when necessary. In the case of smaller animals such as mice and rats, one half to two thirds of the fetuses are examined for skeletal anomalies and the remaining fetuses are examined for soft tissue anomalies. Skeletal examinations are studied by x-ray techniques (particularly of larger animals such as pigs) or by staining the bones to assess the degree of

22

Table 2. Comparative time periods of embryonic and fetal development in humans and experimental animals

	Human	Monkey	Rat	Mouse	Rabbit	Hamster	Guinea pig
Total gestation time	267	166	21–22	18–20	31–34	15.5–16	64–68
Fetuses per litter (number)	1	1	12–13	8–10	6–9	10–14	2–3
Implantation	6–7	9	5–6	7	6	4.5–5	6
Neural plate	18–20	19–21	9.5	8		7.5	13.5
First somite	20–21	20–21	10	8.3		7.7	14.5
Heart — first beats	22		10.2			8	16.5
Pronephrons	22		10				16.5
Anterior neuropore closed	24–25	23–24?	10.5	9	9.5	8.25	15.5
Otocyst closed	25		11.3	9		8.5	16.5
Three branchial arches	26		11.5	9.6		8.25	16.5
Upper limb bud	27–28	25–26	10.5	9.3	10.5	8.25	16.5
Posterior neuropore closed	26–27		11.3	9.5		8.5	16.5?
Lung bud appears	28		12.1	9.6		9	17.5
Lower limb bud appears	29–30	26–27	11.2?	10.3	11	9.75	18.5
Eye pigment	34–35			11.3	14		
Crown-rump length (mm)	37	33	15	13.5	14		
Ossification begins	40–43		17–18	12.5		12.5	
Digit separation	43–47			15.3			28
Heart septation complete	46–47		15.5	13		11	26.1
Eyelids closed	56–58	53	18	16.3	20	13.5	
Palate closed completely	56–58	44–45	16–17	15	19–20	12.25	

Modified after Shepard, T.H. (Ed.), *Catalog of Teratogenic Agents,* 4th ed., John Hopkins University Press, 1983.

ossification or malformation. The most used methods for skeletal staining are alizarin either alone[20] or in combination with alcian blue for cartilage staining.[21] Reduced ossification may indicate retarded development of the fetus. For organ examinations, the fetus is fixed, stained, and cut into millimeter-thin sections, and then examined by stereo microscope. This method was developed by Wilson.[18]

Recently, a new method for examining the viscera for rats doing autopsy under a stereo microscope has been described.[22, 23] The findings of organs and skeletal examinations are classified according to their significance for the viability of the subject examined.

Guidelines recommend various group sizes depending on species. 20 pregnant animals are recommended for rats and 12 for rabbits, and if monkeys are used even smaller groups are accepted. There is no clear motivation for these group sizes. For example, rabbits exhibit much greater variation in individual parameters (including abortion, fetal death, frequency of malformation, etc.) than rats, so for rabbits the test groups should in fact be larger than for rat studies.

In the case of monkeys, the problems are even greater since they usually have only one fetus, thus leading to an all-or-nothing result as regards, e.g., abortion, malformation, etc.[24] For monkeys, the size of the groups should therefore be much larger than for rats and mice.

THE PERINATAL AND POSTNATAL STUDY (BEHAVIORAL TERATOLOGY)

Prenatal exposure to chemicals may lead to a range of functional disturbances in the offspring. For example, lead and methylmercury affect brain development[25, 26] but effects on fertility,[27] the immune system,[28] metabolism of foreign substances,[29] and development as a whole have been observed.[28-30]

"Behavioral teratology" identify changes in behavior due to effects on the central nervous system (CNS) and the peripheral nervous system (PNS). As behavior is affected by the function of other organs such as liver, kidneys, and the endocrine system, toxic effects on these organs in offspring may also be reflected in general changes in behavior.[31]

No single test is able to reflect the entire complex and intricate function of behavior. For testing behavior, therefore, a range of parameters, a "test battery", is used to identify changes in individual functions.[28, 32-33]

METHODS

In principle, behavioral teratology represents an extension to conventional teratology and, because of the great work, normally only one dose level is used. The selected dose level must not have any known toxic effect (recorded in a conventional teratology study) that could interfere with the later testing. The most used animal species are rats and mice.

The guidelines generally recommend groups of 20 animals with dosing from day 15 of gestation to day 21 post gestation i.e. spanning fetogenesis and the entire lactation period (Figure 1). However, the recommended dosing period does not cover all events since the CNS is also susceptible to abnormal development during the period of organogenesis. Consequently, dosing is often started earlier, for example, on day 1 or day 6 of pregnancy.[28,35] After birth, the number of progeny is recorded and the litters are adjusted so that each contains the same number of pups. In order to determine whether the chemical substance tested affects the offspring directly via the mother's milk or indirectly, either via a change in milk production or as a result of a change in the behavior of the exposed mothers, "cross-fostering" may be employed. Cross-fostering is a method where litters from exposed mothers are reared by control mothers and vice versa and this method makes it possible to minimize the factors mentioned above. It is especially important in behavioral teratology to maintain the environmental conditions as constant as possible in order to reduce variation in the results. Well defined experimental conditions like light, noise, temperature, litter size, cross-fostering, and a fixed time schedule for carrying out individual tests are essential for the outcome of the experiment.

In behavioral studies, the length of gestation, litter size, sex distribution, and the weight of the new-born animals are recorded at birth and then weekly. Studies that intend to identify abnormal developments are conducted on individual animals over short or longer periods. In rat, studies last until weaning (3 weeks) although this period does not cover the entire period of brain development as the brain does not attain an approximate adult stage until the age of 6 weeks (corresponding to 12 to 15 years of age in humans).[29]

Methodology employed in behavioral teratology is described in reviews such as Adams and Buelke-Sam,[29] Geller et al.,[36] Johnson and Kochhar,[30] Pryor et al.,[37] Rodier,[38] Spyker,[39] and Tilson et al.[40] Behavioral teratology tests may generally be grouped into tests of physical development, simple reflexes, motor function, development of the senses, spontaneous activity, learning and memory, and functions of the neurotransmitter systems.

IN VIVO SCREENING TESTS

As the capacity for toxicity testing cannot keep up with the number of chemicals in modern society, there is an increasing demand for new toxicological tests of shorter duration, using fewer resources. Especially for "old chemicals", where the patent rights no longer exist, or chemicals introduced into the market years ago, when no or only few toxicity data were required, it is essential to develop "tools" for obtaining data for safety assessment. In recent years such new screening tests for reproductive and developmental toxicity have been developed. By definition, a "screening test" is limited in scope compared to a conventional test. Data from a screening test indicating a possible toxic potential of a substance identify that substance as one of high priority for further evaluation.

A short presentation of two examples of screening tests for reproductive and developmental toxicity is given below.

THE *IN VIVO* TERATOLOGY SCREENING TEST

This test was introduced by Chernoff et al.[41] as an alternative method to the "old, familiar" teratogenicity tests. The hypothesis underlying this test is that most prenatal effects do not just produce specific defects but also are manifested in the postnatal period as a lack of viability and reduced growth. Pregnant mice (rats can be used) are exposed to a test substance from day 8 to day 12 of pregnancy. One dose level is employed (the minimum toxic dose for the mother animal) together with a control group. The mother animals are weighed during the period of exposure. After birth, the litter is weighed on the first and third day. Stillborn young and young that die after birth are dissected and examined for defects.

COMBINED REPEAT DOSE AND REPRODUCTIVE/DEVELOPMENTAL TOXICITY SCREENING TEST

This screening method has been made a guideline test, prepared by the OECD,[7] as a tool in the preliminary evaluation of old chemicals for which little or no information is available. The name implies that this design is more than a reproduction test including repeated dosing of both male and female rats corresponding to that of the "repeated dose (28 days) toxicity test". Until an evaluation of the test system has been made only rats should be used.

The principle of the combined repeat dose and reproductive/developmental toxicity screening test is that the test substance is administered in graduated doses to groups (normally 3 but more can be used) of young mature adult males and females. In contrast to other tests, a clear effect of the test substance is required on the parental generation at the highest dose group. If at a dose level of 1000 mg/kg bw a test fails to produce any effect, studies at other dose levels may not be needed. (What corresponds to that of the limit test in the guideline for reproduction and teratogenicity tests).

Males should be dosed for two weeks before mating, which is considered sufficient for detection of the majority of effects on male fertility and spermatogenesis, and the dosing continues both during the mating period and until the females have terminated pregnancy (total dosing period at least 40 days).

Females of the parental generation should be dosed for two weeks (with the objective of covering at least two complete estrous cycles) in order to elicit any adverse effects on estrous by the test substance. The animals are then mated and the test substance is given through mating and pregnancy and until day 4 of lactation. The number of animals used should be sufficient to obtain at least 8 pregnant females from a 1:1 (one male to one female) mating.

The animals are observed daily for changes in clinical appearance. Body weight is recorded weekly for the parental animals and for offspring at birth and on day 4, and weight gains for the different periods are calculated. Food consumption is measured. The specific parameters of reproduction recorded are: pregnancy rate, duration of pregnancy, number of pups per litter, number of live and dead pups, and number of pups with anomalies. All pups are killed after an observation period of 4 days and examined macroscopically.

The males are used for examination of possible changes in the blood parameters after mating and all animals are sacrificed and investigated for macroscopic changes. Histology is only performed on animals in the highest dosage group and the control group with special attention to gonadal organs. A comparison of findings of such short-term *in vivo* tests with the results of standard teratogenic tests reveals a high correlation, particularly in cases where the test substance produces malformations or lethal effects in standard teratogenic testing. On the other hand, the sensitivity of short-term *in vivo* testing appears to be less in cases where the test substance in standard tests produces fetotoxic effects in form of, e.g., an increased incidence of additional ribs. The use of only eight pregnant animals per group in the combined repeat dose and reproductive/developmental toxicity screening test results in an additional reduction of sensitivity.

The use of laboratory animals for experimental purposes in general raises great concern for animal welfare. Ethical considerations have led to the investment of many resources to find alternative approaches to the "traditional" toxicological test methods. The development and evaluation of *in vitro* tests is in progress. However, for the foreseeable future, data from reproduction and developmental toxicity tests in laboratory animals will contribute information vital to health assessment following exposure to chemical substances.

REFERENCES

1. Kalter, H., "Foreword". In *Chemically Induced Birth Defects*. Ed. J.L. Schardein. James L. Marcel Dekker, Inc., pp V-VI, 1985.
2. Meyer, O., Jakobsen, B.M. & Hansen, E.V., "Identification of embryo-foetal toxicity by means of animal studies". In: *Embryo-Foetal Damage And Chemical Substances*. Working party report, Ministry of Health, The National Food Agency of Denmark, Publication no. 181, pp 77-91, 1989.
3. ECETOC. Identification and assessment of the effect of chemicals on the reproduction and development, *Reprod. Toxicol. Monogr. no. 5, 1980.*
4. Health and Welfare Canada. *The Testing of Chemicals for Carcinogenicity, Mutagenicity and Teratogenicity* (Published by the authority of the Honourable Mare Lalonde, Minister of Health and Welfare Canada) Ottawa, Ontario, 1975.

5. National Academy of Sciences (NAS). *Principles and Procedures for Evaluating Chemicals in the Environment*. Washington, D.C., p 72, 1975.

6. National Academy of Sciences (NAS). *Principles and Procedures for Evaluating the Toxicity of Household Substances*. Washington, D.C., p 72, 1977.

7. OECD Organisation for Economic Cooperation and Development. Guidelines for Testing of Chemicals. Section 4: Health Effects.414 "Teratogenicity", 1981. 417 "One generation reproduction toxicity study", 1983. 418 "Two generation reproduction toxicity study", 1983. *Combined Repeat Dose and Reproductive/Developmental Toxicity Screening Test,* annex 3, OECD meeting, London 1990-04-10.

8. U.S. Environmental Protection Agency (U.S. EPA). Proposed Guidelines for Registration of Pesticides in the U.S.; Hazard Evaluation: Humans and Domestic Animals. *Federal Register.,* 43, 37335-37402, 1978.

9. WHO. World Health Organization. *Principles for the Testing of Drugs for Teratogenicity*. ITS Tech. Ser. no. 364, Geneva, 1967.

10. U.S. Food and Drug Administration (U.S. FDA). Advisory Committee on Protocols for Safety Evaluations: Panel on Reproduction Studies in Safety Evaluation of Food Additives and Pesticides Residues. *Toxicol. Appl. Pharmacol.,* 16, 264-296, 1970.

11. Brown, N.A. and Fabro, S., The value of animal teratogenicity testing for predicting human risk. *Clin. Obstet. Gynaecol.,* 26, 467-477, 1983.

12. Calabrese, E. J., "Teratogenicity: Predictive models". In: *Principles Of Animal Extrapolation*. Calabrese, E. J., (Ed.) John Wiley & Sons, Inc., 1983.

13. Schardein, J.L., Schwetz, B.A. & Kenel, M.F., Species sensitivities and prediction of teratogenic potential. *Environ. Health Perspec.,* 61, 55-67, 1985.

14. Salewski, E., Färbemethod zum makroskopischen Nachweis von Implantationsstelle am Uterus der Ratte. *Arch. Exp. Path. Pharmacol.* 247 (II), 1964.

15. Lamb, J.C., Reproductive toxicity testing: evaluating and developing new testing systems. *J. Am. Coll. Toxicol.,* 4, (2), p 163-171, 1985.

16. EEC. *European Community Directive 79-831*. Toxicological methods of annex XIII, July 1983.

17. Palmer, A.K., The design of subprimate animal studies. In *Handbook of Teratology* 4 (Wilson, J.G. and F.C. Fraser, Eds.). Plenum Press, NY, p 215, 1978.

18. Wilson, J.G. and Warkany, J., *Teratology. Principles and Techniques*. University of Chicago Press, IL, 1964.

19. Wilson, J.G., *Environment and Birth Defects*. Academic Press, NY, 1973.

20. Dawson, A.B., *Stain Technol.,* 1-2, 123, 1926.

21. Whitaker, J. and Dix, K.M., Double staining technique for rat foetus skeletons in teratological studies. *Lab. Anim., 13,* 309-310, 1979

22. Stuckhardt, J.L. and Poppe, S.M., Fresh visceral examination of rat and rabbit fetuses used in teratogenicity testing. *Teratog. Carcinog. Mutagen.,* 4, 181-188, 1984.

23. Sterz H. and Lehmann, H., A critical comparison of the freehand razor-blade dissection according to Wilson with an *in situ* sectioning method for fetuses. *Teratog. Carcinog. Mutagen.,* 5, 347-354, 1985.

24. Wilson J.G., Feasibility and design of subhuman primate studies. In *Handbook of Teratology* 4 (Wilson, J.G. and Fraser, F.C.). Plenum Press, N.Y., p 255, 1978.

25. U.S. Department of Health & Human Services. *Toxicological Profile for Lead.* 1992.

26. WHO, IPCS. *Methylmercury.* Environmental Health Criteria 101. 1990.

27. McLachlan, J.A. et al., Transplacental toxicology: prenatal factors influencing postnatal fertility. In *Developmental Toxicology*. C.A. Kimmel and J. Buelke-Sam, Eds.

28. Neubert, D. and Merker, H.J. (eds.), *New Approaches To The Evaluation Of Abnormal Embryonic Development.* VI. Postnatal manifestations of prenatal lesions. Georg Thieme. Publishers Stuttgart, p 429, 1975.

29. Adams, J. and Buelke-Sam, J., Behavioral assessment of the postnatal animal. Testing and methods development. In: *Developmental Toxicology,* C.A. Kimmel and J. Buelke-Sam (Eds.). Raven Press, N.Y. p 233, 1981.

30. Johnson, E.M., and Kochhar, D.M. (Eds.)., *Teratogenesis and Reproductive Toxicology*. Springer Verlag, 1983.

31. Mitchell C.L. & Tilson, H.A., Behavioral Toxicology In Risk Assessment. Problems And Research Needs. *Crc Criti Rev. Toxicol.*, October 1982.
32. Coyle J. et al., Behavioral teratogenesis. A critical evaluation. In *Advances In The Study Of Birth Defects*, vol. 4, Neural and Behavioral Teratology (Persaud T.V.N., Ed.) MTP Press Limited, p. 222, 1980.
33. Jensch R.P., Behavioral testing procedures. A review. In *Teratogenesis and Reproductive Toxicology* (Johnson E.M. and Kochhar, Eds.), Springer Verlag, 1983.
34. Mitchell C.L. et al., Screening for neurobehavioral toxicity. Factors to consider. In *Nervous System Toxicology* (Mitchell C.L., Eds.), Raven Press N.Y., p. 237, 1982.
35. Vorhees D.V. and Butcher, R.E., Behavioral teratogenicity. *Dev. Toxicol.*, 247-98, 1982.
36. Geller J. et al. Test methods for definition of effects of toxic substances on behaviour and neuromotor junction. *Neurobehav. Toxicol.*, 1(suppl. 1), 1979.
37. Pryor G.T., Kyeno, E.T, Tilson, H.R. and Mitchell, C.L. Assessment of chemicals using a battery of neurobehavioral tests. A comparative study., *Neurobehav. Toxicol. Teratol.*, 5, 91-117, 1980.
38. Rodier P.M., Behavioral teratology. In *Handbook of Teratology* no. 4 (Wilson J.G. and Fraser F.C., Eds.). Plenum Press, N.Y., p 397, 1978.
39. Spyker J.M., Behavioral teratology and toxicology. In *Behavioral Toxicology* (Weiss B. and Laties V.G., Eds.). Plenum Press, N.Y., p. 311, 1975.
40. Tilson H.A., Cabe P.A. and Burn T.A., Behavioral procedures for the assessment of neurotoxicity. In: *Experimental and Clinical Neurotoxicology* (P.S. Spencer and H.H. Schaumburg, Eds.) Williams & Wilkins, p. 758, 1980.
41. Chernoff N. and Kavlock, R.J. An *in vivo* teratology screen utilizing pregnant mice. *J. Toxicol. Environ. Health.*, 10, 541, 1982.
42. Shepard T.H. (Ed.), *Catalog of Teratogenic Agents,* 4 ed. John Hopkins University Press. 1983.

Chapter 4

Animal Models for the Study of Allergy

Otto Melchior Poulsen

CONTENTS

INTRODUCTION

Allergy is now recognized as one of the major diseases in the Western hemisphere and up to 20% of the population may suffer from allergy. Food allergy and inhalation allergy are most frequently the result of IgE-mediated hypersensitivity reactions, whereas contact allergies result from the delayed type cell-mediated hypersensitivity reactions.[1]

Laboratory animals, particularly mice, have been used for decades to study the basic mechanisms of the immune system, and present knowledge of the interaction between cell lines, the function of mediators, as well as the identification and functional characterization of components of the Major Histocompatibility Complex have been derived from studies of selected strains of mice.[1,2] Laboratory animals for the study of allergy may be considered a specialization in this research area. The models are widely used in basic studies of the immunological mechanisms leading to hypersensitivity (allergy) or tolerance,[3] including studies of therapeutic strategies for treatment of allergic reactions, e.g., development of new anti-anaphylactic drugs.[4,5] Furthermore, laboratory animals are used for routine tests of the allergenicity of new compounds, which either may pose a health risk (e.g., many industrial

30

Table 1. Homocytotrophic and heterocytotrophic antibodies

Donor species	Homocytophic antibodies[a]	Heterocytotrophic antibodies[b]
Man[5]	IgE	IgE(guinea pig)
Guinea pig[57,58]	IgE, IgG_{1a}, IgG_{1b}	
Rat[6]	IgE, IgG_{2a}	
Mouse[4,9,43,55]	IgE, IgG_1, IgG_{2a}	IgE (rat)

[a]Homocytotrophic PCA-test: donor and recipient animals belong to the same species.
[b]Heterocytotrophic PCA-test: donor and recipient animals belong to different species.

chemicals such as methylmethacrylate, nickel sulphate, isocyanates are strong contact allergens),[6,7] or are intended for intravenous injection.[8] Finally, laboratory animal models are frequently used in the study of food allergy and the allergenicity of food proteins, and several reviews of the use of laboratory animal models in food allergy research have recently been published.[9–11]

ANIMAL MODELS FOR IgE-MEDIATED HYPERSENSITIVITY

In IgE-mediated hypersensitivity, the specific B-lymphocytes of the sensitized subject produce IgE molecules, which become fixed to IgE receptors on mast cells in the connective tissue or basophilic leukocytes in the blood circulation. At a subsequent challenge, the cross-binding of allergen to several IgE molecules on the surface of these cells results in cell degranulation and release of enzymes and mediators (vasoactive amines, prostaglandins, interleukins, etc.) that induce the biological processes leading to the typical symptoms of immediate allergy (rhinitis, conjunctivitis, urticaria, atopic eczema, gastrointestinal reactions, asthma, etc.).[1]

Immunoglobulins, which can bind to and induce degranulation of mast cells and basophilic granulocytes are frequently called cytotrophic or reaginic antibodies. In humans cytotrophic antibodies are almost exclusively of the IgE immunoglobulin class, whereas in laboratory animals other classes of immunoglobulins (e.g., IgG_{1a}, IgG_{2a}, IgG_{2a} and IgG_{2b}) may also be cytotrophic (Table 1). The most frequently used animal models for IgE-mediated hypersensitivity are:

- Passive cutaneous anaphylaxis test (PCA-test)
- Systemic anaphylactic shock test (SAS-test)
- Models for bronchial anaphylaxis (BA-test)
- Models for gastrointestinal anaphylactic reactions (GA-test)

PASSIVE CUTANEOUS ANAPHYLAXIS TEST (PCA-TEST)

Since Ovary,[12] in the early 1960s, described in great detail the extremely high sensitivity and the resultant potential applicability of the guinea pig PCA test, the PCA test has become increasingly important and several new applications (i.e., different species of laboratory animals) have emerged during the last decades. The major steps in the PCA-test are discussed below.[12,13]

Passive Sensitization

Samples of serum containing allergen-specific cytotrophic antibodies are injected intradermally in the back of non-sensitized recipient animals. Jarrett and co-workers[14-16] demonstrated that persistent high titers of IgE were obtained in rats when low concentrations of allergen (i.e.,

<1.0 μg/animal) were injected intraperitoneally or subcutaneously in combination with an adjuvant, preferably aluminum hydroxide. Later, this profound effect of low dose sensitization was confirmed by numerous research groups using rats,[17] mice,[10,18-22] or guinea pigs.[23-25] Low dose sensitization is now generally recommended for the production of sera with high titers of IgE.

Latent Period

During the latent period, the cytotrophic antibodies become fixed to the mast cells and basophilic granulocytes in the zones of injection of sera. Different latent periods may be used to distinguish between the different classes of cytotrophic antibodies.[13,24,26] In contrast to passive sensitization with IgE, passive sensitization with cytotrophic IgG-antibodies is, in general, not persistent. In mice, a short latent period (<3 hours) will give rise to a PCA-reaction, which is the sum of the IgG- and IgE-mediated reactions, whereas a long latent period (>48 hours) leads to a PCA-reaction, which is now believed to be exclusively IgE-mediated.[9] Similarly, distinction between the different homocytotrophic immunoglobulins of guinea pigs can be obtained by using latent periods of 4 hours for IgG_{1a}, 2 to 7 days for IgG_{1b} and >14 days for IgE.[24,26]

As indicated in Table 1, the heterologous mouse/rat PCA-test is specific for murine IgE,[18,27] and this heterologous PCA-test is now mandatory in the test of allergenicity of compounds to be approved by, for example, the Japanese Food and Drug administration. The cytotrophic properties of IgE molecules are completely lost when the serum is heat-treated at 56°C for 60 min, whereas the cytotrophic IgG molecules are heat stable. Hence, parallel PCA-tests with untreated and heat-treated sera give estimates of the total titer of cytotrophic antibodies (IgG and IgE) and cytotrophic IgG.[22,28]

Challenge

After the latent period, the animals are challenged intravenously with allergen dissolved in saline containing Evans Blue dye. The dye molecules are too large to penetrate through the walls of the blood vessels into the tissues. However, in the zone of mast cell degranulation, the released vasoactive amines increase the permeability of the walls of the blood vessels, which, consequently, become permeable to Evans Blue dye. Hence, a positive PCA-reaction is visualized by the appearance of a blue reaction zone in the skin of the recipient animal.[12]

The PCA-test has been applied in a variety of contexts such as studies on:

- Parameters that influence sensitization, e.g., strain differences in the production of cytotrophic antibodies,[14,17,24,29,30] effects of sensitization route, dose of allergen and use of various adjuvants,[14,15,20,31-34] and effects of anti-inflammatory drugs.[5]
- Parameters that influence responsiveness in the PCA-test, e.g., strain differences[35] and density of reaginic antibodies on mast cells.[36]
- Modulation of the immunological response, e.g., by manipulating the suppressor T-lymphocytes.[5,37]
- Effects of modifications of allergens on their sensitizing potential, e.g., hydrolysis of food proteins,[8,38-42] heat treatment of food proteins,[39,51] and chemical modification of proteins (solvent extraction, esterification, etc).[40]

In principle, the PCA-test merely measures the titer of cytotrophic antibodies, and it is frequently claimed that this test is unethical since the results can be obtained using *in vitro* assays such as Enzyme Linked Immuno Sorbent Assay (ELISA).[25] Although this is true when soluble, partially purified preparations of allergens are studied, the argument does not stand when complex allergen preparations (e.g., cow's milk or heat-denatured soy proteins) are used.[10,43-45]

Table 2. SAS score in mice

Score	Symptoms
0	The mouse shows no reactions or only weak hyperventilation, which may be a psychosomatic reaction against the intravenous injection.
+	The mouse prefers to be stationary and will only move slowly when provoked.
++	The mouse does not move even when provoked. When laid on its back, the mouse has great difficulty in turning to an upright position.
+++	The mouse shows severe whole body cramps. Mice entering this state are immediately killed by dislocation of the neck.

SYSTEMIC ANAPHYLACTIC SHOCK TESTS (SAS-TEST)

Guinea pigs are highly sensitive in the SAS-test. Therefore, this species is frequently recommended for the test. Recent studies, however, have indicated that some inbred mouse strains may have a sensitivity similar to that of guinea pigs.[10] The major steps in the SAS-test[10,26,39,46-48,51] are as follows.

Sensitization

Most frequently sensitization is repeated several times over a period of 2 to 3 weeks. Since the SAS-test is common as a mandatory test of the allergenicity of compounds to be approved for human use,[8] the route of sensitization often reflects the intended route of administration in humans. However, in general, the above mentioned low dose sensitization with the allergen in an adjuvant also leads to good sensitization in this test.

Challenge

After the sensitization period, the animals are challenged intravenously with allergen dissolved in saline.

Scoring Systemic Anaphylactic Reactions

Systemic anaphylactic reactions are observed during a period of 15 to 60 min after challenge. During this period, the reactions often increase in intensity and finally reach fatal anaphylactic shock.

The different laboratory animal species (i.e., guinea pigs, mice, and rats) show different major anaphylactic shock reactions.[23,48] Guinea pigs mainly show pulmonary reaction (e.g., bronchospasm), whereas the whole body reactions in mice and rats are the result of a systemic increase in vascular permeability. Table 2 presents a graduated score of SAS reactions in mice,[46] which can, with minor modifications, be applied to guinea pigs.[26]

One major criticism of the SAS-test may be that intravenous challenge does not reflect a normal route of challenge of allergic humans. It should, however, be emphazied that in most cases the aim of the SAS-test is merely to test the potential allergenicity of, e.g., modified food proteins or drugs. The underlying idea is that if an intravenous injection of a compound in sensitized laboratory animals induces systemic anaphylactic reactions, the compound is likely to induce anaphylactic reactions in allergic persons as well.

Some scientists have argued that the score of the SAS-test correlates with the serum titer of specific IgE, and that the SAS-test should be abandoned, since the results can be obtained by either the PCA-test or ELISA.[25] Some studies have, however, indicated that this correlation is not always apparent. BALB/c mice fed pellets containing bovine milk proteins display strong anaphylactic reactions in the SAS-test when challenged with homogenized bovine milk, but these mice have low or undetectable PCA-titers against bovine milk proteins.[10,34,43,46,47,49] Similarly, children with positive provocation tests frequently have negative skin prick tests and no detectable increase in serum concentrations of milk-specific IgE using the Radio Allergo Sorbent Test.[10,50] Furthermore, it was previously shown that the capability of proteins to induce anaphylactic reactions in the SAS-test is dependent both on the antigenic determinants of the protein and on the colloid chemical environment of the protein, e.g., homogenized bovine milk could induce anaphylactic reactions at a far lower concentration than unhomogenized milk. In contrast, only slight differences were observed between the two types of milk in the PCA test.[10,43] Consequently, the SAS-test should not be replaced by the PCA-test in studies of complex colloid chemical effects on the allergenicity of proteins.

ANIMAL MODELS FOR BRONCHIAL ANAPHYLAXIS TEST (BA-TEST)

These models aim to study anaphylactic reactions in the lungs, which are also an important anaphylactic shock organ in humans.

Guinea pigs mainly show bronchial anaphylactic reactions,[48] so naturally the guinea pigs are most frequently chosen as the laboratory animal model for bronchial anaphylaxis.[4,24,52-58] However, some reports describe the used of mice[45,59] and rats.[60] The major steps in the BA-test are discussed below.

Sensitization

Injection of a low dose of allergen in combination with, e.g., aluminum hydroxide is often used to obtain an efficient sensitization,[24,52,55] but allergen in an aerosol has been used to simulate the route of sensitization, expected to be relevant for human allergy to inhaled allergens (e.g., pollen, flour, house dust mites, laboratory animal allergens, etc). Ovalbumin, which has long be recognized as a strong allergen,[12] has been used as a model allergen by the majority of research groups in this field.[24,45,55,56,58,61]

Challenge

The sensitized animals are challenged with an aerosol containing allergen.

Scoring Anaphylactic Bronchial Reactions

Several different scoring systems have been suggested ranging from the simple visual examination of the pulmonary reactions (i.e., ventilation rate and depth)[24,55] to sophisticated systems with advanced plethysmography and differential pressure transducer equipment for measurement of bronchial activity.[4,53,54,57,58]

Similar to the criticism of the SAS-test, it may be argued that challenge in the BA-test may be replaced with the PCA-test and ELISA for measurements of allergen-specific IgE in sera from sensitized animals. Again, this argument does not stand when combined effects on allergenicity are studied, e.g., the recent demonstration of the adjuvant-like potentiating effects of diesel exhaust,[45] SO_2,[56,61] NO_2,[56] and ozone[56] on the pulmonary sensitization of guinea pigs and mice to inhaled ovalbumin. Particularly, diesel exhaust was demonstrated to have a strong adjuvant effect resulting in IgE-titers similar to the titers obtained with the Bordetella pertussis adjuvant generally used for high titer IgE-production.[14-16]

MODELS FOR GASTROINTESTINAL ANAPHYLACTIC REACTIONS (GA-MODELS)

These models are, in principle, very similar to the BA-models, i.e., the models aim to study anaphylactic reactions in a defined organ. In contrast to the well-established and frequently used BA-models, only a few reports describe the development of GA-models using guinea pigs,[26,62-65] rats[64-70] or mice,[71-72] and these models are often poorly defined and have a low sensitivity. The major steps in the GA-test are discussed below.

Sensitization

Attempts to sensitize laboratory animals orally without the use of an adjuvant have failed in nearly all studies, i.e., tolerance was induced, and it has been suggested[3] that this would always be the case in rodents. Consequently, most papers describe the use of parenteral injection of allergen in combination with an adjuvant (i.e., aluminum hydroxide) to obtain adequate sensitization.

Recently, it was demonstrated that BALB/c mice could be sensitized orally with low doses of homogenized cow's milk without the use of an adjuvant.[10,34,49] In contrast, the mice were not sensitized with untreated bovine milk given orally. One possible explanation may be that homogenized milk itself possesses adjuvant-like properties. Similarly, it was recently demonstrated[26] that animals of an inbred high-responder guinea pig strain (IMM/S 740[52]) could be sensitized orally with an ovalbumin-olive oil emulsion, which in principle resembles homogenized milk.

Challenge

The sensitized animals are challenged orally with high doses of allergen.

Scoring Of Gastrointestinal Anaphylactic Reactions

Until recently, no GA-model was sufficiently sensitive to produce strong anaphylactic reactions that could be scored by visual inspection of the animals. Consequently, the majority of GA-models are based on a detailed histological examination of the intestinal wall to score the anaphylactic reactions. Typical signs of gastrointestinal anaphylactic reactions (mast cell degranulation, edema and/or atrophy of villi) have been demonstrated in the gut of guinea pigs,[62] rats,[66,68-70] and mice.[49]

Pedersen[26] recently described a GA-model in which clearly visible systemic anaphylactic reactions could be induced orally in inbred IMM/S 740 guinea pigs sensitized with ovalbumin. However, these reactions were mainly pulmonary, and no sign of gastrointestinal anaphylactic reactions in the intestinal wall could be demonstrated histologically.

In conclusion, reliable and sufficiently sensitive animal models of human gastrointestinal anaphylactic reactions are still lacking.

ANIMAL MODELS FOR CELL-MEDIATED HYPERSENSITIVITY

Cell-mediated hypersensitivity is directed against complexes between carrier proteins and small compounds, denoted haptens. The carrier proteins are proteins of the individual itself (e.g., serum albumin). When present without carrier proteins, the haptens do not possess allergenic properties, but the immune system of the individual may recognize the structure of the hapten-protein complex as a foreign antigenic determinant. After penetration through the skin barrier, the hapten is picked up by antigen-presenting Langerhans cells in the skin. Inside the cells the hapten is processed (i.e., metabolized) and then presented on the cell surface in association with MHC class II antigens. As a result of an interaction between this hapten-presenting complex and specific T_{helper}-lymphocytes, the lymphocytes will proliferate to memory cells. When at a later stage the hapten is presented again, the memory cells will recognize the hapten-presenting complex and proliferate to cytotoxic T-lymphocytes, which are responsible for the tissue damage connected with this type of hypersensitivity.[1,2]

The symptoms of cell-mediated hypersensitivity are mainly local skin reactions (also called contact allergy or contact dermatitis), but systemic cell-mediated hypersensitivity reactions may frequently occur in conjunction with, e.g., allergy to cow's milk.[50]

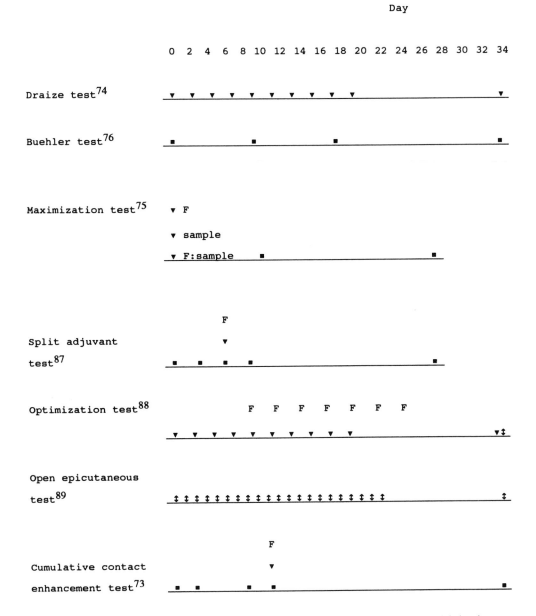

Figure 1. Guinea pig tests for cell-mediated hypersensitivity. ▼ = intradermal injection; ■ = closed patch; ↕ = open patch; F = Freunds Complete Adjuvant.

The guinea pig is the most common species of laboratory animals used for testing potential contact allergens.[2,73] Since Draize[74] published the Draize test, a series of modifications have been proposed (Figure 1). The guinea pig maximization test[75] is today generally accepted and widely applied. In principle, all of the tests involve the following steps.

SENSITIZATION

In three of the tests, sensitization (and challenge) is obtained simply by placing the contact allergen in a vehicle dependent on the solubility of the contact allergen (olive oil, ethanol, acetone, etc.) in an open or closed patch on the clipped and shaven back or neck of the guinea pig. However, the incidence of sensitization (i.e., the number of actually sensitized animals expressed as a percentage of the total number of animals in the sensitization group) in these tests is low. To improve the incidence of sensitization several of the tests in Figure 1 use intradermal injection of Freunds Complete Adjuvant (FCA) given preferably in the neck region. FCA is administered either alone or in combination with the allergen, often conjugated to a carrier protein (e.g., dinitrophenyl-bovine serum albumin). Numerous studies have confirmed that the use of intradermal FCA-injections increases the efficacy of sensitization with contact allergens.[7,44,73,75,76]

CHALLENGE

Challenge is obtained by placing the contact allergen in a vehicle on the skin of the back of sensitized guinea pigs using either open patches (uncovered vehicle) or closed patches (vehicle covered to prevent evaporation and scratch damage in the zone of challenge). In order to prevent falsely positive results (i.e., irritative skin reactions) a preliminary dose-response study is always performed to determine the lowest dose of the test compound that can give rise to irritative skin reactions in unsensitized guinea pigs (i.e., the threshold dose of irritation). In the subsequent test for sensitization capacity of the test compound, the sensitized guinea pigs are challenged at a high dose (denoted the maximization dose), which is still well below the threshold dose of irritation of the compound.

This procedure is frequently believed to produce the strongest possible cell-mediated skin reaction and at the same time to prevent the occurrence of irritative non-allergenic reactions. Consequently, the sensitization capacity of potential contact allergens is rarely tested at several different challenge doses deviating from the maximization dose. However, in a detailed study on different acrylate compounds, it was demonstrated that a clear-cut dose-response relationship does not always prevail between the challenge dose and the strength of the cell-mediated hypersensitivity reactions in the skin.[6,7] The authors suggested that in some cases, challenge at the maximization dose might only underestimate the sensitization potential of the tested compound.

SCORING THE SKIN REACTIONS

Frequently, the number of animals with positive skin reactions as a percentage of the total number of challenged animals is recorded, and the difference between the experimental groups is statistically tested using, e.g., Fisher's Exact Test. However, several papers describe the use of graded score systems.[6,7]

Although the guinea pig maximization test is generally considered reliable for the prediction of contact sensitization potential in humans, Kimber[2] emphasized that the value of the guinea pig tests in human risk assessment is uncertain.

Mice have been widely used in basic studies on the immunological mechanisms involved in cell-mediated hypersensitivity, e.g., factors influencing:

- passive transfer of hypersensitivity[1,2,77]
- response of different cell lines of the immune system[2,37]

The foot pad swelling test[78] has been widely used in this context. Sensitized mice (i.e., inbred BALB/c) are challenged by intradermal injection of allergen in the foot pad of one of the hind legs, whereas the other hind leg serves as a control (saline injected intradermally). A positive cell-mediated hypersensitivity reaction is seen as a swelling of the foot pad during the next days, and the reaction is scored by comparing the volume of the challenged foot with the control foot. The foot pad swelling test may cause a considerable pain and discomfort to the animals, and, consequently, alternative animal models such as the ear swelling test[2,79,80] may be considered more ethical. The principle of the ear swelling test is similar to the foot pad swelling test, i.e., after challenge of sensitized mice the swelling of the challenged ear is compared with the swelling of the control ear.

Kimber and co-workers[2,81-83] have developed a murine local lymph node assay in which challenge of sensitized mice is replaced by studies of isolated lymph nodes. This promising assay was proven well-suited for basic immunological studies of the mechanisms of contact allergy, and the validity of the assay to predict the sensitization potential of allergens has been tested on a wide range of contact allergens. In general, the results were in good agreement with current experience from the human clinic. One major advantage of the local lymph node assay is that sensitization is by way of the relevant route and without the need of an adjuvant.

In the human clinic, the patch test is most frequently used to diagnose cell-mediated hypersensitivity. However, some contact allergens (e.g., monomers and dimers of acrylates such as methylmethacrylates) are so potent that the patch test itself poses a risk of sensitization. Hence, several attempts have been made to develop *in vitro* cytological tests that can replace the patch test. These tests still have a low specificity (i.e., a high number of falsely positive and negative results) and sensitivity, and the tests are still not used for routine diagnosis of contact allergy. However, recent studies on mice have demonstrated ways to increase the specificity and sensitivity of the cytological tests,[44] and in the future the *in vitro* tests may be a good supplement to laboratory animal models in the study of cell-mediated hypersensitivity and in the screening of potential contact allergens.

CONCLUSION

Although the relevance of some animal models for human allergy (e.g., immune regulation of atopic allergy) can be questioned,[3] animal models for both IgE-mediated and cell-mediated hypersensitivity have provided important basic knowledge of the mechanisms involved in allergic reactions, including sensitization and the triggering of allergic reaction. Furthermore, the animal models have provided information of high clinical significance with respect to, for example, the effect of allergen dose and allergen presentation on the development of hypersensitivity vs. the development of tolerance.

Intensive work has been done over the last decade to replace animal models with *in vitro* tests,[44,84,85] but these tests still provide limited information compared with the laboratory animal models. Hence, in some contexts the *in vitro* test may be a useful supplement to laboratory animals, but in general, the animal models in allergy research cannot be replaced with *in vitro* tests.[2,42,86]

REFERENCES

1. Roit, I., Brostoff,J., and Male, D., *Immunology,* Gower Medical Publishing, London, 1985.
2. Kimber, I., Aspects of the immune response to contact allergens: Opportunities for the development and modification of predictive test methods, *Food Chem. Toxicol., 27, 755, 1989.*
3. Björkstein, B. and Ahlstedt, S., Relevance of animal models for studies of immune regulation of atopic allergy, *Allergy, 39, 317, 1984.*
4. Danko, G. and Chapman, R. W., Simple, noninvasive method to measure the antibronchoconstrictor activity of drugs in conscious guinea pigs, *J. Pharmacol. Meth., 19, 165, 1988.*
5. Lewis, A. J., Carlson, R. P., Foster, T. J., Chang, J., Hand, J. M., Unden, B. J., Buckner, C. K., Tio, C., Sisenwine, S. F., and Daniel, W. C., The development of Wy-41,195, an orally effective antiallergic drug in animal models, *Agents Actions T8, 3/4, 308, 1986.*
6. Van der Walle, N. B. and Bensink, T., Cross reaction pattern of 26 acrylic monomers on guinea pig skin. *Contact Dermititis, 8, 376, 1982.*
7. Van der Walle, H. B., Klecak, G., Geleick, H., Bensink, T., Sensitizing potential of 14 mono (meth) acrylate in the guinea pig, *Contact Dermititis, 8, 223, 1982.*

8. Knights, R. J., Processing and evaluation of the antigenicity of protein hydrolysates, in: *Clinical Disorders in Pediatric Nutrition Vol. 4* (ed.), Marcel Dekker, Inc. New York, 1985.

9. Poulsen, O. M., Hau, J., Animal models for the study of allergy, *Scand. J. Lab. Ani. Sci. 16(Suppl. 1), 96, 1989.*

10. Poulsen, O. M., Development and application of two murine models for the study of the allergenicity of cow's milk proteins and -peptides, *Scand. J. Lab. Anim. Sci., 17(Suppl. 1), 1990.*

11. Stokes, C. R., Miller, B. G., Bourne, F. J., Animal models of food sensitivity, in: Brostoff, J. and Challacombe, S.J. (eds). *Food Allergy and Intolerance.* Bailliere Tindall, London. 1987.

12. Ovary, Z., Passive Cutaneous Anaphylaxis. In: *Immunological Methods, Cioms Symposium,* (J.F. Ackroyrd, ed.). Blackwell Scientific Publications, Oxford 1964.

13. Ovary, Z., Local anaphylaxis. 1. Passive Cutaneous Anaphylaxis, in: Williams, C. A. and Chase, M. W. (eds) *Methods in Immunology and Immunochemistry.* Academic Press, London 1976.

14. Jarrett, E. E. E., Stimuli for the production and control of IgE in rats, *Immunol. Rev., 41, 52, 1978.*

15. Jarrett, E. E. E. and Steward, D. C., Rat IgE production. I. Effect of dose of antigen on primary and secondary reaginic antibody response, *Immunology, 27, 365, 1974.*

16. Jarrett, E. E. E., Haig, D. M., McDougall, W., and McNulty, E., Rat IgE production. II. Primary and booster reaginic antibody responses following intradermal or oral immunization, *Immunology, 30, 671, 1976.*

17. Bazin, H. and Pauwels, R., IgE and IgG$_{2a}$ isotypes in the rat, *Prog. Allergy, 32, 53, 1982.*

18. Braga, F. and Mota, I., Homologous passive cutaneous anaphylaxis (PCA) in mice and heterologous PCA induced in rats with mouse IgE, *Immunology, 30, 655, 1976.*

19. Poulsen, O. M. and Hau, J., Murine passive cutaneous anaphylaxis test (PCA) for the "all or none" determination of allergenicity of bovine whey proteins and peptides, *Clin. Allergy, 17, 75, 1987.*

20. Poulsen, O. M. and Hau, J., Dose response assessment of peptide allergenicity using a murine passive cutaneous anaphylaxis test (PCA), in: *Laboratory Animal and Health for All,* Proceedings of the IXth ICLAS International Symposium on Laboratory Animal Science, Bangkok, 1988.

21. Vaz, E. M., Vaz, N. M., and Levine, B. B., Persistent formation of reagins in mice injected with low doses of ovalbumin, *Immunology, 21, 11, 1971.*

22. Watanabe, N. and Ovary, Z., Antigen and antibody detection by *in vivo* methods. A reevaluation of passive cutaneous anaphylactic reactions, *J. Immunol. Methods, 14, 381, 1977.*

23. Lewis, R. M., Immunopathology, in: *Pathology of Laboratory Animals,* eds. K. Benirschke, F.M. Garner, T.C. Jones, 1978, p1948.

24. Lundberg, L., Guinea pigs inbred for studies of respiratory anaphylaxis, *Acta. Path. Microbiol. Scand. sect. C, 87, 55, 1979.*

25. Maekawa, S. and Ovary, Z., Correlation of Murine anti-Dinitrophenyl Antibody content as determined by ELISA, Passive Cutaneous Anaphylaxis and Passive Hemolysis, *J. Immunol. Methods, 71, 229, 1984.*

26. Petersen, D., Applicability of inbred "high-responder" IMM/S 740 guinea pigs as a model for studies of food allergies. (In Danish), The Royal Veterinary and Agricultural University, Copenhagen, Inst. Pharmacology and Pathobiology, *Master's thesis, 1991.*

27. Ovary, Z., Caiazza, S. S., and Kojima, S., PCA reactions with mouse antibodies in mice and rats, *Int. Arch. Allergy Appl. Immunol., 16, 1975.*

28. Parish, W. E., Homologous serum passive cutaneous anaphylaxis in guinea pigs mediated by two τ1 or τ1-type heat-stable globulins and a non-τ1 heat-labile reagin, *J. Immunol., 105, 1296, 1970.*

29. Baeron, M., Couderc, J., Ventura, M., Liacopoulos, P., and Voisin, G.A. Anaphylactic properties of mouse monoclonal IgG2a antibodies, *Cell. Immunol., 70, 27, 1982.*

30. Levine, B. B. and Vaz, N. M., Effect of combination of inbred strain antigen and antigen dose on immune responsiveness and reagin production in the mouse, *Int. Arch. Allergy, 39, 156, 1970.*

31. Andre, C., Bazin, H., and Heremans, J. F., Influence of repeated administration of antigen by the oral route on specific antibody-producing cells in the mouse spleen, *Digestion, 9, 166, 1972.*

32. Bazin H. and Platteau, B., Production of circulating reaginic (IgE) antibodies by oral administration of ovalbumin to rats, *Immunology, 30, 679, 1976.*

33. Hargis, B. J. and Malkiel, S., Production of hypersensitivity in the neonatal mouse, *J. Immunol., 104, 942, 1970.*

34. Nielsen, B. R., Poulsen, O. M., and Hau, J., Reagin production in mice: effect of subcutaneous and oral sensitization with untreated bovine milk and homogenized bovine milk, *In vivo, 3, 271, 1989.*

35. Vaz, N. M. and Ovary, Z., Passive cutaneous anaphylaxis in mice with yG antibodies. IV. Strain differences in susceptibility to mast cell sensitization in vitro, *J. Immunol., 104, 896, 1970.*

36. Watanabe, N. and Kobayashi, A. Sensitivity of passive cutaneous anaphylaxis in rats. I. Inverse relationship between PCA sensitivity and amount of IgE present on mast cells, *Int. Arch. Allergy Appl. Microbiol., 72, 53, 1983.*

37. Chiorazzi, N., Fox, D. A., Katz, D. H., Hapten specific IgE responses in mice. VII. Conversion of IgE "non responder" strains to IgE "responders" by elimination of Suppressor T Cell activity, *J. Immunol., 111, 48, 1977.*

38. Lui, C. T., Das, B. R. and Maurer, P. H., Immunochemical studies of the tryptic, chymotryptic and peptic peptides of heat denatured bovine serum albumin, *Immunochemistry, 4, 1, 1967.*

39. McLaughlan, P., Anderson, K. J., Widdowson, E. M., and Coombs, R. R. A., Effect of heat on the anaphylactic-sensitizing capacity of cows milk, goats milk, and various infant formulae fed to guinea-pigs, *Arch. Dis. Child., 56, 165, 1981.*

40. Matsuda, T., Kato, Y., Watanabe, K., and Nakamura, R., Immunochemical properties of proteins glycosylated through Maillard reaction: ß-lactoglobulin-lactose and ovalbumin-glucose systems, *J. Food Sci., 50, 618, 1985.*

41. Stefanovic, J., Kotulova, D., Bergendi, L., and Huzulakova, I., The passive anaphylactic reaction in guinea pigs elicited by whole and Cathepsin D-degraded antigen, *Folia Microbiol., 19, 71, 1974.*

42. Poulsen, O. M. and Hau, J., Laboratory animals are presently not replaceable in the study of allergy, *ICLAS Bull., 59, 16 1986.*

43. Poulsen, O. M. and Hau, J., Application of a murine anaphylactic shock model. A colloid chemical approach to cow's milk allergy. in: *Laboratory Animal and Health for All,* Proceedings of the IXth ICLAS International Symposium on Laboratory Animal Science, Bangkok, 1988.

44. Robinson, M. K., Optimization of an *in vitro* lymphocyte blastogenesis assay for predictive assessment of immunological responsiveness to contact sensitizers, *J. Invest. Dermatol., 92, 860, 1989.*

45. Takafuji, S., Suzuki, S., Koizumi, K., Tadokoro, K., Miyamoto, T., Ikemori, R. and Muranaka, M., Diesel-exhaust particulates inoculated by the intranasal route have an adjuvant activity for IgE production in mice, *J. Allergy Clin. Immunol., 79, 639, 1987.*

46. Poulsen, O. M., Hau, J., and Kollerup, J., Effect of homogenization and pasteurization on the allergenicity of bovine milk analyzed by a murine anaphylactic shock model, *Clin. Allergy, 17, 449, 1987.*

47. Poulsen, O. M., Hau, J., and Kollerup, J., The effect of homogenization and pasteurization on the allergenicity of bovine milk analyzed by a murine anaphylactic shock model, in: *New Developments in Biosciences: Their Implications for Laboratory Animal Science* (A.C. Beynen and H.A. Solleveld, eds.). Proceedings 3rd FELASA Symposium, Amsterdam, 1987,

48. Treadwell, P. E., Wistar, T., and Rasmussen Jr, A. F. Passive anaphylaxis in mice with homologous antiserum - I. Some quantitative aspects, *J. Immunol., 84, 539, 1960.*

49. Poulsen, O. M., Nielsen, B. R., Basse, A., and Hau, J., Comparison of intestinal anaphylactic reactions in sensitized mice challenged orally with raw untreated milk and homogenized bovine milk, *Allergy, 45, 321, 1990.*

50. Bahna, S.L., Pathogenesis of milk hypersensitivity, *Immunol. Today, 6, 153, 1985.*

51. Heppel, L. M., Cant, A. J., and Kilshaw, P. J., Reduction in the antigenicity of whey proteins by heat treatment: a possible strategy for producing a hypoallergenic infant formula, *Br. J. Nutr., 51, 29, 1984.*

52. Clausen, J. T., Lundberg, L., and Sparck, J. V., Characterization of two strains of selectively bred guinea-pigs, *Acta. Path. Microbiol. Immunol. Scand. sect. C, 91, 377, 1983.*

53. Hulbert, W. C., McLean, T., Wiggs, B., Paré, P. D., and Hogg, J. C., Histamine dose-response curves in guinea pigs, *J. Appl. Physiol., 58, 625, 1985.*

54. Hutson, P. A., Church, M. K., Clay, T. P., Miller, P., and Holgate, S. T., Early and Late-phase bronchoconstriction after allergen challenge of nonanesthetized Guinea pigs, *Am. Rev. Rest. Dis., 137, 548, 1988.*

55. Lundberg, L., Bertelsen, C., Zavaro, A., Samra, Z., and Sompolinsky, D., Experimental allergic conjunctivitis in inbred guinea pig strains with high respectively low bronchial allergic reactivity, *Allergy, 42, 262, 1987.*

56. Matsumura, Y., The effects of ozone, nitrogen dioxide, and sulfur dioxide on the experimentally induced allergic respiratory disorder in guinea pigs, *Am. Rev. Resp. Dis., 102, 430, 1970.*

57. Motojima, S., Yukawa, T., Fukuda, T. and Makido, S., Changes in airway responsiveness and ß- and α-1-adrenergic receptors in the lungs of guinea pigs with experimental asthma, *Allergy, 44, 66, 1989.*

58. Payne, A. N. and de Nucci, G., Anaphylaxis in Guinea Pigs Induced by Ovalbumin Aerosol — In vivo and in vitro methods, *J. Pharmocol. Methods, 17, 83, 1987.*

59. McCaskill, A. C., Hosking, C. S., and Hill, D. J., Anaphylaxis following intranasal challenge of mice sensitized with ovalbumin, *Immunology, 51, 669, 1984.*

60. Ufkes, J. G. R., Ottenhof, M., and Allberse, R. C., A new method for inducing fatal, IgE-mediated, bronchial and cardiovascular anaphylaxis in the rat, *J. Pharmacol. Methods, 9, 175, 1983.*

61. Reidel, F., Krämer, M., Scheibenbogen, C., and Reiger, C. H. L., Effects of SO_2 exposure on allergic sensitization in the guinea pigs, *J. Allergy Clin. Immunol., 82, 527, 1988.*

62. Carrick, B.M. and Alexander, M. D., The effect of milk feeding on specific intestinal protein permeability in the guinea-pig, *Nutr. Res., 2, 603, 1982.*

63. Chubert, A. W., McLaughlan, P., and Coombs, R. R. A., Immediate hypersensitivity reaction to ß-lactoglobulin in the epithelium lining the colon of guinea pigs fed cows milk, *Int. Arch. Allergy Appl. Immunol., 72, 34, 1983.*

64. Koritz, T. N., Suzuki, S., and Coombs, R. R. A., Antigenic stimulation of cow's milk via the oral route in guinea pigs and rats — 1. Measurement of antigenically intact ß-lactoglobulin and casein in the gastrointestinal contents of duodenum, jejunum and ileum, *Int. Arch. Allergy Appl. Immunol., 82, 72, 1987.*

65. Koritz, T. N., Suzuki, S., and Coombs, R. R. A., Antigenic stimulation with cow's milk via the oral route in guinea pigs and rats — 2. Antibodies to ß-lactoglobulin secreted into the alimentary canal and serum, *Int. Arch. Allergy Appl. Immunol., 82, 76, 1987.*

66. Byars, N.E. and Ferraresi, R.W., Intestinal anaphylaxis in the rat as a model of food allergy, *Clin. Exp. Immunol., 24, 352, 1976.*

67. Perdue, M. H., Chung, M., and Gall D. G., Effect of intestinal anaphylaxis on gut function in the rat, *Gastroenterology, 86, 391, 1984.*

68. Roberts, S. A., Reinhardt, M. C., Paganelli, R., and Levinsky, R. J., Specific antigen exclusion and non-specific facilitation of antigen entry across the gut in rats allergic to food proteins, *Clin. Exp. Immunol., 45, 131, 1981.*

69. Stern, M., Pang, K. Y., and Walker, W. A., Food proteins and gut mucosal barrier. II. Differential interaction of cows milk proteins with the mucous coat and the surface membrane of adult and immature rat jejunum, *Ped. Res., 18, 1252, 1984.*

70. Turner, M. W., Boulton, P., Shields, J. G., Strobel, S., Gibson, S., MIller, H. R. P., and Levinsky, R. J., Intestinal hypersensitivity reactions in the rat. I. Uptake of intact protein, permeability to sugars and their correlation with mucosal mast-cell activation, *Immunology, 63, 119, 1988.*

71. Granato, D. A. and Piguet, P. F., A mouse monoclonal IgE antibody anti bovine milk ß-lactoglobulin allows studies of allergy in the gastrointestinal tract, *Clin. Exp. Immunol., 63, 703, 1986.*

72. Malo, C. and Morin, C. L., Establishment of an animal model of ovalbumin sensitized mouse to study protein induced enteropathy, *Gut, 27, 1298, 1986.*

73. Tsuchiya, S., Kondo, M., Okamoto, K., and Takase, Y., Studies on contact hypersensitivity in the guinea pig. The cumulative contact enhancement test, *Cont. Dermat., 8, 246, 1982.*

74. Draize, J. H. Intracutaneous sensitization test in guinea pigs. In: *Appraisal of the Safety of Chemicals in Foods, Drugs and Cosmetics*, Texas, 1959.

75. Magnusson, B. and Kligman, A. M., The identification of contact allergens by animal assay. The guinea pig maximization test, *J. Invest. Dermatol., 52, 268, 1969.*

76. Buehler, E.V., Delayed contact hypersensitivity in the guinea pig, *Arch. Dermatol., 28, 53, 1965.*

77. Landsteiner, K. and Chase, M. W., Experiments on transfer of cutaneous sensitivity to simple compounds, *Proc. Soc. Exp. Biol. Med., 49, 39, 1942.*

78. Singh, B., Lee, K.-C., Fraga, E., Wilkinson, A., Wong, M., and Barton, M. A., Minimum peptide sequences necessary for priming and triggering of humoral and cell-mediated immune responses in mice: use of synthetic peptide antigens of defined structure, *J. Immunol., 124, 1336, 1980.*

79. Asherson, G.L. and Ptak, W., Contact and delayed hypersensitivity in the mouse. I. Active sensitization and passive transfer, *Immunology, 15, 495, 1968.*

80. Gad, S. C. A scheme for the prediction and ranking of relative potencies of dermal sensitizers based on data from several systems, *J. Appl. Toxicol., 8, 361, 1988.*

81. Kimber, I., Hilton, J. and Botham, P. A., Identification of contact allergens using the murine local lymph node assay: Comparisons with the Buehler Occluded Patch Test in guinea pigs, *J. Appl. Toxicol., 10, 173, 1990.*

82. Kimber, I., Hilton, J., Botham, P. A., Basketter, D. A., Scholes, E. W., Miller, K., Robbins, M. C., Harrison, P. T. C., Gray, T. J. B. and Waite, S. J., The murine local lymph node assay: Results of an inter-laboratory trial, *Toxicol. Lett., 55, 203, 1991.*

83. Kimber, I. and Weisenberger, C., Anamnestic responses to contact allergens: Application in the murine local lymph node assay, *J. Appl. Toxicol., 11, 129, 1991.*

84. Gjesing, B., Østerballe, O., Schwartz, B., Wahn, U., Løwenstein, H., IgE antibodies against antigenic components in cow's milk and milk substitutes, *Allergy, 41, 51, 1986.*

85. Skov, P. S., Norn, S., and Weeke, B., A rapid basophil histamine release method, *Eur. J. Resp. Dis., 64(Suppl. 128), 387, 1983.*

86. Schambye, P., Cell toxicology — an alternative to experiments on animals?, *Scand. J. Lab. Anim. Sci., 12, 115, 1985.*

87. Maguire, H. C., The bioassay of allergens in the guinea pig, *J. Soc. Cosmet. Chem., 24, 151, 1973.*

88. Maurer, T., Thoman, P., Weirich, E. G., and Hess, R., The optimization test in the guinea pig. A method for the predicative evaluation of contact allergenicity of chemicals, *Agents Action, 5, 174, 1975.*

89. Klecak, G., Geleike, H., Frey, J. R., Screening of fragrance materials for allergenicity in the guinea pig. I. Comparison of 4 test methods, *J. Soc. Cosmet. Chem., 28, 53, 1977.*

Chapter 5

Animal Models for Cardiovascular Research

Timo Nevalainen

CONTENTS

INTRODUCTION

Cardiovascular diseases present a major challenge to health care systems in the industrialized world. As a consequence, much non-clinical cardiovascular research focuses on modeling human circulatory diseases in experimental animals. Human hearts are similar to other mammalian hearts. They comprise a connective tissue frame, four muscular chambers, an electrical conduction system, and a series of one-way valves. The essential differences are in the coronary and coronary collateral vasculature, which give rise to differences of tolerance to ischemic injury. Many common cardiovascular diseases in humans involve the coronary arteries and/or coronary collaterals in some way.

In the design of experiments using animal models, it is important to consider the validity of the chosen model. Validity means similarity, between man and the chosen model, in basic anatomical structure and physiological or biochemical function, or of disease processes. Other general requirements for animal models are availability at reasonable cost, ease of maintenance and handling, similarity in size, availability as a genetically pure-bred line, and ease of reproduction in captivity.

Availability may be a major limitation on the use of spontaneous animal models for cardiovascular diseases. In the case of induced models, time constraints may also be important. However, the production of animals induced to model chronic human conditions generally takes days, weeks, or months rather than years.

The use of animal models for cardiovascular research has been discussed in many books and articles.[1] Each has taken its own approach, and this article is no exception. Rather than listing the various models available for cardiovascular research, this article will discuss some examples of the characteristics that make certain animal species, stocks, and strains valuable in modeling the most common circulatory diseases in humans. The diseases examined are atherosclerosis, hypertension, and myocardial ischemia.

SPECIFIC CHARACTERISTICS

RODENTS

Surprisingly, the use of mice and rats is less common in cardiovascular research than one might expect. Their small size, which is an advantage in other research fields, may not be so in cardiovascular research. Small size renders them difficult to prepare and operate on; if instruments are used, the miniature size needed may mean extra cost and difficulty. However, some articles on cardiovascular techniques in rats are available.[2]

The main recorded contribution to cardiovascular research using rats has been the establishment of two strains of rats showing hypertension. These are the inbred spontaneously hypertensive rat (SHR) and the Dahl salt-resistant (R) and salt-sensitive (S) strains.[3]

The inbred SHR-strain is an excellent model of hypertension in humans. All the animals develop hypertension by the fifth week of life, blood pressure increases as the animals age, and males are affected more than the females. This strain is not only responsive to anti-hypertensive drugs, but also exhibits complications similar to those observed in humans.[4]

Initially neither human essential hypertension nor the SHR-rat have any associated pathological features other than increased peripheral resistance. In both cases, there is a strong genetic component, cardiovascular complications appear late and salt has an aggravating effect on blood pressure.[4] An obese sub-strain of the SHR-rat is one of the few that exhibits hyperlipemia, increased serum cholesterol, and atherosclerosis.[2] In another sub-strain known as arteriolipidosis-prone rat (ALR), the absorption of cholesterol is twice that of SHR-strain.[5] The possibility of using small rodent species as models of atherosclerosis has been widely studied, but with disappointing results thus far.[6]

Finding controls for the SHR-strain has been a problem. The Wistar-Kyoto (WKY) strain, which is widely used for this purpose, is genetically ill-defined. Its validity for this purpose may therefore be doubtful.[3] Two inbred strains of cross-bred SHR- and WKY-rats have recently been established. SHR-rats are both hypertensive and hyperactive, while WKY-rats exhibit neither characteristic. Of the new strains, WK-HT is hypertensive but not hyperactive, and WK-HA is hyperactive but has normal blood pressure. Together, with the SHR- and WKY-strains, these offer new possibilities for studying the relationship between hypertension and hyperactivity.[7]

The Dahl-rats are the result of selective inbreeding. In Dahl salt-sensitive (S) rats, the age at which a high salt diet is started determines the degree of hypertension. If it begins when the rat is being weaned, blood pressure will exceed 200 mmHg within three weeks. If the high-salt diet is started at the age of three months, blood pressure will increase to 185 mmHg in 1 to 2 months. It is worth noting that S-rats become hypertensive even if fed a normal diet containing 1% NaCl; but this occurs in months rather than weeks.[8]

The blood pressure response to salt in the Dahl-rats seems to be inherited as a polygenetic trait. The blood pressure responses to other forms of induced hypertension are altered, as well as that to salt.[8] Intensive work on breeding transgenic animals is likely to provide new models, especially in rodent species where the main emphasis of transgenics is focused.

RABBIT

The rabbit was the first animal species to be used as a model of atherosclerosis almost 90 years ago. Since then, the species has been used so widely that the rabbit is a symbol of atherosclerosis research. The validity of using New Zealand White stock for atherosclerosis studies has been questioned;[9] but it seems that the rabbit as a species is regaining popularity in research work. This is because of the introduction of several new genetic variants, and because of the tendency of researchers to accept shorter induction times and more physiological regimes to produce the lesions.[6]

Rabbits do not suffer from atherosclerosis spontaneously, although young rabbits may develop spontaneous mediomineralization in the thoracic aorta.[10] Rabbits are extremely sensitive to lipid-rich diets, but the lesions induced are more like those seen in lipid storage disorders.[11] Those were once considered to be merely a disadvantage in the modeling context, but the mechanisms of their development are now thought to be more important than their physiological characteristics.[6] The rabbit used most commonly in studies of diet-induced lesions is the New Zealand stock.

Some effective regression studies of atherosclerosis have been carried out on rabbits, and we now know that in those animals advanced atherosclerotic lesions show marked improvement through feeding regimens designed to reduce blood lipid levels.[12] There is also ample evidence to show that lesions in humans may regress under similar regimens.[13]

New rabbit strains are being substituted for New Zealand stock as models of atherosclerosis. The use of variants further expands the possibilities for studying the relationship between lipids and lesion behavior.[6] The Watanabe strain of rabbits is a spontaneous model of human familial hypercholesteremia in that it shows a high level of low density lipoprotein (LDL).[14] The progression of spontaneous lesions in these animals can be prevented using drugs.[15]

Another new strain, the St. Thomas rabbit, also develops atherosclerotic lesions on a standard diet, and shows higher levels of several lower-density lipoproteins. The establishment of cholesterol hyper-responsive (AX/JU) and hypo-responsive (II VO/JU) strains has been carried out by the Jackson Laboratory.[6]

DOG

The dog has a long history as a model for cardiovascular research; it was already being used in circulatory studies by William Harvey in the 17th century. Since then, the species has continued to be widely used in cardiovascular studies. The reasons for this are mainly practical: for a long time the dog was the only full-grown animal of between 10 and 30 kg, which was readily available; and it was relatively easy to work with.

In addition to induced models of hypertension, inherited essential hypertension has recently been described in the dog.[16] The dogs concerned were bred from two unrelated dogs with essential hypertension. Half of the offspring seem to be hypertensive, the rest are borderline cases or normal. These animals appear to be salt-sensitive compared to normal dogs.

Given the key role of the dog in cardiovascular research, it is unfortunate that the coronary collateral circulation of the dog differs in several aspects from that of humans. In terms of fatal arrhythmias during coronary occlusion, these are more likely to occur in animals with only a few collaterals, such as in humans or the pig, than in animals with an abundance of collaterals, as in the dog and the rat, or a lack of them, as in ungulates.[17-19] This difference is a major one, and makes dogs the non-preferred model for studies related to myocardial ischemia.

It is not only the number of collaterals between the major coronary arteries that differs between species, but also the location of the collaterals, and the resulting blood flow during compromised blood supply. During occlusion of a coronary artery, dogs in general have greater sub-epicardial protection than swine, which usually demonstrate more uniform ischemia.[20]

A few studies have been made on atherosclerosis in dogs.[16] Dogs must, however, be considered unsatisfactory models for the disease, because no spontaneous lesions develop, induced lesions are rarely located in the major arteries and they are predominantly medial.

SWINE

The first famous scientist to study circulation in swine was Leonardo da Vinci almost 500 years ago. Yet it is only recently that swine have become popular in cardiovascular research. The features that may have contributed to such a slow change of attitude are the size of mature farm pigs, their rather uncooperative behavior, and difficulties in anesthesizing them. Swine are now considered a valuable species for cardiovascular research. In addition to circulatory system of good size, both farm pigs and miniature breeds share many features in common with humans.

The coronary vasculature of the pig is more like that in humans than, for instance, the dog. In pigs, the right coronary artery and the left anterior descending artery each supply 40% of myocardium, while in dogs the corresponding percentages are 40 and 15, respectively.[19]

The presence or absence of coronary collaterals is essential to ischemic arrhythmias and injury. In this respect, there are striking differences between species. The pig heart normally has only a few sub-endocardial collaterals, while dogs have three to four sub-epicardial anastomes.[17-19]

The abundant canine collaterals can be rapidly recruited during coronary occlusion, but in pigs this functional protection against arrhythmia and myocardial injury is missing. This difference means that the consequences of ischemia other than arrhythmia are technically easier to evaluate in the dog. The incidence of fatal arrhythmias during acute coronary occlusion typically low in dogs is almost 100% in swine. Furthermore, the incidence of ventricular fibrillation is lower in anesthetized than in conscious swine.[21]

The best evidence of the importance of collaterals is the drop in mortality due to arrhythmia in swine after the induction of collaterals.[22-24] Gradually increasing stenosis of a coronary artery seems to be the most potent stimulus for collateral growth in swine as well as dogs.

Progressive stenosis of the left anterior descending (LAD) coronary artery during growth and maturation in swine induces extensive development of collaterals in the corresponding myocardium, while progessive stenosis of the left circumflex coronary (LCX) artery in adult miniature pigs has been shown to have the same result in this much smaller vascular bed.[24-26] Collateral dependency of the LAD vascular bed can be established in 8 to 13 weeks by gradual stenosis of the proximal LAD artery. In this model, the myocardium can be either totally dependent or independent on the collateral circulation. Furthermore, this model closely mimics the disease in humans and circumvents the difficulties of defining collateral dependency encountered in other animal models.[24]

Swine can be used as models of atherosclerosis. In both the pig and humans, spontaneous atherosclerotic lesions begin early in life, and advanced lesions may contain large quantities of lipids. In both species, the most severe lesions occur in the aorta and the coronary and cerebral arteries. In addition to spontaneous changes, atherosclerosis can be induced by lipid-rich diets.[6,27]

CONCLUDING REMARKS

In cardiovascular studies the researcher has, in theory, a variety of animal models at his disposal. In practice the situation may be quite different, since many choices are excluded because of, for example, unavailability, cost, size, or low incidence of the condition to be studied.

In some studies, using advanced techniques or devices intended for human use, a certain size is a prerequisite. This is also true when small sample sizes or volumes will not suffice. Then the scientist has often to choose between dogs and swine. If prepubertal animals are not suitable and there is no way of handling large animals, only miniature pigs and dogs are available.

In hypertension research, rodent models have been used most often. Other species have not been well-enough established as models. For athersceloris research, the prefered model species are rabbits and swine, particularly special strains of rabbits, which exhibit spontaneous changes. Even though primate models may be valid, they are unavailable to most scientists. The similarity of pigs and humans as regards collaterals is an important validation of the pig model in studies on myocardial ischemia.

REFERENCES

1. Gross, D. R., *Animal Models in Cardiovascular Research*, Martinus Nijhoff Publishers, Boston, 1985.
2. Petty, C., *Research Techniques in the Rat*, Charles C. Thomas, Springfield, Illinois, 1982.

3. Gill, T. S. III. and Harrington, G. M., The rat in biomedical research, in *Health Benefits of Animal Research,* Gay, W. I., Ed., Foundation for Biomedical Research, 1985.
4. Spontaneously hypertensive (SHR) rats: guidelines for breeding, care and use, *ILAR News* 19, G3-G20, 1976.
5. Yamori, Y., Kotamura, Y., Nara, Y., and Iritani, N., Mechanism of hypercholesteremia in arteriolipidosis-prone rats (ALR), *Jpn. Circ. J.* 45, 1068, 1981.
6. Armstrong, M. L. and Heistad, D. D., Animal models of atherosclerosis, *Atherosclerosis,* 85, 15, 1990.
7. Hendley, E. D., Holets, V. R., McKeon, T.W. and McCarty, R., Two new Wistar-Kyoto rat strains in which hypertension and hyperactivity are expressed separately, *Clin. Exp. Hypertens. (A),* 13, 939, 1991.
8. Rapp, J. A., Dahl salt-susceptible and salt-resistant rats, *Hypertension,* 4, 753, 1982.
9. Vesselinovitch, D., Animal models of atherosclerosis, their contributions and pitfalls, *Artery,* 5, 193, 1979.
10. Fox, R. R., The rabbit as a research subject, in *Health Benefits of Animal Research,* Gay, W. I., Ed., Foundation for Biomedical Research, 1985.
11. Hadjiisky, P., Bourdillon, M. C., and Grosgogeat, Y., Modeles experimentaux d'atherosclerose, *Arch. Mal. Coeur. Vaiss.,* 84, 1596, 1991.
12. Wissler, R. W. and Vesselinovitch, D., Can atherosclerotic plagues regress? Anatomical and biochemical evidence from nonhuman animal models, *Am. J. Cardiol.,* 65, 33F, 1990.
13. Blankenhorn, D. H., Nessim, S. A., Johnson, R.L., Sanmarco, M. E., Azen, S. P., and Cashin-Hempill, L., Benefical effects of combined colestin-niacin therapy on coronary atherosclerosis and coronary venous bypass grafts, *JAMA,* 257, 3233, 1987.
14. Havel, R. J., Yamada, N. Y., and Shames, D. M., Watanabe hyperlipemic rabbit: Animal model for familial hypercholesteremia, *Arteriosclerosis,* 9(Suppl I), 33, 1989.
15. Nagano, Y. and Kita, T., Studies on atherosclerosis with an animal model, *Nippon Ronen Igakkai Zasshi,* 29, 249, 1992.
16. Bovee, K. C., Littman, M. P., Saleh, F., Beeuwkes, R., Mann, W., Koster, P. and Kinter, L. B., Essential hereditary hypertension in dogs: A new animal model, *J. Hypertens.,* 4(Suppl 5), S172, 1986.
17. Lumb, G. D. and Singletary, H. P., Blood supply to the atrioventricular node and bundle of His: A comparative study in pig, dog and man, *Am. J. Pathol.,* 41, 65, 1962.
18. Schaper, W., Jageneau, A., and Xhonneux, R., The development of collateral circulation in the pig and dog heart, *Cardiologia,* 51, 321, 1967.
19. Schaper, W., *The Collateral Circulation of the Heart,* Elsevier, North Holland, Amsterdam, 1971.
20. Mc Donough, K. H., Dunn, R. B., and Griggs, D. M. Jr., Transmural changes in porcine and canine hearts after circumflex artery occlusion, *Am. J. Physiol.,* 246, H601, 1984.
21. Nevalainen, T. O., Hartikainen, J. E. K., Ahonen, E. A. T., Voipio, H. M., and Hakumäki, M. O. K., A conscious porcine model for sudden cardiac death, *Scand. J. Lab. Anim. Sci.,* 13, 109, 1986.
22. Blumgart, H. L., Zoll, P. M., Freedberg, A. S. and Gilligan, D. R., The experimental production of intercoronary arterial anastomoses and their functional significance, *Circulation,* 1, 10, 1950.
23. Eckstein, R. W., Effect of exercise and coronary artery narrowing on coronary collateral circulation, *Circ. Res.,* 5, 230, 1957.
24. Millard, R. W., Induction of functional coronary collaterals in the swine heart, *Basic Res. Cardiol.,* 76, 468, 1981.
25. White, F. C., and Bloor, C. M., Coronary collateral circulation in the pig: Correlation of collateral flow with coronary bed size, *Basic Res. Cardiol.,* 76, 189, 1981.
26. Roth, D. M., Maruoka, Y., Rogers, J., White, F. C., Longhurts, J. C., and Bloor, C. M., Development of collateral circulation in the left circumflex ameroid-occluded swine myocardium, *Am. J. Physiol. (Heart Circ. Physiol.,22),* 253, H1279, 1987.
27. Luginbuhl, H., Rossi, G. L., Ratcliffe, H. L., and Muller, R., Comparative atherosclerosis, in *Advanced Veterinary Science and Comparitive Medicine,* Brandly, C. A., Cornelius, C. E., Simpson, C. F., Eds., Academic Press, New York, 1977.

Chapter 6

Animal Models in Gastroenterology

Karl Johan Öbrink

CONTENTS

INTRODUCTION

The gastrointestinal tract is not only a locus for food digestion and absorption; it also plays an important role in endocrinology and immunology.[1] It should furthermore be remembered that the gut is filled with numerous bacteria, mostly having a symbiotic function with the host organism, and often essential for normal metabolism. With respect to digestion, gastrointestinal research is concerned with mainly two facts of function: secretion-absorption and motility. Secretion-absorption includes stimulatory and inhibitory mechanisms (nervous and humoral) and ion and molecular transport mechanisms. Motility depends on nervous and hormonal influences and involves smooth muscle functions. Both facts are usually studied in the same types of animal model.

The functional anatomy differs between mammals and other species, but also among the mammalians there are fundamental differences in the gastrointestinal tract, e.g., between ruminants and non-ruminants. Only in very special contexts are ruminants used as a model for humans.

In a large number of experiments, mostly chronic, the different gastrointestinal organs have been made accessible and/or modified by surgical procedures so as to make observations possible. Examples of such techniques will be mentioned in the following. The majority of them were developed rather long ago but are still used (see for instance Babkin[2] and Gregory[3]).

Models for normal function are numerous and mostly easy to develop. In fact, all animal experiments used in basic gastroenterology research can be looked upon as such models. Where gastrointestinal diseases are concerned, however, only few spontaneous disease models seem to be directly applicable to humans.

USEFUL MODELS IN STUDIES OF THE GASTROINTESTINAL TRACT

TEETH

Although primates are often considered essential in odontological research, other animal species have also been used successfully. Caries and periodontitis are two diseases that have been studied in animal models: caries in rats, hamsters, and dogs[4] and periodontitis especially in dogs.[5]

SALIVARY GLANDS

The salivary glands have been examined extensively in many species, but cats and dogs predominate. In the majority of cases, the salivary ducts have been cannulated and for chronic experiments permanent fistulas can be prepared.[2,3]

STOMACH

Secretion physiology involves both stimulation mechanisms and production of gastric juice. In humans, it is usually necessary to intubate the patient with a stomach tube that is passed through the esophagus in order to collect gastric juice. In animals, this can be accomplished by means of fistulas from the stomach through the abdominal wall. There are three main types of fistula models: whole stomach fistulas, Pavlov pouches, and Heidenhain pouches. There is a vast amount of literature available on these preparations and excellent overviews were presented long ago by Babkin[2] and Gregory.[3] The majority of these preparations have been made on dogs, but cats, pigs, and even chickens[6] have been used.

Of the whole stomach fistula, special mention should be made of the rumen fistula, which is a wide-hole opening that makes observation of the physiological processes in the rumen possible.[7,8] The Pavlov pouch is made from part of the greater curvature of the stomach without cutting the vagus nerves that run in the subserosal layers of the stomach wall. The Heidenhain pouch is also made from part of the greater curvature but is completely separated from the main stomach, thus being deprived of vagal innervation. A variation of the Heidenhain pouch is the fully transplanted subcutaneous pouch.

The stimulation of gastric secretion is normally divided into three phases: a cephalic phase, a gastric phase, and an intestinal phase. The first is stimulated by the vagus nerve after smell or sight of food or other indications of a coming meal, and to study this experimentally, animals have been prepared for sham feeding. The original and mostly used procedure has been to bring the middle part of the esophagus out to the lower surface of the neck, thus causing the food that the animals eat and chew to fall out through the esophageal stoma. The food will consequently not reach the stomach.[2,3]

The gastric and the intestinal phase is largely a hormonal event heavily involving the antral mucosa. This has been shown in a great number of experiments where the antrum, and other parts of the stomach and duodenum, have been either removed or excluded from normal contacts in the alimentary tract. For information about many different operations, the reader is referred to Gregory.[3]

Many of the studies on ion and water transport have been performed in isolated or semi-isolated organs or tissues, for instance the gastric flap,[9,10] where a piece of gastric mucosa is exposed during an acute experiment. It has an intact blood and nerve supply and is mostly made in dogs and cats. A rat model useful for studies of the microcirculation of the mucosa and its relation to secretion has been developed by Holm-Rutili.[11] Other useful preparations are the isolated gastric mucosa model (mostly made in frogs or guinea pigs)[12,13] and the isolated gastric gland model (mainly made in rabbits, dogs, rats, or humans).[14] Even isolated parietal cells from different species including humans have been widely used.[15]

MODELS FOR GASTRIC AND DUODENAL ULCERS

The ulcer disease is still not well understood. The ulcer itself is merely a symptom of underlying disturbances. A great number of experimental animal models have been suggested and used for therapeutical evaluations. The techniques have aimed either at removing the normal alkaline protection against the gastric acid or at causing severe stress.

Many years ago a classical but still useful survey was published by Ivy and co-workers.[16] In this survey, several well-known and often used models can be found, e.g., the Shay rat, which is made by placing a ligature around the pylorus. After a few days, the rats will develop gastric ulcer. Another model is the Mann-Williamson dog,[16,17] where the duodenum including the pancreatic and bile ducts is transplanted to the lower ileum and the jejunum is connected to the stomach. Several modifications based on the same principle have been reported. Stress-induced ulcers can be provoked in many ways, restraint techniques being the most commonly used. It should, however, be made very clear that these methods need thorough ethical consideration. An important factor of ulcer etiology is infection by Helicobacter pylori. Several new animal models for the study of this new area have been reported, e.g., using gnotobiotic piglets, gnotobiotic dogs, primates,[18] and, recently, small rodents.[18,19]

SMALL INTESTINE
The physiology and pathophysiology of the small intestine has mostly been studied in intestinal loops. A piece of the gut is cut out and both ends sutured to the abdominal wall. In chronic experiments, the remainder of the intestine is sutured end to end.[3] Modern applications are found in many reports.[20,21]

LARGE INTESTINE
Similar principles for study as described for the small intestine also hold for studies of the large intestine. This organ, however, shows malfunctions that are of major clinical importance and therefore great efforts have been made in trying to establish suitable animal models. There have appeared several reviews of models of inflammatory bowel diseases.[22-24] A spontaneous animal model for chronic colitis is found in Cotton-Top Tamarins (a South American marmoset),[25] but possibilities for experiments on these animals are restricted as they constitute an endangered species.

Experimental ulcerative colitis has been provoked in guinea pigs, rabbits, and hamsters by dextran sulphate sodium (DSS), but the best result seems to have been reached with mice that were given DSS in drinking water.[26]

PANCREAS AND LIVER
The exocrine pancreas and bile can be reached by cannulating the pancreatic and bile ducts and connecting the cannula to the abdominal surface. This mostly involves a duodenal stoma. The different anatomies of the ducts in different species should be observed. Some have a common duct ending in the duodenum, while others have separate or multiple ones. Classical procedures are described by Gregory,[3] but modern induction of pancreatitis in small rodents is also possible.[27]

REFERENCES

1. Johnson, L.R. (Ed.), *Physiology of the Gastrointestinal Tract* (2 volumes), Raven Press, New York, 1981.
2. Babkin, B.P., *Secretory Mechanism of the Digestive Glands*, 2nd ed., P.B. Hoeber Inc., New York, 1950.
3. Gregory, R.A., *Secretory Mechanisms of the Gastro-Intestinal Tract*, Edward Arnold (Publishers) Ltd, London, 1962.
4. Gardner, A.F., Dark, B.H. and Keary, G.T., Dental caries in domesticated dogs, *J. Amer. Vet. Med. Assoc.*, 140, 433, 1962.
5. Page, R.C. and Schroeder, H.E., *Periodontitis in Man and Other Animals. A Comparative Review*, Karger, Basel, 1982.

6. Burhol, P.G., Gastric Secretion in the Chicken. *Scand. J. Gastroenterol.*, 6(Suppl. 11), 1971.
7. Hecker, J.F., *Experimental Surgery on Small Ruminants,* Butterwords, London, 1974.
8. Björnhag, G. and Jonsson, E., Replaceable gastrointestinal cannulas for small ruminants and pigs, *Livest. Prod. Sci.,* 11, 179, 1984.
9. Moody, F. and Durbin, D., Effects of glycine and other instillates on concentration of gastric acid, *Am. J. Physiol.*, 209, 122, 1965.
10. Öbrink, K.J. and Waller, M., The transmucosal migration of water and hydrogen ions in the stomach, *Acta Physiol. Scand.*, 63, 175, 1965.
11. Holm-Rutili, L. and Öbrink, K.J., Rat gastric mucosal microcirculation *in vivo, Am. J. Physiol.*, 248, G741, 1985.
12. Hogben, C.A.M., The chloride transport system of the gastric mucosa, *Proc. Natl. Acad. Sci. USA*, 37, 393, 1951.
13. Flemström, G., Sodium transport and impedance properties of the isolated frog gastric mucosa at different oxygen tensions, *Biochim. Biophys. Acta,* 225, 35, 1971.
14. Berglindh, T. and Öbrink, K.J., A method for preparing isolated glands from the rabbit gastric mucosa. *Acta Physiol. Scand.* 96, 150, 1976.
15. Mårdh, S., Cabero, J.L. and Li, Z.-O., Effects of gastrin on isolated parietal cells, In *The Stomach as an Endocrine Organ*, Håkanson, R. and Sundler, F. Eds. Elsevier Science Publishers (Biomedical division), 1991, 253.
16. Ivy, A.C., Grossman, M.I. and Bachrach, W.H., *Peptic Ulcer,* The Blakiston Company, Philadelphia, 1950.
17. Mann, F.C. and Williamson, C.S., The experimental production of peptic ulcer, *Ann. Surg.*, 77, 409, 1923.
18. Dick-Hegedus, E. and Lee, A., Use of a mouse model to examine anti-Helicobacter pylori agents, *Scand. J. Gastroenterol.* 26, 909, 1991.
19. Karita, M., Kouchiyama, T., Okita, K. and Nakazawa, T., New small animal model for human gastric Helicobacter pylori infection: Success in both nude and euthymic mice, *Am. J. Gastroenterol.*, 86, 1596, 1991.
20. Lundgren, O., Studies on blood flow distribution and countercurrent exchange in the small intestine, *Acta Physiol. Scand.,* Suppl. 303, 1967.
21. Flemström, G., Garner, A., Nylander, O., Hurst, B.C. and Heylings, J.R., Surface epithelial HCO_3^- tranport by mammalian duodenum *in vivo, Am. J. Physiol.*, 243, G348, 1982.
22. Strober, W., Animal models of inflammatory bowel disease — An overview. *Dig. Dis. Sci.*, 30, 12 (Suppl), 1985, 35.
23. Onderdonk, A.B., Experimental models for ulcerative colitis. *Dig. Dis. Sci.*, 30, 12, (Suppl), 1985, 405.
24. Stenson, W.F., Animal models of inflammatory bowel disease. In *Inflammatory Bowel Diseases*, Rachmilewitz, D. and Zimmerman, J., Eds., Kluwer Academic Publishers. The Netherlands, 1990, 71.
25. Madara, J.L., Podolsky, D.K., King, N.W., Sehgal, P.K., Moore, R. and Winter, H.S., Characterization of spontaneous colitis in Cotton-Top Tamarins (*Saguinus oedipus*) and its response to Sulfasalazine. *Gastroenterology*, 88, 13, 1985.
26. Okayasu, J., Hatakeyama, S., Yamada, K.M., Ohkusa, T., Inagaki, Y. and Nakaya, R., A novel method in the induction of reliable experimental acute and chronic ulcerative colitis in mice. *Gastroenterology*, 98, 694, 1990.
27. Schmidt, J. Rattner, D.W., Lewandrowski, K., Compton, C.C., Mandavilli, U., Knoefel, W.T. and Warshaw, A.L., A better model of acute pancreatitis for evaluating therapy, *Ann. Surg.*, 215, 44, 1992.

Chapter 7

Animal Models in Reproductive Physiology

Harry Donnelly and Jann Hau

CONTENTS

INTRODUCTION

This chapter has been restricted to female reproduction and the emphasis has been put on comparative aspects of morphology and physiology. The reason for this is that we aim to give the reader information on which to base the choice of optimal animal species for studies of reproductive physiology. Thus, it is not the intention to discuss individual models, spontaneous or induced, for disorders associated with reproduction. Emphasis has been placed on laboratory rodents and although non-human primates are very often the optimal model for humans, especially when studying menopause and menstruation, the numbers used are small in comparison with other groups and are limited by public opinion. The reproductive physiology of farm animals has been extensively studied in its own right rather than as a model for humans. For this reason, less emphasis has been placed on this group of animals.

The first part of the chapter focuses on comparative anatomy, because this is often important for research projects in which the aim is to have structural similarity between the human and the animal model. The latter half of the chapter deals with comparative endocrinology and physiology, which is equally important when choosing the most appropriate animal model.

FEMALE REPRODUCTIVE ORGANS

OVARY

In the Mustelidae and Muridae, the ovary is enclosed in a thin, fluid-filled transparent capsule or bursa composed of loose connective tissue, blood vessels, nerves, and a few smooth muscle fibers and lined on its inner and outer surfaces by mesothelium. In these animals, the periovarian space communicates with the abdominal cavity only through a narrow channel.

In rabbits, guinea-pigs, and primates, the ovary is located in a more open ovarian bursa. This consists of a thin peritoneal fold of the mesosalpinx that is attached to the upper oviduct

0-8493-4390-9/94/$0.00+$.50
© 1994 by CRC Press Inc.

54

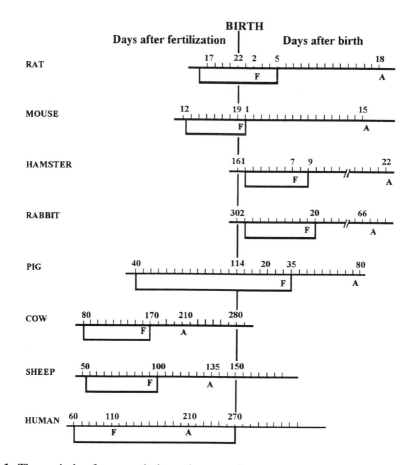

Figure 1. The periods of oogenesis in various species are represented by the rectangles; A indicates the appearance of the first antral follicles and F the beginning of follicular growth. The first spontaneous ovulations after birth occur as follows: rat = 35 to 40 days; mouse = 30 to 35 days; hamster = 25 to 30 days; rabbit = 3 to 4 months (induced); pig = 7 months; cow = 1 year; sheep = 6 to 7 months; woman = 11 to 14 years. (Adapted from Bleer, T.G. *Reproduction in Mammals: 1 — Germ Cells and Fertilization*, edited by C.R. Austin and R.V. Short, p. 17. Cambridge University Press, Cambridge, 1982.

and is derived from the broad ligament. In mammals, oogenesis begins early in fetal life and ends months to years later in the sexually mature adult. Eggs originate from a small number of stem cells, the primordial germ cells, that have an extragonadal origin.

Primordial germ cells are first recognized in humans among the endodermal cells of the yolk sac and migrate to the genital ridges in the 6th week of embryonic development. In the mouse, they are found sequentially in four different sites, first in the extraembryonic tissues of the yolk sac and allantois, then in the hindgut epithelium. Following this, they are found in the dorsal mesentery of the gut and finally reach the developing gonads on day 10 to 11. When they reach the surface epithelium of the gonad, the primordial germ cells move into the cortex and together with the supporting epithelial cells give rise to the cortical sex cords.

In the rat, hamster, and rabbit, oogenesis continues into the post-natal period but, in general, most if not all definitive ova are formed by birth and de-novo oogenesis does not occur later (Figure 1). The development of the primordial follicle into a mature Graafian follicle is a gradual process but is often divided into a number of stages, illustrated in Figure 2.

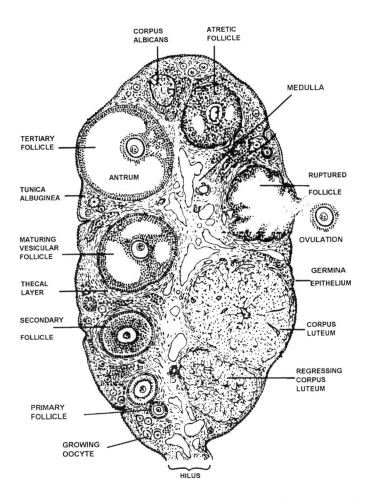

CORPUS
ALBICANS

ATRETIC
FOLLICLE

MEDULLA

TERTIARY
FOLLICLE

ANTRUM

RUPTURED

FOLLICLE

TUNICA
ALBUGINEA

OVULATION

MATURING
VESICULAR
FOLLICLE

GERMINA
EPITHELIUM

THECAL
LAYER

SECONDARY

CORPUS
LUTEUM

FOLLICLE

REGRESSING
CORPUS
LUTEUM

PRIMARY
FOLLICLE

GROWING
OOCYTE

HILUS

Figure 2. Composite diagram of the stages of follicular development, ovulation, corpus luteum formation, and regression. (Redrawn from Freeman, M.E., *The Physiology of Reproduction*, edited by E. Knobil and J. Neill et al., p. 1893. Raven Press, New York, 1988.)

During the human ovarian cycle, a continuous trickle of developing pre-antral follicles occurs throughout the cycle as growth of these does not require gonadotrophin support and the pre-antral follicles do not secrete significant amounts of steroids. Studies of follicular growth in sheep and pigs indicate that it is under both endocrine and paracrine control. Local factors include steroids, growth factors such as epidermal growth factor (EGF)/transforming growth factor α (TGFα), fibroblast growth factor (FGF) follicle regulatory protein (FRP) and insulin-like growth factor-1 (IGF-1). It is suggested that in development, the follicles in these species pass through a stage at which they are responsive to growth factors following which endocrine control mechanisms become more important.[3] The human ovarian cycle consists of an antral phase, ovulation, and the luteal phase. Together, these occupy one complete ovarian cycle. This distinguishes humans from many species including laboratory rodents. In these species most or all antral growth occurs while the luteal phase of the previous crop of follicles is still proceeding. So, in these species the complete antral phase, ovulation, and complete luteal phase occupy longer than one complete ovarian cycle. The tonic levels of gonadotrophins in the luteal phase in these species is adequate to maintain antral growth of the follicles. This follicular growth during the luteal phase also means that in these species, follicular estrogen secretion will occur in the luteal phase of the cycle. Follicular growth also continues during pregnancy and pseudopregnancy in the mouse,[4,5] and during pregnancy in the rat.[6] The absence of follicular estrogen in the higher primate is replaced by the estrogenic secretion of the corpus luteum.

OVIDUCT, UTERUS, AND VAGINA

The oviduct leads from the vicinity of the ovary to the uterine lumen and is divided into four regions: the infundibulum with its fimbrae, the ampulla, the isthmus, and the utero-tubal junction, which in primates has extramural and intramural portions. There is considerable species variation in the length and degree of coiling of the oviduct. It is uncoiled in primates, relatively straight in the rabbit and extensively coiled in the mouse, rat, and guinea-pig. Adjacent to the ovary, the oviduct begins at the infundibulum whose structure is related to that of the ovarian bursa. Where the bursa is poorly developed, for example in the rabbit, guinea-pig, and ungulates, the infundibulum is equipped with a fringe of long finger-like processes, the fimbrae, which make close contact with the surface of the ovary. In the muridae, where the ovary is enclosed in a peri-ovarian sac, the fimbrae are not well developed and have limited contact with the ovary. The situation in primates is intermediate between these two extremes. Changes in the contractility and appearance of the fimbrae occur during the ovarian cycle. (For a review of those occurring in the primate, see Brenner and Maslar.[7])

The utero-tubal junction where the oviduct enters the uterus shows wide variation in structure from species to species. In primates, the junction is divided into an extramural portion and an intramural section, which passes through the wall of the uterus. It is very complex in some species such as the pig and comparatively simple in others such as the carnivores.

There are four anatomical types of uterus based on the relationship between their two parts, the body and the horns. Primates have a simplex uterus, which is divided into a fundus, a body, and a cervix. The lumen in the fundus is distinctly bicornuate. In the duplex uterus, the horns are completely separated and may open into the vagina through separate cervices (rabbit) or the horns may be joined at the cervix and have a single os cervicis (mouse, rat, and guinea-pig). In the bicornuate uterus of the pig and the insectivores, the horns are mostly separate but fused caudally to form a small uterine body that has a single cervix. Carnivores and some ungulates have a bipartite uterus with a substantial uterine body and the horns showing varying degrees of fusion, there is again a single cervix. In cats, dogs, and ruminants, a septum partially bisects the uterine body.

The vaginal epithelium undergoes cyclical changes during the ovarian cycle. These are less pronounced in the human than in rodents where the epithelium shows marked changes that may be used as an indicator of the stage of the cycle. At estrus, it is markedly cornified and devoid of leucocytes. The cornified layer is shed at the end of estrus and the wall is invaded by leucocytes. Guinea-pigs have a membrane closing the vagina that ruptures spontaneously during estrus and parturition. In rats, the vaginal opening occurs near the time of the first ovulation and may be used as an index of puberty.

GAMETE AND ZYGOTE TRANSPORT

Semen is deposited into the vagina close to the cervix in primates and the rabbit. However, in rodents, pigs, and horses, it is ejaculated directly into the lumen of the uterus and thus the spermatozoa do not have to pass through the cervix.

Very shortly after ejaculation in primates, the seminal plasma coagulates. Within 1 hour, the coagulum is completely liquefied by proteolytic enzymes in the ejaculate and the spermatozoa are fully mobile. In rodents, the coagulate forms a copulatory or vaginal plug that persists for about 24 hours. This may be used as an indicator that mating, but not necessarily conception, has occurred.

Table 1. Length of the ovarian cycle in various species

Species	Total length (days)	Follicular phase (days)	Luteal phase (days)
Human	24–32	10–14	12–15
Mouse and rat[1]	13–14	2	11–12
Mouse and rat[2]	4–5	2	2–3
Rabbit[1]	14–15	1–2	13
Pig	19–21	5–6	15–17
Sheep	16–17	1–2	14–15

[1]Following mating with a sterile male or artificial stimulation of the cervix.
[2]Spontaneous cycle length.

In most species, fertilization will only occur in the oviduct but under experimental conditions it may take place in the uterus in rabbits [8] and humans and, of course, *in vitro*. [9–11] There are differences in the details of ovum transport through the oviduct between species, but for most mammals, transit time is from 3 to 4 days and for most species this remains the same whether the ova are fertilized or not. Ova remain capable of fertilization and giving rise to a normal embryo that develops through to birth for only a short period after ovulation. The estimated fertile life of some mammalian ova range from up to 24 hours for the human to 6 to 8 hours in the rabbit. If fertilization is delayed beyond this point, then development of the embryo may be initiated but is likely to be abnormal and of limited duration.

In some species, zygotes can survive in the oviduct at a time when they cannot survive in the uterus. [12] The secretions of the epithelial cells of the oviduct maintain the growth and well-being of the developing embryo and in non-primates, premature entry of the ova into the uterus is detrimental to their further development. This does not seem to be the case with primates. With humans, the successful pregnancies resulting from intra-uterine deposition of ova fertilized *in vitro* confirm that oviductal secretions are not required for ovum development. [13]

OVARIAN CYCLES

The mammalian ovarian cycle is an example of a highly integrated series of neuroendocrinological events and the underlying control mechanisms have been the subject of extensive research. With the exception of women, a repeated series of cycles is not usual but instead, only a few cycles may occur between successive pregnancies. Indeed, in many small rodents, there is a postpartum estrus within 24 hours of parturition at which fertile mating is possible and frequently occurs.

One complete estrous cycle is the interval between successive ovulations where each ovulation is preceded by a phase of estrogen dominance. Since the estrogen is derived from the follicle, the period before ovulation is often called the follicular phase of the cycle. Correspondingly, the post ovulatory phase of the cycle is often called the luteal phase because progesterone is derived from the corpus luteum.

Mammalian estrous cycles are of three types: first, those in which ovulation is induced by cervical stimulation during copulation. This is followed by a spontaneous luteal phase (rabbit, cat, ferret, and camel). Second, those in which ovulation is spontaneous but the stimulus of copulation is required to induce the luteal phase (rat, mouse); and finally, those in which both ovulation and the luteal phase are spontaneous (primates marsupials, goats, horses, pigs, cattle, and sheep).

The duration of the ovarian cycle for various species and their constituent phases are shown in Table 1. Differences are obvious both in the absolute length of the cycle and in the relative duration of its follicular and luteal phases but here is nevertheless an underlying fundamentally similar organization.

A unique feature of the ovarian cycle in the higher primates (*Cercopithecidae, Hylobatidae, Pongidae, Hominidae*) is the periodic shedding of the endometrium, menstruation, which occurs towards the end of the luteal phase of the cycle when progesterone levels have declined. By convention, the first day of menstrual bleeding is considered to be the first day of the primate cycle. In the higher primates, the ovarian cycle is often termed the menstrual cycle.

MENSTRUAL CYCLE

In common with other mammalian species, the principal endocrinological event in the primate ovarian cycle is the marked gonadotrophin surge, which occurs between 24 and 40 hours before ovulation. In the first half of the cycle, there is increasing synthesis of estradiol by the developing follicle and this is reflected in rising concentrations of this steroid in the peripheral circulation; progesterone is, however, at very low levels. The sudden initiation of the pre-ovulatory surge in gonadotropin is accompanied by a rapid increase in estradiol followed by a drop.

After ovulation, the rapidly developing corpus luteum secretes increasing quantities of progesterone and serum levels of this hormone rise rapidly until the mid-point of the luteal phase of the cycle when they begin to decrease. Large amounts of estrogens are also produced by the corpus luteum and the change with time in serum estrogen levels is similar to that of progesterone in the human other primates.

During the luteal phase, the levels of LH and FSH are lower than those observed during the follicular phase. However, they begin to rise again at the end of the cycle and attain concentrations typical of the follicular phase during the first few days of the next cycle.

New world monkeys (*Callitricidae, Cebidae*) do not menstruate and their steroid hormone levels, transport, and tissue receptor binding appear to be quite different from those typical of the higher primates.[14]

Plasma levels of gonadotrophins show an ultradian rhythm in primates and many other mammals. This pulsatile release of LH and FSH, with a period of about 1 hour, has been found in ovariectomized rhesus monkeys and in agonadal or postmenopausal humans. The frequency of the pulses does not change during the follicular phase or during the pre-ovulatory gonadotrophin surge of the cycle. During the LH surge, there is an increase in the amplitude of the pulses. However, this is not reflected in changes in the levels of steroid hormones in the circulation.

The frequency of the gonadotrophin pulses is reduced during the luteal phase and, unlike the follicular phase, there is a pulsatile release of progesterone in response.

CONTROL OF GONADOTROPHIN SECRETION

The synthesis and release of both FSH and LH is regulated by a single gonadotrophin releasing hormone, GnRH (LHRH or LRF-luteinizing hormone), which is a deca-peptide produced by neurons in the hypothalamus. The pulsatile secretion of the gonadotropins from the pituitary reflects the pulsatile release of GnRH into the pituitary portal circulation. In the rhesus monkey (and other species), the origin of the pulse generator appears to be in the mediobasal hypothalamus, which contains the arcuate nucleus and the periventricular structures immediately adjacent.

The pulsatile secretion of GnRH has been shown to be necessary for the production of normal patterns of LH and FSH secretion as well as maintaining normal follicle development. Although there is a marked reduction of the GnRH pulse frequency during the luteal phase of the cycle, repetitive menstrual cycles can occur when driven by pulsatile GnRH administration at an unchanging follicular phase frequency. In contrast, slowing of the frequency disrupts normal follicular development and abolishes ovulation.

McNeilly et al.[15] have reviewed the factors involved in selection of a follicle for ovulation using the ewe as a model. In this species, the growth of large oestrogenic follicles with the potential to ovulate is controlled by the plasma levels of FSH. Basal levels, but not pulses of LH, are essential for this response. The withdrawal of FSH from other developing follicles during the follicular phase of the cycle is not sufficient reason for selection nor is there evidence for the secretion of a growth supressing factor(s) by the selected follicle. LH pulses may induce atresia of non-selected follicles and the follicle selected may be the one that can survive the fall in plasma FSH and the large increase in LH pulses during the follicular phase.

During the primate's menstrual cycle, the regulation of gonadotrophin output is controlled mainly, if not exclusively, by the secretory products of the ovary. Plasma concentrations of FSH and LH increase after ovariectomy or the menopause principally because of the removal of estradiol and a rapid decline in gonadotrophin levels can be produced by restoring estradiol levels to those seen in the follicular phase of the cycle. Progesterone, given in large doses to ovariectomized rhesus monkeys, however, has little if any effect in reducing raised gonadotropin levels. These negative feedback effects of estradiol have two important features: (1) only low levels are needed to suppress LH and FSH secretion and (2) the effects are very rapid.

The preovulatory surge in gonadotrophin secretion results from the positive feedback effects of estradiol. To act in this way, in the rhesus monkey, estradiol must rise above about 150 pg/ml and must remain elevated for at least 36 hours.[16]

Although progesterone and many of its analogs block spontaneous and estrogen-induced gonadotrophin surges, the pre-ovulatory increase in progesterone may be required for the full development of the gonadotrophin surge.[17]

The relative roles of hypothalamic and pituitary mechanisms in mediating the feedback actions of the ovarian steroids remain controversial and attempts to extrapolate results from rodent studies to other mammals, including humans, may have introduced confusion and controversy.

In the rat, mouse, and guinea-pig, for example, gonadotrophin surges occur only in the female. Although the system is present in the fetus and/or neonate of either sex, it is rendered inoperative in males by the action of testicular hormones secreted during the critical phase of intrauterine or early postnatal development.[18] This "masculinization" of the hypothalamus does not occur in the same way in primates and the capacity for generating a gonadotrophin surge exists in normal male monkeys and men and can be demonstrated in castrated adult male primates. Similarly, female rhesus monkeys exposed to high levels of testosterone in the uterus show menstrual cycles as adults after puberty.[19]

In the rat, it has been shown that the tonic and surge modes of gonadotrophin secretion are regulated by different areas of the hypothalamus. The tonic mode is controlled by endocrine neurones whose cell bodies are located in the arcuate nucleus of the medial basal hypothalamus. The surge mode, however, requires input from the pre-optic area and the suprachiasmatic nuclei (SCN). However, in the monkey, unlike rodents, the gonadotrophin surge is not coupled to the light/dark cycle and the pre-optic area and SCN may be obliterated without affecting the surge.[18]

It would seem, however, that both the negative and positive feedback effects of estradiol on gonadotrophin secretion occur at the level of the pituitary. The blocking action of progesterone on estradiol-induced gonadotrophin surges in women may occur in the central nervous system.[20] In contrast, its enhancing effect when administered simultaneously with estradiol appears to be at the pituitary.[21]

The duration of the menstrual cycle is determined by two components, the time taken for follicle development with its production of estradiol and the corpus luteum and its continuing production of progesterone. Under the influence of basal gonadotrophin secretion, it takes about 14 days for the developing Graafian follicle to produce enough estradiol to initiate the preovulatory surge of gonadotrophin. The corpus luteum has a functional life-span of 14 days and during this time the development of new follicles is inhibited by progesterone.

In most nonprimate mammals, including rat, guinea-pig, ruminants, and the pig, luteolysis is brought about by the secretion of prostaglandin $F_{2\alpha}$ (PGF2α) by the uterus during the late luteal phase of the cycle[22–24] In ruminants, episodes of PGF2α release occur at intervals of about 6 hours as a result of a positive feedback loop in which oxytocin, secreted by the corpus luteum, acts on the uterus to stimulate PGF2α secretion.[25]

In primates, the uterus does not appear to be involved in luteolysis since hysterectomy in women[26] or rhesus monkeys[27] does not affect the ovarian cycle. The high levels of estrogens produced by the corpus luteum, however, may be luteolytic, their action being mediated by local release of prostaglandins[28] They may also reduce pituitary LH secretion and so reduce luteotropic support leading to luteolysis.[29] Oxytocin of ovarian origin released in response to estrogens may also play a role in spontaneous luteolysis in the rhesus monkey.[30]

Following luteolysis, the inhibitory influence of progesterone on follicle development is removed and a new cycle may begin. In the 1930s, it was discovered that extracts of bovine testis could inhibit the appearance of "castration cells" in the pituitary following irradiation of the testis. The active principle was termed "inhibin".[31] Historically, inhibin was regarded as a testicular hormone involved in the regulation of pituitary FSH by a negative feedback mechanism without affecting LH. Inhibin and the structurally related activin peptides form part of a larger superfamily that includes transforming growth factor (TGF)-ß[32] Extensive recent research, reviewed by Mather et al.[33] has shown that the major role of these hormones in reproduction is that of paracrine and/or autocrine regulatory factors of gonadal, pituitary, and placental function. Inhibin, which is produced in the gonads, is capable of specifically regulating FSH release by the pituitary but along with the activins, it also acts locally in the ovary to modulate steroidogenesis, regulate follicular determination and growth, and oocyte maturation.[33] Inhibin B, or activin B are produced by the pituitary[34] along with follistatin, the activin-binding protein. Follistatin inhibits activin stimulation or basal release of FSH from pituitary cultures; however, when bound to equimolar amounts of activin, the complex has neither stimulatory or inhibitory activity.[35] During pregnancy, a major source of inhibin is the placenta and the addition of an antiserum to inhibin to placental cell cultures increased hCG and GnRH release without changes in human placental lactogen.[36]

OVARIAN CYCLES AND PSEUDOPREGNANCY IN THE MOUSE, RAT, AND RABBIT

The ovarian cycles of the rat and mouse have one distinctive feature, the cycle differs in length depending on whether or not the females mate. The estrous cycle in the unmated female is only 4 to 5 days, largely because the luteal phase of the cycle is very brief and the corpora lutea only become transiently functional producing progestagens — a small amount of progesterone but mainly 20α OH-progesterone. If the female has an infertile mating at the time of ovulation, then the luteal phase of the cycle is extended to 11 to 12 days instead of the normal 2 days — this is often called pseudopregnancy. The stimulus of the cervix at mating sets up a diurnal release of prolactin from the pituitary, in addition to the normally occurring nocturnal peak. This forms an essential part of the luteotrophic complex in these species. Without it, luteal life is abbreviated from the normal extended period. Pseudopregnancy may also be induced in the rabbit and in these species, it can be used to study the endocrinology of early pregnancy without the presence of a fetus.

Potential encounters with mates will be restricted to the hours of darkness for nocturnally active rodents. This selective pressure has led to the development of an estrous cycle that is closely synchronized to the daily light/dark cycle. In the rat and mouse (and other rodents) the timing of the gonadotrophin peak, which triggers ovulation, is extremely precise, always happening at the same time of day. For rats, this is between 1600 and 1800 hours on the day of pro-estrus when the animals are housed under a "normal" 12:12 L:D photoperiod with light from 06.00 to 18.00. Reversal of the L:D cycle causes this time period and ovulation and estrous behavior to shift through 12 hours. Light intensity also affects the estrous cycle of the mouse, increased intensity prolonging its length and the period of vaginal cornification.[37] Studies of hormone profiles in rodents show that the relationship between estradiol, FSH, and LH are similar to those of the menstrual cycle in primates. Apart from the time scale, there are only two obvious differences; a marked surge in progesterone, which begins during the LH surge and peaks soon after it, and a prolactin surge which is coincident with the LH surge. This surge originates in the interstitial tissue of the ovary and not in the follicle. It has important effects on sexual behavior but although it is not essential for the LH surge it does seem to facilitate the action of estradiol.

In "induced" ovulators, the gonadotrophin surge is activated by a neuro-endocrine reflex that involves the transmission of impulses up the spinal cord to the hypothalamus and the activation of GnRH producing neurones. However, in most species, the gonadotrophin surge occurs independently from copulation and the system is activated solely by the action of ovarian hormones. There is a major role for the CNS in providing a GnRH supply and acting as a target for steroid modulation. The CNS also mediates the effects of environmental factors such as coital stimuli, olfactory cues, and light on the regulation of reproductive activity. The CNS also acts to allow social factors to influence reproduction. These are most readily observed in humans.

A female rabbit caged alone shows little evidence of a cycle. Blood levels of estrogens are high, progestagens are low, and ovulation cannot be detected, yet the ovary contains waves of developing antral follicles as in a continuous follicular phase. Stimulation of the cervix is an essential component of the cycle and 10 to 12 hours after stimulation the doe will ovulate and have a luteal phase or "pseudopregnancy" lasting 10 to 12 days. If a vasectomized male is left with her, she will show a 14 day cycle with a 2 day follicular phase and a 12 day luteal phase.

As in the rat and mouse, stimulation of the cervix is a source of sensory input to the CNS which in this case involves a surge of LH that will rescue and advanced antral follicles from atresia and cause them to ovulate. This phenomenon of induced ovulation occurs in other species such as the cat and ferret and there is some suggestion that it occurs in humans as well.

IMPLANTATION, RECOGNITION, AND MAINTENANCE OF PREGNANCY

Implantation has been studied in detail in recent years, in particular in the human, the mouse, and the cow, both *in vivo* and *in vitro*. During implantation the blastocyst, which must be at the "expanded" stage, makes contact with the endometrium that has undergone hormone dependant changes that will enable implantation.

The trophoectoderm and epithelium become firmly adherent and although the consequences of attachment vary considerably in detail, there is a common feature; the initial close contact between trophoectoderm and uterine epithelium induces vascularisation and differentiation in the underlying endometrial stroma tissue so that it eventually becomes the maternal component of the placenta. The attachment of embryos to the uterine epithelium occurs in two stages, apposition and adhesion.[38] In rats and mice, apposition occurs as the uterine lumen closes around the embryos[39] but in the rhesus monkey, the expansion of the blastocyst is mainly responsible for establishing initial contact between the trophoblast and epithelium.[40] At this early stage of attachment, the embryos may be dislodged from the uterus by gentle perfusion. Adhesion of the trophoblast cells develops as the apposition phase progresses and leads to an increasingly intimate contact between the membranes of the blastocyst and the endometrial cells.

The process of penetrating the epithelium and establishing a vascular relationship with the mother varies considerably from species to species and is described in detail by Weitlauf.[41]

In some species, including the primates, guinea-pig, and the ferret, the conceptus penetrates the epithelium between adjacent cells and invades the underlying stroma — invasive implantation. The initial attachment occurs at the "ectoplasmic pads" of the syncytial trophoblast and in the rhesus monkey, the syncytial trophoblastic processes go on to invade the basal lamina of the endometrial blood vessels

The rat and mouse show displacement penetration[39,42] in which there is death and detachment of the uterine epithelium at the site of attachment. This brings the embryo into contact with the basal lamina and the trophoblast undermines adjacent epithelial cells enlarging the area of contact with the embryo. The basal lamina is then breached by ectoplasmic processes of underlying decidual cells.[43]

In other species, such as the rabbit,[44] epithelial integrity is more or less retained and it becomes incorporated within the placenta - non-invasive or fusion implantation. Attachment occurs between the syncytial trophoblast and individual epithelial cells. The epithelial cells are converted into a syncytium and the resulting "pegs" of trophoblast extend to the basal lamina, which they penetrate followed by the endometrial blood vessels. The free-living phase of embryos that show non-invasive implantation is relatively long when compared with other embryos. For example, attachment does not occur until 16 days after mating in the sheep (non-invasive) but occurs at 4 to 5 days after mating in the mouse and rat. Consequently, invasive embryos tend to be smaller at attachment.

The period during which the uterus is receptive for implantation of the free-living blastocyst is short and results from the programmed sequence of the actions of estrogen and progesterone on the endometrium.[45]

Studies with the mouse suggest that there appear to be three essential steps. Firstly, the priming of the uterus with estrogen during pro-estrus maximises the sensitivity of the uterus to the induction of deciduomata. Subsequently, exposure of the uterus to progesterone during the first 4 days of pregnancy prepares it to respond to further exposure to estrogen, which is necessary for the onset of implantation. Finally, the induction of the changes in the endometrium needed for implantation results from a second exposure to estrogen on day 4 of pregnancy, called the nidatory peak. Suitable priming of the uterus with steroid hormones is essential for successful implantation. Under estrogen domination, the uterus cannot accommodate an implanting embryo. For rodents and lagomorphs, such a uterus is hostile to the embryo.

In women who participated in an *in vitro* fertilization program, implantation failure was associated with a lower progesterone to estradiol ratio . Experiments with mice showed that the inhibitory effects of estradiol could be overcome by concomitant administration of progesterone.[46] If, however, rats and mice are deprived of the normal "nidatory" peak of estradiol, which occurs during the luteal phase of the cycle, while maintaining progesterone levels, the embryos enter the uterus as usual but do not implant and the blastocyst may spend several days in the uterus in this quiescent state. If a single injection of estrogen is given at this stage, then embryonic metabolism increases, attachment rapidly occurs, and decidualization is initiated.

Exposure of the uterus to estrogen results in a stimulation of glandular secretion that includes the zona lysing enzyme as well as glucose, amino acids, and ions, which cause embryonic activation. It also makes the epithelial cells responsive or sensitive to the blastocyst so that they can transmit evidence of its attachment to the underlying stromal cells.[47]

These enabling changes in the uterus occur throughout the endometrium and are accompanied by localized changes that occur in response to a stimulus or signal(s) from the embryo. In the mouse and rabbit, the development of edema, which is the first change associated with implantation, can occur while the blastocyst is still enclosed in the zona pellucida. Therefore, this signal would seem not to require contact between the trophoblast and the uterine epithelium.[48,49]

The nature of the signal from the embryo has been the subject of extensive research and many factors have been investigated including physical stimulation, carbon dioxide produced by the blastocyst, steroids, histamine, and prostaglandins. Platelet activating factor (PAF), which is an ether phospholipid, is synthesized by the embryo and may be important in the implantation process.[50] More controversial is the Early Pregnancy Factor (EPF), which was proposed following the observation that lymphocytes from pregnant mice were less active in the rosette inhibition test using a standard anti-lymphocyte serum than those from non-pregnant animals.[51] The use of the term EPF has implied the existence of a novel, pregnancy-specific protein with the unique capacity to induce increased rosette inhibition titers. Recent results, however, argue against this and suggest that a complex of molecules and interactions, involving particularly thioredoxin or thioredoxin-like molecules, are responsible for the EPF phenomenon.[52] This mechanism may act as an immunological response modifier of the maternal immune system.[53]

Other peptide and protein growth factors such as insulin-like growth factor and epidermal growth factor and its receptor have been suggested to exert an autocrine/paracrine role in trophoblast function.[54]

The cellular and biochemical responses of uterine tissue following exposure to either semen or the products of conception show clear parallels with the immune and inflammatory responses in other epithelial tissues. The uterine epithelial cells in the mouse have a marked capacity to produce cytokines, mainly colony stimulating factor-1 (CSF-1),[55] granulocyte macrophage-CSF (GM-CSF), and Interleukin-6 (IL-6)[56] and the role of these in implantation has been reviewed by Vinatier et al.[57]

The output of GM-CSF and IL-6 increases greatly following an exposure to semen,[58] which initiates the recruitment and activation of local leucocytes within the uterus as the primary step in its preparation for implantation.[59] Additionally, the increased production of GM-CSF and IL-6 occurring in response to a seminal component originating in the seminal vesicle is controlled by estrogen, being maximal at estrus when the uterine epithelium is most likely to be exposed to semen. It has been proposed that the enhanced output of cytokines, in particular GM-CSF and IL-6 in response to seminal plasma, initiates a cascade phenomenon within the cytokine network inter-linking uterine cells, and as pregnancy progresses, the influence of this network is extended to include the conceptus.[60] GM-CSF and IL-6 along with colony stimulating factor-1 (CSF-1) and leukemia inhibitory factor are produced by the uterine epithelium under the regulation of both progesterone and estrogen.[61] It has been postulated that these, together with other inflammatory cytokines such as the interferons (IFN) and tumour necrosis factor (TNF), participate in an elaborate cytokine network that allows communication between the developing conceptus and its mother.[62] Blastocyst implantation in the mouse depends on a transient burst of expression of LIF in the endometrial glands on the fourth day of pregnancy.[63] The signal for LIF expression is maternal in origin and may be regulated by estradiol.[64] In the mouse, production of CSF-1 by the uterus increases many thousand-fold during pregnancy and any loss of ability to produce this and other cytokines results in increased loss of embryos as, for example, with homozygous op/op mice which are deficient in CSF-1. The offspring from a CBA x DBA/2 cross have an impaired ability to produce GM-CSF in the placenta and this results in their abortion.[65] CSF-1 is also synthesised by the glandular epithelial cells of the pregnant human endometrium and by first trimester human trophoblasts giving rise to significant increases of CSF-1 in maternal serum and endometrium during the first trimester of pregnancy. These data suggest that CSF-1 may be involved in the regulation of cell proliferation and differentiation in the human endometrium and in the regulation of placental function by autocrine and/or paracrine mechanisms.[66,67]

As well as their role in implantation, CSF-1 and other lympho-hematopoietic growth factors may act as paracrine growth factors for the developing embryo and may be the mediators of the synchrony between the pre-implantation embryo and the steroid primed endometrium.[68]

Delayed implantation can occur in rats and mice as a result of the natural suppression of endogenous estrogen secretion in females that are suckling young of the previous litter and have conceived following a post-partum mating. With the rat, the delay is related to the number of young suckled and does not normally occur if the litter size is less than five; implantation can be induced by a single injection of estrogen. With mice, the delay in implantation depends on three or more pups suckling for at least the first three days of pregnancy. Gonadotrophin secretion is inhibited[69] and estrogen levels remain low. The delay again can be terminated by the injection of estrogen or the removal of the pups. In the rat, estrus and ovulation are also delayed during lactation and the duration of this delay is dependant on litter size.[70,71] During lactation, prolactin levels are raised in response to suckling and, in consequence, progesterone secretion continues from the corpus luteum.[72] Follicular growth does not appear to continue during suckling presumably due to the inhibition of FSH release from the pituitary.[69]

Infertility during lactation has been seen in a number of nonhuman primates including the gorilla, chimpanzee, baboon, and various macaques. An effect of lactation on reproduction also occurs in several New World primates (spider, howler, and squirrel monkeys) but not in the marmoset. Most studies have been carried out on the rhesus monkey and these show that the absence of follicular development during lactational infertility is associated with low plasma estradiaol levels that persist for about 150 days post-partum.[73,74] Plasma levels of FSH and LH are also reduced during lactation; FSH levels increase progressively, reaching follicular phase levels by 6 to 10 months post-partum, whereas LH is suppressed for 9 months post-partum and only attains normal follicular phase levels by around 12 months.[75] Levels of prolactin are elevated throughout lactation[75,76] but the consequent maintenance of corpus luteum function and resulting progesterone secretion do not appear to be responsible for the suppression of gonadotrophin secretion.[77] In women, breast-feeding delays the resumption of ovarian cyclicity but the duration of the delay is highly variable. As in other primates, this period of post-partum amenorrhea is associated with raised levels of prolactin but the amount of prolactin released in response to suckling and the basal level decrease with time post-partum and during lactation. The plasma levels of FSH increase to normal values within three weeks post-partum, whereas LH levels remain suppressed in most women throughout lactational amenorrhea. It is still not clear whether the elevated levels of prolactin play a significant role in the inhibition of LH release and ovarian activity. As in other species, it may only play a minor role and the principal effect is a direct suckling induced inhibition of GnRH/LH release. The link within the hypothalamus between the incoming neural signal due to suckling and the GnRH pulse generator remains unclear.[72]

Implantation is initiated during the luteal phase of the ovarian cycle and the prolongation of the life of the corpus luteum is essential for the establishment of pregnancy in many mammals. In species, including humans and other primates, the luteal phase is spontaneously prolonged for 14 to 16 days whether or not mating has occurred. In primates, LH is required for the maintenance and function of the corpus luteum[78–82] but, unlike the rat, prolactin is not.[83]

In the unmated rat and mouse, the luteal phase is relatively brief and, except for a brief period shortly after ovulation, the corpora lutea do not secrete enough progesterone to maintain a decidual reaction. The stimulus of mating in the rat activates a pituitary secretion of prolactin that is characterized by daily diurnal and nocturnal surges. This mode of prolactin secretion continues for 12 to 13 days and prolongs the normal brief luteal phase of the estrous cycle into either a pseudopregnancy, which is about half the length of a pregnancy if fertilization does not occur, or well into the first half of normal gestation. If a recently mated mouse encounters an unfamiliar male, implantation may be inhibited[84] due to blockade of luteotrophic support from the pituitary.[85] The effect is mediated by a male pheromone and females are apparently able to discriminate between males on the basis of differences in the major histocompatibility complex.[86]

The endocrinological control of the life span and function of the corpus luteum appears to be similar in other rodents except for the hamster where LH and FSH are required in addition to prolactin for the normal secretion of progesterone.[87]

Because the rabbit is a reflex ovulator, corpora lutea are only found after mating, cervical stimulation, or hormonal induction of ovulation. If the stimulus to ovulation is not a fertile mating, then a pseudopregnancy results and the corpora lutea secrete progesterone for 16 to 17 days.[88] During this time, normal luteal function is maintained by LH stimulated follicular secretion of estrogens.[89]

Both LH and prolactin are required for normal luteal function in dogs,[90,91] whereas in pigs the corpora lutea are capable of function without gonadotrophin support.[92] Although LH appears to be the primary luteotrophin in ewes and cows, controversy remains regarding the role of prolactin in the regulation of luteal function in domestic ruminants.[93]

In primates, the large farm animals, and even in the rat, mouse, and rabbit, the prolonged luteal phase, and therefore progesterone dominance, is not as long as pregnancy itself. If the pregnancy is to continue, the conceptus must circumvent or neutralize the mechanisms by which corpus luteum regression normally occurs. Of these, the best understood way of extending the life of the corpus luteum is the luteotrophic stimulus in which pituitary luteotrophins are secreted at the time of mating — as in the rat — and this maintains the corpus luteum for the first half of pregnancy. During the second half of pregnancy, luteotrophins are secreted by the placenta. Another common mechanism is for the conceptus to produce an inhibitor of the luteolytic action of PGF2α produced by the uterus — as in the sheep. This substance is likely to be interferon α, which blocks the expression of the endometrial oxytocin receptor essential for luteolysis.[25] Human interferon α (IFNα) shows clear homology with ovine trophoblast protein 1 (oTP-1) and bovine trophoblast protein 1 (bTP-1) both of which are secreted by the pre-implanting trophoblast and have luteotrophic or antileutolytic properties. In both the cow and ewe, IFN seems to play a key role in maintaining early corpus luteum function and early pregnancy.[94,95] Other lymphokines, such as the interleukins, may also play important roles in reproduction through their interaction with hormones.[96]

In humans and higher primates, the principal luteotrophic factor in early pregnancy is chorionic gonadotrophin (CG). Synthesis of hCG occurs in the implanting blastocyst and is continued in the syncytiotrophoblast (cells) from which it is released into the maternal circulation. The central role of CG as a luteotrophin has been substantiated in women[79] and in monkeys.[82] In addition, although no interaction between IFNα and other trophoblast products has yet been demonstrated, IFNα has been demonstrated to stimulate hCG secretion by a cancer cell line *in vitro*.[97]

The life of the corpus luteum is not always prolonged; in marsupials, its life span in the pregnant and non-pregnant animal is similar and the gestation period is about the same length as the estrous cycle. In the ferret and dog, the luteal phase is of similar length to the gestation period; therefore, there is no need to prolong the life of the corpus luteum.

The requirement for progesterone continues throughout pregnancy and an essential proportion of this steroid continues to be provided by the corpora lutea, which are under the control of the maternal pituitary since removal of either the ovary or pituitary results in abortion. In other species, pregnancy clearly does not depend totally on steroids secreted by pituitary-ovarian interactions since at varying periods during pregnancy, one or both may be removed without inducing abortion (Table 2).

The maintenance of luteal function in pregnancy is largely regulated by the continued secretion of a luteotrophic complex of hormones from the pituitary as hypophysectomy always

Table 2. The effect of ovariectomy and hypophysectomy on the maintenance of pregnancy

| Species | Gestation period (days) | Approximate stage of pregnancy when procedure carried out | | | |
| | | Ovariectomy | | Hypophysectomy | |
		1st half	2nd half	1st half	2nd half
Woman	267	+	+	+	+
Rhesus monkey	165	+	+	+	+
Mouse	20	-	-	±	+
Hamster	16	-	-	-	+
Rat	21	-	±	-	+
Guinea-pig	65	±	+	+	+
Rabbit	31	-	-	-	-
Cat	65	-	±		±
Ferret	42	-	±	-	±
Dog	62	-		-	±
Sheep	148	-	+	-	+
Goat	150	-	-	-	-

+ = fetusus survive; ± = some fetuses survive; - = abortion or resorption

results in abortion. In the rabbit, for example, the corpus luteum degenerates after hypophysectomy and prolactin plus FSH and possibly low levels of LH are necessary to support luteal function.

In other animals, for example the rat and mouse, it appears that the pituitary is only necessary at the beginning of pregnancy since placental luteotrophins are able to compensate for its removal later on. Prolactin and LH are the chief components of the pituitary luteotrophic complex during the first half of gestation in the rat and they are supplemented during the second half by a placental luteotrophic complex.[98] Both a rat placental lactogen (rPL)[99,100] with prolactin like activity and a chorionic gonadotrophin (rCG) with LH like properties[101,102] have been identified. Hypophysectomy at this stage is without effect, whereas the ovary is required all through pregnancy.

In some species, the placenta may assume some of the endocrine functions of the ovary and this is best seen in species such as the primates (humans) where ovariectomy does not terminate pregnancy. Within two weeks of fertilization, the human fetus synthesises hCG, which maintains the progestagenic activity of the corpus luteum. Within a further two weeks, it is also synthesising all the steroid hormones required for pregnancy and although the corpus luteum remains active for the whole of pregnancy, it can be dispensed with after only 4 to 5 weeks and plays only a trivial part in total progesterone output at later stages. In other animals like the rat, mouse, rabbit, and hamster, the placenta never secretes sufficient progesterone to maintain pregnancy in the absence of the ovaries.

Many different species have been used as animal models in the study of the biological importance of pregnancy-associated serum proteins. Some of the best known human pregnancy proteins like hPL and hCG show strong structural similarity to pituitary hormones whereas others are very different like, for example, alpha-fetoprotein (AFP) (which has been extensively studied in animal models, the mouse in particular).

Since 1970, a number of human pregnancy-associated serum proteins have been detected and described. Among these proteins are human pregnancy-specific beta1-glycoprotein (SP-1), steroid-binding β-globulin (SP-2),[103] pregnancy zone protein (PZP),[104] placental protein 5 (PP5),[105] PP10, PP12, and PP14,[106] respectively. Pregnancy-associated plasma protein-A

(PAPP-A) and pregnancy-associated plasma protein -B (PAPP-B)[107] and Fetal Antigens 1 and 2 (FA1 and FA2)[108] have also been detected. The new pregnancy proteins have been the object of intensive studies, but their potential physiological significance and effect remain, to a large extent, unknown. The presence of AFP, CG, and PL has been described in different mammalian species, but few analogous proteins immunologically cross-reacting with the more recently described human proteins have been documented in animals lower than primates.

Proteins showing immunological cross-reaction with human pregnancy zone protein (PZP) have been demonstrated in serum from several monkey species.[109,110] Although the grivet monkey PZP seems to be very similar to human PZP, the serum concentration in the nonpregnant animal is at the same level as the PZP concentration in pregnant women at midterm. Moreover, the two proteins respond differently to exogenous estrogens, which cause a marked reduction in the serum concentration of the protein in the monkey, whereas they cause a rise in PZP concentration in women.[110] Thus, the grivet does not seem to represent an appropriate model for the study of PZP. An immunologically cross-reacting protein has been reported in the beagle dog,[111] and in the dog PZP has been suggested to act as an acute phase reactant.[112] Using antisera against dog PZP, we have recently described serum levels during pregnancy in the mink, where PZP does not appear to be pregnancy specific.[113] A series of pregnancy-associated murine proteins (PAMPs) have been studied and used as models for human proteins.[114–117]

Pregnancy is generally accepted to be a physiological state associated with mild immunosuppression and many of the pregnancy proteins have been suggested to be immunosuppressive. A special branch of reproductive physiology has focused on the immunological aspects of pregnancy and numerous reports have suggested mechanisms for how the fetus, which may be considered a foreign allograft, avoids immunological rejection. The mouse has been the most popular species in reproductive immunology research. Space does not permit us to go into detail with the different hypotheses, but recent studies suggest that IFN, which has well-documented immunomodulatory properties may be an important factor in the regulation of the maternal-fetal graft relation. In the mouse, both acute and chronic graft-vs.-host disease are associated with and increase in IFNα production. In contrast with human maternal blood and tissues, fetal blood, fetal organs, placenta, membranes, and decidua all contained significant amounts IFNα.[118] Investigations involving human embryos have indicated that the capacity for successful implantation following *in vitro* fertilization (IVF) is related to their secretion of greater amounts of immunosuppressive factors measured by concanavalin A and phytohemagglutinin lymphocyte proliferation assays. IFNα secretion was also measured but no significant differences were found between embryos that implanted successfully and those that failed.[119]

No maternal immune response against the pre-implanting embryo has been described, but following implantation, there are many reports showing that the immune system of the maternal organism recognizes the allogenic fetus. Maternal immunoglobulins are transported across the placental barrier by specific receptors providing the neonate immunological protection. The normal fetomaternal immune relationship has recently been reviewed by Billington.[120]

The contact between the maternal organism and the fetus occurs predominantly through the placenta, which develops from the chorion, formed by the trophoblast, and other fetal membranes. It is a vital organ for the successful completion of pregnancy, acting both as an endocrine organ that produces luteotrophins and as a means of exchange of physiologically important molecules including oxygen and nutrients of which carbohydrates are the most important. The placenta is moreover important as an anchor for the fetus, providing buoyancy and freedom of movement and growth during development. Although the placenta has fundamentally similar functions in different species of mammals, it exhibits a remarkable variation in structure from one species to another. When choosing animal models for the interaction between fetus and mother, it may be of importance to use a species with the same degree of intimacy between the fetal and maternal circulations as in the human. Table 3

68

Table 3. Tissues separating maternal and fetal blood

Designation	Endo-thelium	Epi-thelium	Maternal blood	Tropho-blast	Endo-thelium	Typical examples
Epitheliochorial	+	+		+	+	Ungulates
Endotheliochorial	+	-		+	+	Carnivores
Hemo-chorial						
"mono"	-	-		+	+	Guinea pig, man
"di"	-	-		++	+	Rabbit
"tri"	-	-		+++	+	Rat, mouse

(modified from Bjorkman[121]) gives an overview of the species differences in this respect . It is interesting that the small laboratory rodents have placental structures that make them more obvious models for the human than other species of domestic animals.

PARTURITION

Parturition has been studied in greatest detail in the sheep and the human and although the underlying mechanism is possibly the same in all species, the means by which it is activated will vary according to the various endocrine strategies employed to maintain pregnancy. The sheep is representative of those animals that are dependant on the placenta rather than the corpus luteum for steroid hormone production in the later stages of pregnancy. The fetus has a dominant role in timing the onset of parturition[122] through the maturation of its pituitary-adrenal axis.[123] Cortisol from the fetal adrenal gland initiates changes in the output of steroid hormones and prostaglandins from the placenta, decidua, and fetal membranes. In response to changes in steroids, there is an increase in myometrial responsiveness to agonists such as prostaglandins and oxytocin and changes in the cervix all of which culminate in birth. The part played by the primate fetus in initiating parturition is less clear as experiments involving fetal hypophysectomy or adrenalectomy in rhesus monkeys gave equivocal results[124,125] although there is evidence for a functional pituitary-adrenal axis and an increase in the level of adrenal steroid production in late pregnancy.[126–128] The development of the neuroendocrine system of the sheep and its role in intrauterine development and the onset of birth have been reviewed by Brooks et al.[129] In humans, little evidence has been found to suggest that the role of cortisol in parturition is analogous to that in the sheep.[130]

In species such as the mouse, rat, rabbit, goat, and cow, where the maintenance of pregnancy is dependant on the continued secretion of progesterone from functional corpora lutea, the onset of parturition is associated with their regression and a rapid decline in the level of circulating progesterone. As in the sheep, the goat fetus signals the onset of parturition through increased adrenal cortisol output[131,132] which results in increased production of prostaglandins by the uterus. These then exert a luteolytic effect on the corpora lutea resulting in decreased progesterone output. Regression of the corpora lutea may also result from withdrawal of placental lactogen. Prostaglandins may or may not have a similar luteolytic effect in other species. In rats, near term, the fall in progesterone levels may result from an increase in the conversion of progesterone to 20α dihydro-progesterone[133] and its accelerated secretion.[134]

Expulsion of the fetus is achieved by coordinated contractions of the myometrium assisted later in labor by involuntary contractions of striated muscle in the abdominal wall. In the rabbit, the myometrium under progesterone dominance is refractory to stimulation by oxytocin and prostaglandin F2α (PGF2α) and parturition is preceded by a decrease in the concentration of progesterone in the plasma and myometrium and by removal of the "progesterone-block" to myometrial excitability.[135] The role of progesterone in other species is less clear. For example, in the sheep, maternal plasma concentration of progesterone may not fall until the time of parturition or may remain raised until delivery of the placenta as they do in primates[131,133,136] where there is no evidence that systemic progesterone withdrawal is a prelude to parturition.[137–140]

Parturition is normally associated with an increase in maternal plasma estrogen levels, and although estrogens promote the responsiveness of the uterus to a variety of agonists including oxytocin and PGF2α in most species, this increase in estrogen does not seem to be a prerequisite to birth in the sheep or primates.[130] In the rat, however, estrogen inhibits myometrial activity perhaps by influencing relaxin production.[141]

The cervix will resist the contractions of the uterus and the large increase in intra-uterine pressure that accompany them, retaining the fetus in the uterus unless its structure changes to become soft and compliant. The process by which this occurs is not well understood but prostaglandins seem to be important factors controlling "cervical ripening". Not only this, but they also are effective in inducing myometrial contractions. PGF2α and PGE2 are of major importance during parturition and arachadonic acid is their common precursor. The availability of arachadonic acid is probably rate limiting and its formation depends on the enzyme phospholipase A2. This enzyme is found largely in an inactive form, bound to membranes in lysosomes of the decidua and fetal membranes and actors that control PG synthesis may act by altering the stability of these membranes.[142]

Prostaglandins have come to be regarded as the final common mediators of parturition through their regulation of myometrial contractility. Their synthesis and role in the onset of parturition is discussed in detail by Challis and Olson,[130] who draw attention to the great dissimilarities in the effects of steroid hormones on prostaglandin production by intra-uterine tissues in sheep and humans.

Oxytocin is present in both maternal and fetal circulations and since it is unlikely that it crosses the placenta, it appears to be secreted independently by both mother and fetus.[143,144] Oxytocin receptors are present in the myometrium and decidua of rats and humans and these are sensitive to regulation by steroid hormones, progesterone decreasing, and estrogen increasing their number.[145] The number of receptors increases dramatically in humans shortly before and at the onset of labor[146] and as a result there is a greater increase in the sensitivity of the myometrium to oxytocin than there is in the circulating levels of the hormone.[146]

Oxytocin stimulates the production of PGF2α and PGE$_2$ from human and rat decidua[148,149] but blocking prostaglandin synthesis in the rat did not prevent oxytocin from stimulating myometrial contraction,[148] suggesting that it promotes uterine contractility directly and indirectly via prostaglandins.

REFERENCES

1. Baker, T.G., Oogenesis and ovulation. In: *Reproduction in mammals:1 — Germ Cells and Fertilization*, edited by C.R. Austin and R.V. Short, p.17. Cambridge University Press, Cambridge, 1982
2. Freeman, M.E., The ovarian cycle of the rat. In: *The Physiology of Reproduction,* Edited by E. Knobil and J. Neill et al., p. 1893. Raven Press Ltd., New York, 1988
3. Hunter, M.G., Biggs, C., Faillace L.S., and Picton H.M., Current concepts of folliculogenesis in monovular and polyovular farm species. *J. Reprod. Fert., Suppl.* 45:21, 1992.
4. Gidley-Baird, A.A., White, B.M., Hau, J. and Poulsen, O.M., Initiation and control of ovulation in the mouse luteal phases. Effects of gonadotrophins and gonadotrophin releasing hormone. *Acta Endoctinol. (Copenh)*, 113:576, 1986.

5. Gidley-Baird, A.A., White, B.M., Hau, J. and Poulsen, O.M., Initiation and control of ovulation in the mouse luteal phases. Effects of oestrogen, progesterone and prolactin. *Acta Endoctinol. (Copenh),* 113:582, 1986.

6. Taya, K. and Sasamoto, S., Induction of ovulation by exogenous gonadotrophin during pseudopregnancy, pregnancy or lactation in rats. *J. Reprod. Fertil.* 51:467, 1977.

7. Brenner, R.M. and Maslar, I.A., The primate oviduct and endometrium. In: *The Physiology of Reproduction,* edited by E. Knobil and J. Neill et al.,p. 303, Raven Press Ltd., New York, 1988.

8. Chang, M.C., Développement de la capacité fertilisatrice des spermatozoïdes du lapin à l'intérieur du tratus génital femelle et fécondabilité des oeufs de lapine. In: *La Fonction Tubaire et Ses Troubles: Physiologie, Explorations, Pathologie, Thérapeutique,* p. 40, Masson & Cie, Paris, 1955.

9. Estes, W.L. Jr. and Heitmeyer, P.L., Pregnancy following ovarian implantation. *Am. J. Surg.,* 24:563, 1934.

10. Preston, P.G., Transplantation of the ovary into the uterine cavity for the treatment of sterility in women. *J. Obstet. Gynacol. Br. Emp.,* 60:862, 1953.

11. Iklé, F.A., Schwangerschaft nach des Ovars in den Uterus. *Gynaecologia,* 151:95, 1961.

12. Adams, C.E., Egg survival relative to maternal endocrine status. In: *Ovum Transport and Fertility Regulation,* edited by M.J.K. Harper, C.J. Pauerstein, C.E. Adams, E.M. Coutinho, H.B. Croxatto, and D.M. Paton,p 425. Scriptor, Copenhagen, 1976.

13. Harper, M.J.K., Gamete and Zygote transport. In: *The Physiology of Reproduction,* edited by E. Knobil and J. Neill et al., p 103. Raven Press Ltd., New York, 1988, chap. 4.

14. Knobil, E. and Hotchkiss, J., The Menstrual Cycle and Its Neuroendocrine Control. In: *The Physiology of Reproduction,* edited by E. Knobil & J. Neill et al., p. 1971. Raven Press Ltd., New York, 1988.

15. McNeilly, A.S., Crow, W., Brooks, J., and Evans, G., Luteinizing hormone pulses, follicle-stimulating hormone and control of follicle selection in sheep. *J. Reprod. Fert., Suppl.* 45:5, 1992.

16. Karsch, F.J., Weick, R.F., Butler W.R., Dierschke, D.J., Krey L.C., Weiss, G., Hotchkiss, J., Yamaji, T., and Knobil, E., Induced LH surges in the rhesus monkey: Strength-duration characteristics of the estrogen stimulus. *Endocrinology,* 92:1740, 1973.

17. Liu, J.H., and Yen, S.S.C., Induction of midcycle gonadotrophin surge by ovarian steroids in women: A critical evaluation. *J. Clin. Endocrinol. Metab.,* 57:797, 1983.

18. Karsch, F.J., The hypothalamus and anterior pituitary gland. In: *Reproduction in Mammals:3. Hormonal Control of Reproduction,* 2nd ed., edited by C.R. Austin and R.V. Short, p. 1. Cambridge University Press, Cambridge, 1984.

19. Johnson, M., and Everitt, B. (1988): The Regulation of Gonadal Function. In: *Essential Reproduction,* 3rd ed., p. 101. Blackwell Scientific Publications Ltd., Oxford, 1988.

20. Pohl, C.R., Richardson, D.W., Marshall, G., and Knobil, E., Mode of action of progesterone in the blockade of gonadotrophin surges in the rhesus monkey. *Endocrinology,* 110:1454, 1982.

21. Wildt, L., Hutchinson, J.S., Marshall, G., Pohl, C.R., and Knobil, E., On the site of action of progesterone in the blockade of the estradiol-induced gonadotrophin discharge in the rhesus monkey. *Endocrinology,* 109:1293, 1981.

22. Keyes, P.L., Gadsby, J.E., Yuh, K.C.M., and Bill, C.H., The corpus luteum. In: *Reproductive Physiology IV. International Review of Physiology, Volume 27,* edited by R.O. Greep, p57. University Park Press, Baltimore, 1983.

23. Niswender, G.D., Schwall, R.H., Fitz, T.A., Farin, C.H., and Sawyer, H.R., Regulation of luteal function in domestic ruminants: New concepts. *Recent Prog. Horm. Res.,* 41:101, 1985.

24. Rothchild, I., The regulation of the mammalian corpus luteum. *Recent Prog. Hormon. Res.,* 37:183, 1981.

25. Flint, A.P.F., Stewart, H.J., Lamming, G.E., and Payne, J.H., Role of oxytocin receptor in the choice between cyclicity and gestation in ruminants. *J. Reprod. Fertil., Suppl.* 45:53, 1992.

26. Beling, C.G., Stewart, M.L., Marcus, S.L. and Markham, S.M., Functional activity of the corpus luteum following hysterectomy. *J. Clin. Endocrinol. Metab.,* 30:30, 1970.
27. Neill, J.D., Johansson, E.D.B., and Knobil, E., Failure of hysterectomy to influence the normal pattern of cyclic progesterone secretion in the rhesus monkey. *Endocrinology,* 84:464, 1969.
28. Auletta, F.J., Agins, H., and Scommegna, A., Prostaglandin F mediation of the inhibitory effect of estrogen on the corpus luteum of the rhesus monkey. *Endocrinology,* 103:1183, 1978.
29. Schoonmaker, J.N., Bergman, K.S., Steiner, R.A., and Karsch F.J., Estradiol-induced luteal regression in the rhesus monkey: Evidence for an extraovarian site of action. *Endocrinology,* 110:1708, 1982.
30. Auletta, F.J., Paradis, D.K., Wesley, M., and Duby, R.T., Oxytocin is luteolytic in the rhesus monkey (*Macaca mulatta*). *J. Reprod. Fertil.,* 72:401, 1984.
31. McCullagh, D.R., Dual endocrine activity. *Science,* 76:19, 1932.
32. Burt, D.W., Exolutionary grouping of the transforming growth factor-beta superfamily. *Biochem. Biophys. Res. Commun.,* 184(2):590, 1992.
33. Mather, J.P., Woodruff, T.K., and Krummen, L.A., Paracrine regulation of reproductive function by inhibin and activin. *Proc. Soc. Exp. Biol. Med.,* 201:1, 1992.
34. Roberts, V.J., Peto, C.A., Vale, W., and Sawchenko, P.E., Inhibin/activin subunits are costored with FSH and LH in secretory granules in the rat anterior pituitary gland. *Neuroendocrinology,* 56(2):214, 1992.
35. Shimonaka, M., Inouye, S., Shimisaki, S., and Ling, N., Follistatin binds to both activin and inhibin through the common beta-subunit. *Endocrinology ,* 128:3313, 1991.
36. Petraglia, F., Sawchenko, P., Lim, A., Rivier, J., and Vale, W., Localization, secretion, and action of inhibin in human placenta. *Science,* 237:187, 1987.
37. Donnelly, H., and Saibaba, P., Light Intensity and the oestrous cycle in albino and normally pigmented mice. *Lab. Anim.,* 27: 385-390, 1993.
38. Enders, A.C., Mechanisms of implantation of the blastocyst. In: *Biology of Reproduction: Basic and Clinical Studies,* edited by J.T. Velardo and B.A. Kasprow, p 313. Symposium on Reproductive Biology, Sponsored by Third Pan American Congress of Anatomy, 1972.
39. Enders, A.C., and Schlafke, S., A morphological analysis of the early implantation stages of the rat. *Am. J. Anat.,* 120:185, 1967.
40. Enders, A.C., Hendrickx, A.G., and Schlafke, S., Implantation in the rhesus monkey: Initial penetration of endometrium. *Am. J. Anat.,* 167:275, 1983.
41. Weitlauf, H.M., Biology of Implantation. In: *The Physiology of Reproduction,* edited by E. Knobil and J. Neill et al., p. 231. Raven Press Ltd., New York, 1988.
42. Finn, C.A., and Lawn, A.M., Transfer of cellular material between the uterine epithelium and trophoblast during the early stages of implantation. *J. Reprod. Fertil.,* 15:333, 1968.
43. Enders, A.C., and Schlafke, S., Comparative aspects of blastocyst-endometrial interactions at implantation. In: *Maternal Recognition of Pregnancy,* CIBA Foundation Symposium No. 64 (new series), p3. Excerpta Medica, New York, 1979.
44. Enders, A.C., and Schlafke, S., Penetration of the uterine epithelium during implantation in the rabbit. *Am. J. Anat.,* 132:219, 1971.
45. Harper, M.J., The implantation window. *Baillieres Clin. Obstet. Gynaecol.,* 6(2):351, 1992.
46. Gidley-Baird, A.A., O'Neill, C., Sinosich, M.J., Porter, R.N., Pike, I.L., and Saunders, D.M., Failure of implantation in human in vitro fertilization and embryo transfer patients: the effects of altered progesterone/estrogen ratios in humans and mice. *Fertil. Steril.,* 45:69, 1986.
47. Johnson, M., and Everitt, B., Implantation and the Establishment of the Placenta. In: *Essential Reproduction,* 3rd ed., p. 224. Blackwell Scientific Publications Ltd., Oxford, 1988.
48. McLaren, A., Can mouse blastocysts stimulate a uterine response before loosing the zona pellucida? *J. Reprod. Fertil.,* 19:199, 1969.
49. Hoos, P.C., and Hoffman, L.H., Temporal aspects of rabbit uterine vascular and decidual responses to blastocyst stimulation. *Biol. Reprod.,* 23:453, 1980.

50. Ryan, J.P., O'Neill, C., Ammit, A.J. and Roberts, C.G., Metabolic and developmental responses of preimplantation embryos to platelet activating factor (PAF). *Reprod. Fert. Dev.* 4, 387, 1992.

51. Morton, H., Hegh, V., and Clunie, G.J.A., Immunosuppression detected in pregnant mice by rosette inhibition test. *Nature*, 249:459, 1974.

52. Clarke, F.M., Identification of molecules and mechanisms involved in the 'early pregnancy factor' system. *Reprod. Fertil. Dev.*, 4(4):423, 1992

53. Morton, H., Cavanagh, A.C., Athanasas-Platsis, S., Quinn, K.A., and Rolfe, B.E. (1992): Early pregnancy factor has immunosuppressive and growth factor properties. *Reprod. Fertil. Dev.*, 4(4):411, 1992.

54. Hofmann, G.E., Drews, M.R., Scott, R.T. Jr., Navot, D., Heller, D. and Deligdisch, L., Epidermal growth factor and its receptor in human implantation trophoblast: immunohistochemical evidence for autocrine/paracrine function. *J. Clin. Endocrinol. Metab.* 74, 981, 1992

55. Pollard, J.W., Apparent role of the macrophage growth factor, CSF-1, in placental development. *Nature*, 330(6147):484, 1987

56. Robertson, S.A., Mayrhofer, G., and Seamark, R.F., Uterine epithelial cells suthesize granulocyte macrophage colony stimulating factor and interleukin-6 in pregnant and non-pregnant mice. *Biol. Reprod.*, 46(6):1069, 1992

57. Vinatier, D., Tiffet, O., Dufour, P., Tiberghien, B., Maunoury-Lefebvre, C.,and Monnier, J.C., Cytokines et grossesse: physiologie. *J. Gynecol. Obstet. Biol. Reprod. Paris*, 21(5):535,1992.

58. Robertson, S.A., and Seamark, R.F., Granulocyte macrophage colony stimulating factor (GM-CSF) in the murine reproductive tract: stimulation by seminal factors. *Reprod. Fertil. Dev.*, 2(4):359, 1990

59. Finn, C.A., (1986): Implantation, menstruation and inflammation. *Biol. Rev.*, 61:3213, 1990.

60. Robertson, S.A., and Seamark, R.F., Granulocyte-macrophage colony stimulating factor (GM-CSF): one of a family of epithelial cell-derived cytokines in the preimplantation uterus. *Reprod. Fertil. Dev.*, 4(4):435, 1992.

61. Robertson, S.A., Brannstrom, M., and Seamark, R.F., Cytokines in rodent reproduction and the cytokine-endocrine interaction. *Curr. Opin. Immunol.*, 4(5):585, 1992.

62. Tabibzadeh, S., Human endometrium: an active site of cytokine production and action. *Endo. Rev.*, 12:272, 1991.

63. Stewart, C.L., Kaspar, P., Brunet, L.J., Bhatt, H., Gadi, I., Kontgen, F., and Abbondanzo, S.J., Blastocyst implantation depends on maternal expression of leukaemia inhibitory factor. *Nature*, 359(6390):76, 1992

64. Fry, R.C., The effect of leukaemia inhibitory factor (LIF) on embryogenesis. *Reprod. Fertil. Dev.*, 4(4):449,1992.

65. Chaouat, G., Menu, E., Clark, D.A., Dy, M., Minkowski, M., and Wegmann, T.G., Control of fetal survival in CBA x DBA/2 mice by lymphokine therapy. *J. Reprod. Fertil.*, 89:447, 1990.

66. Pampfer, S., Tabibzadeh, S., Chuan, F.C., and Pollard, J.W., Expression of colony stimulating factor 1 (CSF-1) messenger RNA in human endometrial glands during the menstrual cycle: molecular cloning of a novel transcript that predicts a cell surface form of CSF-1. *Mol. Endocrinol.*, 5(12):1931, 1991.

67. Daiter, E., Pampfer, S., Yeung, Y.G., Barad, D., Stanley, E.R., and Pollard, J.W., Expression of colony stimulating factor 1 in the human uterus and placenta. *J. Clin. Endocrinol. Metab.*, 74(4):850, 1992.

68. Pampfer, S., Arceci, R.J., and Pollard, J.W., Role of colony stimulating factor-1 (CSF-1) and other lympho-hematopoietic growth factors in mouse pre-implantation development. *Bioessays*, 13(10):535, 1991.

69. Gidley-Baird A.A., Endocrine control of implantation and delayed implantation in rats and mice. *J. Repro. Fertil. Suppl.*, 29:97, 1981.

70. Rothchild, I., The corpus luteum-pituitary relationship: The association between the cause of luteotrophin secretion and the cause of follicular quiescence during lactation: the basis for a tentative theory of the corpus luteum-pituitary relationship in the rat. *Endocrinology,* 67:9, 1960.

71. van der Shoot, P., Lankhorst R.R., de Roo, J.A., and de Greef, W.J., Suckling stimulus, lactation and suppression of ovulation in the rat. *Endocrinology,* 103:949, 1978.

72. McNeilly, A.S., Suckling and the Control of Gonadotrophin Secretion. In: *The Physiology of Reproduction,* edited by E. Knobil & J. Neill et al., p. 2323. Raven Press Ltd., New York, 1988.

73. Short, R.V., Lactation — The central control of reproduction. In: *Breast-Feeding and the Mother, Ciba Foundation Symposium, No. 45,* p73. Elsevier, Excerpta Medica, Amsterdam and Oxford, 1976.

74. Williams, R.F., and Hodgden, G.D., Mechanism of lactational anovulation in primates: Nursing increases ovarian steroidogenesis. In: *Factors Regulating Ovarian Function,* edited by G.S. Greewald and P.F. Terranova, p 17. Raven Press, New York, 1983.

75. Plant, T.M., Schallenberger, E., Hess, D.L., McCormack, J.T., Dufy-Barbe, L., and Knobil, E., The influence of suckling on estrogen induced gonadotrophin discharges in the female rhesus monkey (*Macaca mulatta*). *Biol. Reprod.,* 23:760, 1980.

76. Schallenberger, E., Richardson, D.W., and Knobil, E., Role of prolactin in the lactational amenorrhoea of the rhesus monkey (*Macaca mulatta*). *Biol. Reprod.,* 25:370, 1981.

77. Dierschke, D.J., Yamaji, T., Karsch, F.J., Weick, R.F., Weiss, G., and Knobil, E., Blockade by progesterone of estrogen-induced LH and FSH release in the rhesus monkey. *Endocrinology,* 92:1496, 1973.

78. Vande Wiele, R.L., Bogumil, J., Dyrenfurth, I., Ferin, M., Jewelewicz, R., Warren, M., Rizkallah, T., and Mikhail, G., Mechanisms regulating the menstrual cycle in women. *Rec. Prog. Horm. Res.,* 26:63, 1970.

79. Hanson, F.W., Powell, J.E., and Stevens, V.C., Effects of hCG and human pituitary LH on steroid secretion and functional life of the human corpus luteum. *J. Clin. Endocrinol. Metab.,* 32:211, 1971.

80. Rice, B.F., Hammerstein, J., and Savard, K., Steroid hormone formation in the human ovary. II Action of gonadotrophins *in vitro* in the corpus luteum. *J. Clin. Endocrinol. Metab.,* 24:606., 1964.

81. Stouffer, P.L., Nixon, W.E., Gulays, B.J., and Hodgen, G.D., Gonadotrophin sensitive progesterone production by rhesus monkey luteal cells *in vitro*: A function of age of the corpus luteum during the menstrual cycle. *Endocrinology,* 100:506, 1977.

82. McDonald, G.J., Effect of hCG antiserum (A/S) on ovulation and corpus luteum function in the monkey, *Macaca fascicularis. Proceedings of the IVth Annual Meeting of the Society for the Study of Reproduction,* Abstr. 16, 1971.

83. Baird, D.T., Control of luteolysis. In: *The Luteal Phase,* edited by S.L. Jeffcoate, p 25. John Wiley & Sons, Chichester, 1985.

84. Bruce, H.M., A block to pregnancy in the mouse caused by proximity of strange males. *J. Reprod. Fertil.,* 1:96, 1960.

85. Ryan, K.D., Schwartz, N.B., Changes in serum hormone levels associated with male-induced ovulation in group-housed adult female mice. *Endocrinology,* 106:959, 1980.

86. Potts, W.K., Manning, C.J., Wakeland, E.K., Mating patterns in seminatural populations of mice influenced by MHC genotype. *Nature,* 352:619, 1991.

87. Greenwald, G.S., Endocrinology of the Pregnant Hamster. In: *The Hamster, Reproduction and Behavior,* edited by H.I. Siegel, p. 53. Plenum Press, New York and London, 1985.

88. Hilliard, J., Scaramuzzi, R.J., Penardi, R., and Sawyer, C.H., Serum progesterone levels in hysterectomized pseudopregnant rabbits. *Proc. Soc. Exp. Biol. Med.,* 145:151, 1974.

89. Bill, II, C.H., and Keyes, P.L., 17β-estradiol maintains normal function of corpora lutea throughout pseudopregnancy in hypophesectomized rabbits. *Biol. Reprod.,* 28:608, 1983.

90. Concannon, P.W., Effects of hypophesectomy and of LH administration on luteal phase plasma progesterone levels in the beagle bitch. *J. Reprod. Fertil.,* 58:407, 1980.

91. Concannon, P.W., Reproductive physiology and endocrine patterns of the bitch. In: *Current Veterinary Therapy VIII Small Animal Practice,* edited by Robert W. Kirk, p886, 1983.

92. du Mesnil du Buisson, F., and Leglise, P.C., Effet de l'hypophesectomie sur les corps jaunes de la truie. Resultants preliminaires. *C. R. Acad. Sci.,* 257:261, 1963.

93. Niswender, G.D., and Nett, T.M., The Corpus Luteum and Its Control. In: *The Physiology of Reproduction,* edited by E. Knobil and J. Neill *et al*, p. 489. Raven Press, New York, 1988.

94. Stewart, H.J., Guesdon, F.M.J., Payne, J.H., Charleston, B., Vallet, J.L., and Flint, A.P.F., Trophoblast interferons in early pregnancy of domestic ruminants. *J. Reprod. Fertil., Suppl.* 45:59, 1992.

95. Jenkin, G., Oxytocin and prostaglandin interactions in pregnancy and at parturition. *J. Reprod. Fertil, Suppl.* 45:97, 1992.

96. Chard, T., Interferon as a fetoplacental signal in human pregnancy. In: *Placental Communications: Biochemical, Morphological and Cellular Aspects*, edited by L. Cedard, E. Alsat, J.-C. Challier, G. Chaouat, A. Malassiné. Colloque INSERM/John Libbey Eurotext Ltd., 199:117, 1990

97. Iles, R.K., and Chard, T., Enhancement of ectopic β-human chorionic gonadotrophin expression by interferon-α. *J. Endocrinol.,*123:501, 1989.

98. Linkie, D.M., and Niswender, G.D., Characterization of rat placental luteotrophin: Physiology and biochemical properties. *Biol. Reprod.,* 8:48, 1972.

99. Kelly, P.A., Shiu, R.P.C., Robertson, M.C., and Friesen, H.G., Characterization of rat chorionic mammotrophin. *Endocrinology,* 96:1187, 1975.

100. Robertson, M.C., and Friesen, H.G. The purification and characterization of rat placental lactogen. *Endocrinology,* 97:621, 1975.

101. Haour, F., Tell, G., Sanchez, P., and Debre, R., Mise en evidence et dosage d'une gonadotrophine chorionique chez le rat (rCG). *C.R. Acad. Sci., Ser. D,* 282:1183, 1976.

102. Jayatilak, P.G., Glasser, L.A., Warshaw, M.L., Herz, Z., Gruber, J.R., and Gibori, G., Relationship between luteinizing hormone and decidual luteotrophin in the maintenance of luteal steroidogenesis. *Biol. Reprod.,* 31:556, 1984.

103. Bohn, H., Nachweis und Charakterisierung von Schwangerschaftsproteinen in der menschlichen Placenta, sowie ihre quantitative immunologische Bestimmung im Serum schwangerer Frauen. *Arch. Gynak.,* 210, 440, 1971.

104. Smithies, O., Zone electrophoresis in stach gels and its application to studies of serum proteins. *Adv. Prot. Chem.,* 14, 65, 1959.

105. Bohn, H., Isolation and characterization of placental specific proteins SP1 and PP5. *Prot. Biol. Fluid.,* 24, 117, 1976.

106. Bohn, H., New pregnancy related proteins in humans and their analogues in animals. In: *Pregnancy Proteins in Animals, Proceedings of the International Meeting Copenhagen, Denmark, April 22-24, 1985,* edited by J. Hau, p. 247. Walter de Gruyter, Berlin, New York, 1986.

107. Lin, T-M., Halbert, S.P., Kiefer, D., Spellacy, W.N. and Gall, S. J., Characterization of four human pregnancy-associated plasma proteins. *Am. J. Obstet. Gynec.,* 118:223, 1974.

108. Fay,T., Jacobs, I., Teisner, B., Poulsen, O., Chapman, M., Stabile, I., Bohn, H., Westergaard, J.G. and Grudzinskas, J.G. (1988): Two fetal antigens (FA1 and FA2) and endometrial proteins (PP12 and PP14) isolated from amniotic fluid: characterization and distribution in fetal and maternal tissues. *Eur. J. Obstet. Gynecol. Reprod. Biol.,* 29:73, 1988.

109. Bohn, H. and Ronneberger, H., Immunologischer Nachweis von Schwangerschaftsproteinen des Menschen im Serum trachtiger Tiere. *Arch. Gynak.,* 215, 277, 1973.

110. Teisner, B., Folkersen, J., Svendsen, P., Hau, J. and Hindersson, P., Demonstration of an analogue to human pregnancy zone protein in the African green monkey. *J. Med. Primatol.,* 8, 298, 1979.

111. von Schoultz, B., Stigbrand, T., Martinsson, K. and Holmgren, N., Demonstration of analogues to the human pregnancy zone protein in animals. *Acta endocrinol.,* 81, 379, 1976.

112. Strom, H., Alexandersen, S., Poulsen, O.M. and Hau, J., Canine pregnancy zone protein, an acute phase reactant in degenerative joint disease? In: *Pregnancy Proteins in Animals, Proceedings of the International Meeting Copenhagen, Denmark, April 22-24, 1985,* edited by J. Hau, p. 213. Walter de Gruyter, Berlin, New York, 1986.

113. Hau, J., Anderden, L.L.I., and Bohn, H., Plasma levels of pregnancy associated alpha2 glycoprotein during pregnancy in the mink. *Lab. Anim.,* 27:161, 1993.

114. Hau, J., Svendsen, P., Teisner, B. and Svehag, S-E., Studies of pregnancy-associated murine serum proteins. *J. Reprod., Fert.,* 54, 239, 1978.

115. Hau, J., Westergaard, J.G., Svendsen, P., Bach, Annelise and Teisner, B., Comparison between pregnancy-associated murine protein-2 (PAMP-2) and human pregnancy-specific beta1-glycoprotein (SP-1). *J. Reprod. Fert.,* 60:115, 1980.

116. Hau, J., Svendsen, P., Teisner, B. and Brandt, Jette, Pregnancy-associated murine protein 3 (PAMP-3): Characterization and serum levels. *Biol. Reprod.,* 24:163, 1981.

117. Hau, J., Westergaard, J.G., Svendsen, P., Bach, Annelise and Teisner, B., Comparison of pregnancy-associated murine protein-1 and human pregnancy zone protein. *J. Reprod. Immunol.,* 3, 341, 1981.

118. Chard, T., Craig, P.H., Menabawey, M., and Lee, C., Alpha interferon in human pregnancy. *Br. J. Obstet. Gynaecol.,* 93:1145, 1986.

119. Jones, K.P., Warnock, S.H., Urry, R.L., Edwin, S.S., and Mitchell, M.D., Immunosuppressive activity and alpha interferon concentrations in human embryo culture as an index for successful implantation. *Fertil. Steril.,* 57(3):637, 1992.

120. Billington, W.D., The normal fetomaternal immune relationship. *Baillieres Clin. Obstet. Gynaecol.* 6, 417, 1992.

121. Björkman, N., Comparative Structural and Functional Features of the Mammalian Placenta. In: *Pregnancy Proteins in Animals, Proceedings of the International Meeting Copenhagen, Denmark, April 22-24, 1985,* edited by J. Hau. Walter de Gruyter, Berlin, New York, 1986.

122. Liggins, G.C., Fairclough, R.J., Grieves, S.A., Kendall, J.Z., and Knox, B.S., The mechanism of initiation of parturition in the ewe. *Recent Prog. Horm. Res.,* 29:111, 1973.

123. Liggins, G.C., The foetal role in the initiation of parturition in the ewe. In: *Foetal Autonomy* (Ciba Foundation Symposium), edited by G.E.W. Wolstenholme and M. O'Connor, p218, Churchill, London, 1969.

124. Chez, R.A., Hutchinson, D.L., Salazar, H., and Mintz, D.H., Some effects of fetal and maternal hypophysectomy in pregnancy. *Am. J. Obstet. Gynecol.,* 108:643, 1970.

125. Mueller-Heubach, E., Meyers, R.E., and Adamsons, K., Effects of adrenalectomy on pregnancy length in the rhesus monkey. *Am. J. Obstet. Gynecol.,* 112:221, 1972.

126. Seron-Ferre, M., Taylor, N.F., Lindholm, V., Voytek, C., and Jaffe, R.B., Metaphysical changes in fetal adrenal steroidogenesis throughout gestation in the rhesus monkey. In: *Perinatal Endocrinology,* edited by E. Albrecht and G. Pepe, p. 129. Perinatology Press, Ithica, N.Y., 1985.

127. Walsh, S.W., Norman, R.L., and Novy, M.J., *In utero* regulation of rhesus monkey fetal adrenals: effects of dexamethasone, adrenocorticotrophin, thyrotropin-releasing hormone, prolactin, human chorionic gonadotropin, and melanocyte-stimulating hormone on fetal and maternal plasma steroids. *Endocrinology,* 104:1805, 1979.

128. Walsh, S.W., Regulation of progesterone and estrogen production during the rhesus monkey pregnancy. In: *Perinatal Endocrinology,* edited by E. Albrecht and G. Pepe, p. 219. Perinatology Press, Ithica, N.Y., 1985.

129. Brooks, A.N., Currie, I.S., Gibson, F., and Thomas, G.B., Neuroendocrine regulation of sheep fetuses. *J. Reprod. Fertil., Suppl.,* 45:69, 1992.

130. Challis, J.R.G., and Olson, D.M., Parturition. In: *The Physiology of Reproduction,* edited by E. Knobil and J.Neill *et al.,* p. 2177. Raven Press Ltd., New York, 1988.

131. Thorburn, G.D., Physiology and control of parturition. In: *Physiology and Control of Parturition in Domestic Animals,* edited by F. Ellendorf, p. 1. Elsevier, Amsterdam. 1979.

132. Thorburn, G.D., Challis, J.R.G., and Robinson, J.S., Endocrine control of parturition. In: *Biology of the Uterus,* edited by R.M. Wynn, p. 653. Plenum, New York, 1977.

133. Thorburn, G.D., and Challis, J.R.G., Control of parturition. *Physiol. Rev.,* 59:863, 1979.

134. Wiest, W.G., Progesterone and 20α-hydroxypregn-4-en-3-one in plasma, ovaries and uteri during pregnancy in the rat. *Endocrinology,* 87:43, 1970.

135. Challis, J.R.G., Davies, I.J., and Ryan, K.J., The concentrations of Progesterone, estradiol-17β in the myometrium of the pregnant rabbit and their relationship to the peripheral plasma steroid concentrations. *Endocrinology,* 95:160, 1974.

136. Challis, J.R.G., Endocrinology of late pregnancy and parturition. *Int. Rev. Physiol.,* 22:277, 1980.

137. Lanman, J.T., Parturition in non-human primates. *Biol. Reprod.,* 16:28, 1977.

138. Winterer, J., Palmer, A.E., Cicmanec, J., Davis, E., Harbaugh, S., and Loriaux, D.L., Endocrine profile of pregnancy in the patas monkey (Erythrocebus patas). *Endocrinology,* 116:1090, 1985.

139. Smit, D.A., Essed, G.G.M., and de Haan, J., Predictive value of uterine contractility and the serum levels of progesterone and oestrogens with regard to preterm labour. *Gynecol. Obstet. Invest.,* 18:252, 1984.

140. Hanssens, M.C.A.J.A., Selby, C., and Symonds, E.M., Sex steroid hormone concentrations in preterm labour and the outcome of treatment with ritodrine. *Br. J. Gynaecol.,* 92:698, 1985.

141. Downing S.J., Lye, S.J., Bradshaw, J.M.C., and Porter, D.G., Rat myometrial activity in vivo: effects of estradiol-17ß and progesterone in relation to cytoplasmic progesterone receptors. *J. Endocrinol.,* 78:103, 1978.

142. Johnson, M., and Everitt, B., Parturition. In: *Essential Reproduction,* 3rd edition, p. 294. Blackwell Scientific Publications Ltd., Oxford, 1988.

143. Forsling, M., The neurohypophyseal hormones. In: *Physiology and Control of Parturition of Domestic Animals,* edited by F. Ellendorf, p43. Elsevier, Amsterdam, 1979.

144. Alexander, D.P., Britton, H.G., Forsling, M.L., Nixon, D.A., and Ratcliffe, J.G., Pituitary and Plasma concentrations of adrenocorticotrophin, growth hormone, vasopressin and oxytocin in fetal and maternal sheep during the latter half of gestation and the response to haemorrhage. *Biol. Neonate,* 24:206, 1972.

145. Fuchs, A-R., Periyasamy, S., Alexandrova, M., and Soloff, M.S., Correlation between oxytocin receptor concentrations and responsiveness to oxytocin in pregnant rat myometrium: Effects of ovarian steroids. *Endocrinology,* 113:742, 1983.

146. Fuchs, A-R., Fuchs, F., Husslein, P., and Soloff, M.S., Oxytocin receptors in the human uterus during pregnancy and parturition. *Am. J. Obstet. Gynecol.,* 150:734, 1984.

147. Soloff, M.S., Oxytocin receptors and the mechanisms of oxytocin action. In: *Oxytocin: Clinical and Laboratory Aspects,* edited by J.A. Amico and A.G. Robinson, p.259. Elsevier, New York, 1985.

148. Riemer, R.K., Goldfein, A.C., Goldfein, A., and Roberts, J.M., Rabbit uterine oxytocin receptors and *in vitro* contractile response: Abrupt changes at term and the role of eicosanoids. *Endocrinology,* 119:699, 1986.

149. Fuchs, A-R., Fuchs, F., Husslein, P., Soloff, M.S., and Fernstrom, M.J., Oxtocin receptors and human parturition: A dual role for oxytocin in the initiation of labor. *Science,* 215:1396, 1982.

Chapter 8

Animal Models in Fetal Physiology

Anthony M. Carter

CONTENTS

0-8493-4390-9/94/$0.00+$.50

INTRODUCTION

The foundations of fetal physiology were laid by Sir Joseph Barcroft at Cambridge,[1] Donald Barron at Yale, and Geoffrey Dawes at Oxford. As a result of their work, the sheep became the most widely accepted model in fetal physiology, a bias that is reflected in the organization of this chapter. At first, experiments were performed with the ewe anesthetized and the fetus exteriorized.[2] Subsequently, techniques were developed for catheterization of the umbilical vessels through a small incision in the uterine wall,[3] enabling samples of fetal blood to be collected at intervals over periods of days or weeks. This was to usher in a new era in which the study of the chronically instrumented, unstressed sheep fetus became the norm. There was, however, a transitional period in which the fetus was studied in utero but in acute experiments. It was during this transition that the microsphere technique was established for the measurement of organ blood flows in the fetus[4, 5] and detailed descriptions of current surgical procedures began to appear. These developments coincided with the emergence of a new clinical discipline, perinatology. There ensued a reduction in neonatal mortality and morbidity that owed much to methods of diagnosis and treatment evaluated in, or suggested by, experiments on sheep.

THE SHEEP AS AN EXPERIMENTAL ANIMAL

BREEDING

Fetal physiologists are dependent on a steady supply of time-dated pregnant sheep and most maintain their own flock or make appropriate arrangements with a local farm. There are several excellent texts on sheep husbandry[6] and the management of experimental sheep.[7] To ensure a constant supply of pregnant sheep throughout the spring, ewes are introduced to the ram from late September (Northern hemisphere) and for the next 3 to 4 months. A harness containing a colored crayon is strapped to the ram's chest, so that when a ewe is tupped her fleece is marked. The flock is inspected once a day to note which ewes have been freshly tupped.[2] The estrous cycle is 16 to 17 days in sheep, so most ewes will be tupped during the first two weeks after they have been introduced. Vaginal sponges impregnated with medroxyprogesterone acetate are often used to synchronize estrus. They are kept in for 2 weeks and mating occurs about 40 h after the sponge has been removed.[7] Some sheep have a second, shorter breeding season that enables work to be resumed in the autumn. To obtain pregnancies out of season, hormone treatment is necessary, possibly in conjunction with artificial alteration of the daylight pattern.[8]

ANESTHESIA

Animals should be shorn and acclimatized to the laboratory environment for several days before surgery. The ewe must be fasted for 24 h in order to avoid rumen distension during surgery (bloat), but should not be deprived of water. General anesthesia of the ewe and fetus can be maintained with 1 to 2% halothane in 40% N_2O and 60% O_2 (v/v). A respirator should be coupled to the anesthetic system to assist and control ventilation. To enable insertion of an endotracheal tube, anesthesia can be induced with intravenous sodium thiopental. Some authors favor the use of halothane alone and induce anesthesia with halothane administered by mask.[9] Alternatively, surgery can be performed under epidural anesthesia with 1% (w/v) tetracaine hydrochloride, supplemented with intravenous ketamine for sedation and a local anesthetic for fetal skin incisions.[10] Dissociative anesthesia induced and maintained by a continuous intravenous infusion of ketamine is a further possibility.[11]

SURGERY

A complete surgical scrub of the animal should be done and all surgical procedures carried out under stringent aseptic conditions.[9] The abdomen is opened by midline incision. A trochar is introduced to make a stab wound through the flank and catheters and leads threaded through the trochar sheath. Electrocautery is recommended for incisions in the uterus and fetal skin. The myometrium and endometrium are incised in an area free of cotyledons. The membranes are then cut and the cut edges fixed to the uterine wall with Babcock clamps. If the procedure requires delivery of the fetal head or trunk for surgery, an assistant should suspend the uterus by the clamps to minimize loss of amniotic fluid. The Babcock clamps can then be adjusted to attach the uterus and membranes to the fetal skin. Once surgery has been completed, the hysterotomy is closed with a continuous overlay, taking care to pick up the chorionic and amniotic membranes. This is followed by a continuous Lembert suture to appose the serosal tissue and ensure strong healing without adhesion. The abdominal wall is closed with a continuous suture, followed by single sutures to provide additional support. The skin is closed with single sutures or wound clips and the stab wound with a purse-string suture through the skin. Maternal catheters may be tunnelled subcutaneously to exit through this or a separate stab wound.

POSTOPERATIVE CARE

Animals should be housed individually and we favor using the recovery period to accustom the ewe to the metabolic cage or cart in which the studies will be performed (Figure1). Four points deserve attention when maintaining the chronically instrumented fetus:[9] (1) the encouragement of proper feeding postoperatively and provision of excellent animal care; (2) antibiotic treatment; (3) the daily check and flushing of catheters; and (4) sterile handling of catheters, stopcocks, and flushing solutions.

Postoperative Feeding

To lessen the risk of maternal ketoacidosis, the ewe should be encouraged to stand and eat as soon as possible after surgery. Most animals start to eat before they can stand. A careful record should be kept to ascertain that the ewe continues to eat, drink, urinate and defecate. Animals that refuse food may be in pain and should be given an analgetic such as flunixin. If feeding is discontinued for more than 24 h, sodium propionate can be given by mouth to counteract the development of ketoacidosis and atonia of the rumen. Failure to defecate may indicate painful post-surgical complications, such as torsion of the small intestine, and an immediate put down should be considered.

Antibiotic Treatment

Antibiotic coverage should be given on the day of surgery and for the next 3 days. We give a combination of streptomycin and penicillin to the ewe as an i.m. injection and administer an antibiotic to the fetus through the amniotic and venous lines. Many authors consider it unnecessary to give antibiotics by the intravenous route, as the fetus ingests amniotic fluid and can absorb antibiotics through the gut. If fetuses are lost due to infection, the organisms responsible should be identified to ensure the adequacy of the current antibiotic treatment.

Checking and Handling of Catheters

The exteriorized end of the catheters can be closed with sterile plastic stopcocks and stored in plastic bags or in a cloth pouch stitched to the flank of the ewe. Alternatively, the tip of each catheter can be sealed with a metal pin during storage. Sterile handling of catheters and stopcocks is essential.

Catheters should be flushed daily with heparinized saline solution. It is advisable first to withdraw blood from the catheter, thereby removing any clots that it may contain. Blood samples should be taken from maternal and fetal arterial catheters to assess blood gas status and acid-base balance. Values should be corrected to body temperature, normally 39°C for the ewe and 39.5°C for the fetus.

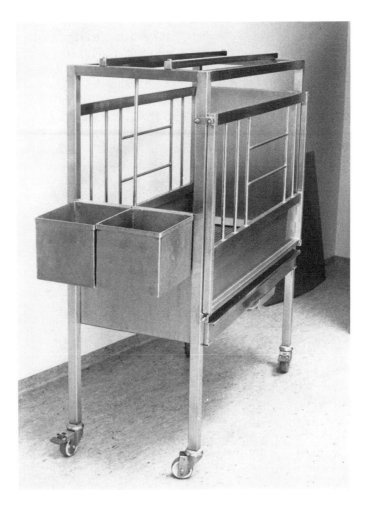

Figure 1A. Metabolic cage used to accommodate the chronically catheterized ewe and sheep fetus. (Photograph courtesy of Dr. Per Svendsen, Odense University.)

Maternal and fetal blood gases, pH, arterial blood pressure and heart rate are usually stable within 48 h of surgery.[9] However, other physiological functions take longer to stabilize,[12] and a recovery period of at least 5 days is to be recommended.

ZOONOSES
Animal care personnel should be acquainted with the common symptoms of disease[7, 13, 14] and all personnel should be aware of the risk of zoonotic infection. Several outbreaks of Q fever have been associated with the use of sheep in perinatal research. The birth fluids and placentas of infected sheep contain enormous amounts of *Coxiella burnetii* and there is massive contamination of the environment at the time of parturition.[15]

INSTRUMENTATION

CATHETERS
The most common catheter materials are polyvinyl and silastic tubing. To avoid kinking, a composite catheter is often used, in which the inner polyvinyl catheter is protected for most of its length by an outer catheter of polyvinyl or polyethylene.[16] Catheters should be color-coded to facilitate identification.

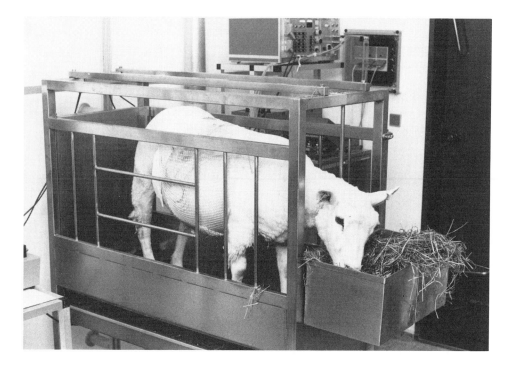

Figure 1B. The animal should be at a comfortable working height. (Photograph courtesy of Dr. Per Svendsen, Odense University.)

Umbilical Blood Vessels

The umbilical vessels send branches across the chorioallantoic sac to supply 40 to 100 discrete cotyledons. To catheterize these vessels, a small incision is made in the uterus, chorion, and amnion and the membranes pulled out until umbilical vessels of about 1 mm diameter are encountered. A fine catheter is inserted into the vessel and advanced into the main umbilical artery or vein.[17] To ensure that the catheter is threaded in the right direction, it is advisable first to search for a sizeable vessel, then to find a tributary and catheterize that.

Lower Body Blood Vessels

The descending aorta and inferior vena cava can be accessed from the corresponding femoral vessels. A useful alternative, requiring less exposure of the fetus, is to insert the catheters through the pedal artery and vein.[18] The vein should be approached from the outside of the foot, where it is quite superficial. The artery lies deeper, close to the bone, and is accompanied by one or two veins. The length of catheter required for the tip to reside in the descending aorta or caudal vena cava equals the length of the foot at all gestational ages.[90]

Upper Body Blood Vessels

Preductal aortic blood can be obtained from a catheter advanced from a radial artery into the brachiocephalic artery or ascending aorta, and a catheter can be advanced from a forelimb vein into the superior vena cava.[19] The carotid artery and jugular vein may be catheterized after exposure of the head and neck. However, they can be accessed through a small uterine incision made directly above the vessels of the fetal neck.[20]

Amniotic Cavity

An amniotic catheter is a useful route for administration of antibiotics. Moreover, registration of amniotic fluid pressure provides an essential reference for fetal arterial blood pressure, especially when measured by an external transducer, since the posture of the ewe is constantly changing. To ensure patency of this catheter, it should be provided with multiple side holes and the tip protected by a length of outer tubing with side holes.

Maternal Blood Vessels

Catheters can be placed in the femoral vessels or in a pedal artery and vein[18] and advanced to the maternal descending aorta and inferior vena cava.

ELECTRODES

The leads for recording or stimulating electrodes are usually made from teflon-coated stainless steel wire, which conducts current between points where the coating has been scraped away. Sets of leads, two for recording and one for reference, can usefully be assembled in a length of polyvinyl tubing.

Leads may be sewn to the fetal sternum, nuchal muscle, and uterine wall, respectively, to record fetal EKG, muscle tone, and uterine EMG. To record the fetal electrocorticogram, electrodes are implanted biparietally on the dura through burr holes made with a dental drill. Electroocular recordings are obtained from electrodes implanted through the orbital ridge of the zygomatic bone.[21]

FLOW PROBES

To measure ventricular output, a cuff-type electromagnetic flow transducer can be placed around the main pulmonary trunk,[22] ascending aorta[23] (Figure 2), or both vessels.[24] These procedures require thoracotomy, which is performed in the third intercostal space. Electromagnetic flow transducers may also be applied to the inferior and superior venae cavae and the intra-abdominal portion of the umbilical vein.[25] To achieve controlled reduction of fetal placental blood flow, Anderson and associates[26] placed a cuff occluder around the distal aorta immediately downstream of an electromagnetic flow sensor. Recently, a transit-time ultrasonic flow probe has been used to measure blood flow in the umbilical artery of the sheep fetus.[27]

FETAL CIRCULATION AND RESPIRATION

The fetal cardiovascular system and its responses to stressful stimuli have been studied extensively by microsphere measurements of regional blood flow.[4] These studies usually yield information on fetal oxygen consumption and on oxygen delivery from the placenta and its distribution to various organs.[28] To enable more detailed studies of the respiration and metabolism of individual organs, by analyzing venous outflow, techniques have been developed for the catheterization of the coronary sinus,[29] sagittal sinus,[30] renal vein,[31] portal vein,[32] and right and left hepatic veins[18] (Figure 3). Cardiac function has been evaluated by placing flow probes and snares around the aorta, main pulmonary artery, and ductus arteriosus. Techniques used to examine baroreflex and chemoreflex control of the fetal cardiovascular system include recording of the traffic in afferent neurons, nerve transection, and receptor denervation.[33]

An important advance in obstetrics has been the introduction of techniques for the noninvasive assessment of fetal and placental hemodynamics. It is possible to estimate volume flow in the umbilical vein by a combination of real-time ultrasonography and the pulsed Doppler ultrasound technique.[34,35] However, the predominant approach in clinical practice has been to analyze arterial blood flow velocity waveforms. The sheep fetus is a useful model in which to evaluate the results of Doppler waveform analysis by comparison with direct measurements of pressures, flows, and resistances made with intravascular catheters and electromagnetic or transit-time flow probes.[27, 36]

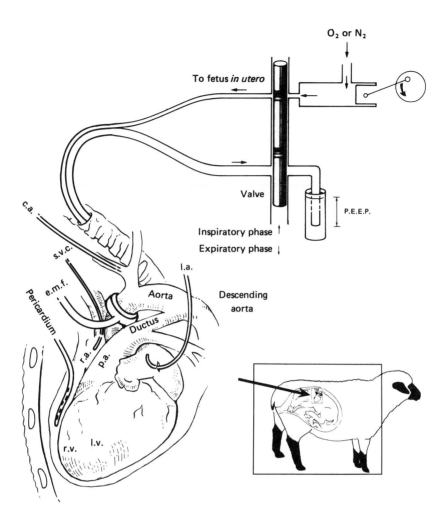

Figure 2. Instrumentation of the sheep fetus for studies of left ventricular function. An electromagnetic flow sensor (e.m.f.) was placed on the ascending aorta to measure ventricular output. Catheters were placed in the pericardium, the right atrium (r.a.) via the superior vena cava (s.v.c.) and the left atrium (l.a.). The right ventricle (r.v.), left ventricle (l.v.) and pulmonary artery (p.a.) are indicated. Also shown is a system used to ventilate the fetus in utero. (From Morton, M. J., Pinson, C. W., and Thornburg, K. L., *J. Physiol.*, 383, 413, 1987. With permission.)

THE FETAL LUNG AND FETAL BREATHING

MATURATION OF THE LUNG

The development of a stable, distensible lung depends in part on structural changes and in part on surfactant synthesis and secretion. The current viability of infants delivered prematurely, with very low birth weights, reflects increased understanding of these processes. The dependence of lung maturation upon the interplay of corticosteroids, other hormones and growth factors has been examined in detail in fetal sheep.[37]

FETAL BREATHING

Although full distension of the lungs first occurs at birth, the human fetus exhibits a regular pattern of breathing movements from the 26th week of gestation until term.[38] The movement

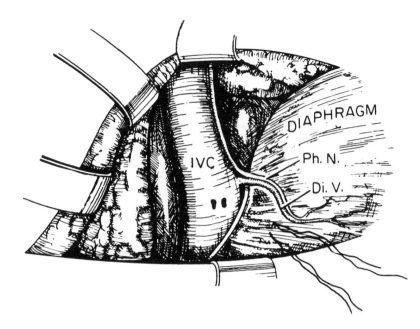

Figure 3. Surgical approach to the intrathoracic portion of the inferior vena cava (IVC), through a right thoracotomy, to enable catheterization of the right and left hepatic veins. The attachment of the diaphragmatic vein (DiV) to the IVC was the landmark for catheter insertion into the IVC to enter the hepatic veins. The location of the puncture sites is shown. PhN is the phrenic nerve. (Bristow, J., Rudolph, A. M., and Itskovitz, J. *J. Develop. Physiol.*, 3, 255, 1981. With permission.)

to and fro of fluid in the airways that is occasioned by these contractions of the diaphragm is thought to be of importance for lung maturation. In addition, fetal breathing has attracted attention because improved understanding of how respiration is controlled in the perinatal period might lead to a reduction in the incidence of cot deaths. The control of fetal breathing involves inhibitory processes that are unique to this stage of life. A significant advance that may lead to identification of the pathways responsible is the development of a stereotaxic atlas of the brain for the sheep fetus at 108 and 120 days gestation.[39] With this in hand, discrete areas of the brain stem can be precisely located and the effect of small electrolytic lesions on respiratory function investigated.[40]

BEHAVIORAL STATE

Towards the end of gestation, the sheep fetus exhibits periodic alterations in behavioral state that are reflected in the electrocorticogram (ECoG). A low voltage ECoG is associated predominantly with rapid eye movement (REM) sleep, interspersed with periods of active wakefulness. The high voltage ECoG is associated with a loss of eye movements and increased postural tone, as during quiet sleep in the adult. Fetal breathing is episodic and associated with low voltage electrocortical activity, while high voltage episodes are virtually apneic (Figure 4).

The existence of episodic variations in fetal activity has important implications for the design of study protocols. If behavioral state is to be taken into account, the fetus must be appropriately instrumented for registration of ECoG, electro-ocular activity, nuchal EMG, and tracheal pressure. In many types of study, behavioral state can be disregarded, but it is worth noting that cerebral oxidative metabolism increases during the high voltage electrocortical state[41] and that there is a fall in arterial blood pressure and a change in regional blood flow distribution on transition from high to low voltage electro-cortical activity.[42]

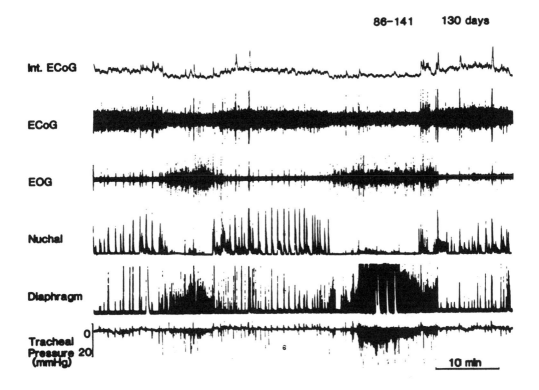

86–141   130 days

Int. ECoG

ECoG

EOG

Nuchal

Diaphragm

Tracheal
Pressure
(mmHg)

0

20

10 min

Figure 4. Polygraph record from a sheep fetus at day 130 of gestation, showing periodic alterations in behavioral state that are reflected in the electrocorticogram (ECoG). A low voltage ECoG is associated predominantly with rapid eye movements, registered in the electrooculogram (EOG). High voltage ECoG is associated with a loss of eye movements and increased postural tone, as registered in the electromyogram from the nuchal muscle. Fetal breathing (tracheal pressure and diaphragm electromyogram) is episodic and associated with low voltage electrocortical activity. (Johnston, B. M., Bennet, L., and Gluckman, P. D., in *Advances in Fetal Physiology: Reviews in Honor of G. C. Liggins*, Gluckman, P. W., Johnston, B. M., and Nathanielsz, P. W., Eds., Perinatology Press, Ithaca, 1989, chap. 11. With permission.)

In the human fetus, behavioral states have been defined on the basis of fetal body movements, eye movements, and heart rate patterns.[43] In contrast to the sheep fetus, human fetuses do exhibit breathing activity during quiet sleep, although the frequency and amplitude of these movements differ from those seen during REM sleep. Recent work indicates that the baboon may be a more appropriate model than the sheep for studies of respiratory control in the fetus.[44]

CENTRAL NERVOUS SYSTEM DEVELOPMENT

When clinically evaluated, infants born with growth retardation demonstrate accelerated neurological development,[45] yet they are at increased risk of neurological handicap later in life. This paradox raises important questions about neural maturation and has led to the development of a range of techniques for the assessment of brain function, including recording of somatosensory and brainstem auditory evoked potentials.[46]

Electrophysiological and neurochemical events during asphyxia have been examined by stereotactic implantation of electrodes and microdialysis tubing in the fetal hippocampus, followed by power spectral analysis of the ECoG and analysis of the dialysate to measure changes in extracellular concentrations of ions and neurotransmitters.[47]

FETAL METABOLISM AND ENDOCRINOLOGY

PLACENTAL EXCHANGE

The fetus acquires oxygen and nutrients for intermediary metabolism and growth via the placenta, and it disposes of carbon dioxide and other waste products by the same route. The factors influencing placental exchange of respiratory gases are well understood,[48] largely due to experimental work in sheep. The regulation of placental glucose transfer has been studied extensively in this model.[49] However, the placental barrier of the sheep differs from that of man in fine structure, being epitheliochorial rather than hemochorial, and has several peculiarities of function. Non-esterified fatty acids (NEFA), for example, cross the ovine placenta in only trace amounts,[50] whereas maternal plasma is an important source of fetal NEFA in man. The guinea pig is a better model in which to examine the consequences of maternal hyperlipidemia, which is a feature of diabetic pregnancy.[51]

FETAL FLUID BALANCE

Fetal water balance is thought to be dependent largely on the regulation of water transfer across the placenta.[52] The composition of amniotic fluid, allantoic fluid, and fetal urine can be followed over long periods following catheterization of the fluid sacs and urinary bladder.[12] Catheterization of the fetal bladder is also a prerequisite for studies concerning the maturation of renal function and the endocrine control of fluid and electrolyte balance in the fetus.[31, 53]

HORMONES AND FETAL METABOLISM

The endocrine control of fetal metabolism has been extensively studied in the sheep[54] because of the ease with which exogenous hormones can be administered through indwelling catheters and blood samples obtained for the determination of plasma concentrations of metabolites and hormones. Additional information has been gleaned by ablation techniques, notably pancreatectomy.[55] The pregnant ewe and her fetus yield ample amounts of tissue for the investigation of cellular function by immunocytochemistry, *in situ* hybridization techniques, and Northern blotting, as well as cell culture.

FETAL GROWTH

CONTROL OF FETAL GROWTH

Fetal growth and fetal nutrition are inextricably linked. There is a significant reduction in the concentrations of most essential amino acids in the plasma of small-for-gestational-age (SGA) human fetuses,[56] an imbalance that may be causally related to intrauterine growth restriction (IUGR). Amino acid extraction across the placenta and fetal liver of the sheep can be studied by placing catheters in an umbilical artery and vein and in the left hepatic vein.[57]

INTRAUTERINE GROWTH RESTRICTION

SGA infants have a higher morbidity and mortality than those with a birth weight appropriate for gestational age.[58] Hitherto, much research has been directed towards an understanding of the mechanisms responsible for the neurological sequelae of IUGR, which range from cerebral palsy to behavioral disturbances.[58] A new focus for research on IUGR is suggested by recent epidemiological evidence of a strong link between low birth weight and adult cardiovascular disease.[59] The mechanisms whereby fetal adaptations to a poor intrauterine environment predispose to adult hypertension are as yet unknown. There exist several animal models of IUGR[60] that may prove useful in exploring these relationships.

Carunclectomy

The sheep placenta is comprised of 40 to 100 discrete cotyledons; the fetal villi develop in apposition to the endometrial caruncles, which are present in the uterus of the non-pregnant ewe. The number of cotyledons formed can be reduced by excising most of the caruncles before tupping. This procedure (carunclectomy) results in the birth of small lambs[61] and has been used to study metabolism in growth retarded fetuses.[62] The carunclectomy model has been criticized, however, because ultrasound analysis of umbilical artery flow velocities suggests that growth restriction is not related to a restriction in fetal placental circulation, as in the most frequently observed type of human IUGR.[63]

Embolization of the Umbilical Circulation

Techniques that restrict fetal growth late in gestation may be more relevant to studies of human type II IUGR. One such model depends upon reducing fetal placental blood flow by embolization. It is possible to cause a 33% reduction in fetal placental blood flow by repeated injection of large numbers of microspheres into the umbilical circulation. Over a period of 9 days, this can cause a 20% reduction in fetal weight.[64] An important feature of this model is the increase in placental resistance and resultant alteration in the umbilical artery flow velocity profile, which is an early feature of human IUGR.[65]

THE PHYSIOLOGY OF BIRTH

If the mechanisms that lead to the onset of labor were understood, it might be possible to reduce the incidence of premature delivery, with its attendant complications, which remains a major problem in clinical obstetrics. The chain of endocrine events that culminates in parturition in sheep is known in great detail.[66, 67] Maturation of the fetal hypothalamic-pituitary-adrenal axis plays a pivotal role, as established by the work of Sir Graham (Mont) Liggins.[68] An increase in responsiveness to adrenocorticotrophic hormone within the adrenal cortex of the fetus leads to a surge in cortisol secretion. Fetal cortisol increases the activity of placental 17α-hydroxylase, causing increased conversion of progesterone to estrogen. This precipitates synthesis of prostaglandin $F_{2\alpha}$ by the fetal chorioallantois and leads ultimately to myometrial contraction.

Unfortunately, the human placenta does not express the enzyme 17α-hydroxylase, nor has fetal cortisol been implicated in the initiation of human parturition. This is a timely reminder that extrapolation from animal models to humans is fraught with uncertainty.

OTHER ANIMAL MODELS

The inability of non-esterified fatty acids to cross the sheep placenta, dissimilarities between the breathing patterns of ovine and human fetuses, and the absence of an essential role for fetal cortisol in human parturition are examples that caution against extensive reliance on a single model for the human fetus. In view of the seasonal nature of research in many sheep laboratories, it is surprising that no consensus has emerged on an alternative model for out-of-season experiments.

PRIMATES

The rhesus monkey was used earlier to demonstrate how blood circulates through the intervillous space of the hemochorial placenta,[69] and techniques have been described for instrumentation of the fetuses of rhesus monkeys[70] and baboons.[71] Primates have usually been studied under anesthesia or with the mother lightly sedated.[72] Recently, techniques have been described for the measurement of fetal tracheal fluid pressure, heart rate, and electroencephalogram in fetuses of unrestrained baboons.[44, 73] This is a promising model for the study of behavioral state and fetal breathing patterns. However, primate preparations are costly and, therefore, unlikely to gain wide currency.

UNGULATES

The fetuses of farm animals are of intrinsic interest to veterinarians and there are some exceedingly good comparative studies on conscious cattle, horses, and pigs.[74, 75] The fetus of the llama has been examined for adaptations to oxygen limitation at high altitude.[76]

LAGOMORPHS AND RODENTS

Rabbits and rats have been used to examine maternal adaptations to pregnancy and to assess the effects of drugs on maternal placental blood flow. However, the fetuses are too small for studies of function above the tissue level.[77]

The Guinea Pig

Gestation lasts ~70 days in the guinea pig and the fetus weighs >100 g at term. Techniques have been described for the catheterization of blood vessels and determination of organ blood flows in acute experiments.[78, 79] Extradural electrodes for ECoG recording have been implanted in guinea pig fetuses and the preparations maintained for 7 to 12 days postoperatively.[80] This suggests that it might ultimately be possible to study chronically catheterized guinea pig fetuses. The guinea pig should be an attractive alternative to the sheep, since it has a hemochorial placenta and, therefore, already is widely used for studies of placental function.[81, 82]

The Capybara

A close relation of the guinea pig, the capybara, offers the advantage of a hemochorial placenta and a large fetus. A colony of these animals is, however, expensive to maintain in a temperate climate, since they are semiaquatic and require a supply of tepid, running water.[91]

CURRENT TRENDS IN FETAL PHYSIOLOGY

Improved neonatal care has led to a dramatic decrease in the mortality of preterm infants, but not all survivors are healthy babies. In Sweden, a country with approximately 100,000 births per year, perinatal mortality was estimated to have been reduced by nearly 4,000 in a period of 12 years, but at the cost of almost 300 extra cases of cerebral palsy.[83] Such trends have directed research towards understanding the physiology and pathophysiology of the immature fetus and to developing techniques for the study of the sheep fetus in mid-gestation.[84-87]

Research on the control of fetal growth continues apace. In a clinical context, the SGA infant remains a major concern. There is, for example, a strong association between poor intrauterine growth and the incidence of spastic cerebral palsy.[88] Additionally, the recent demonstration of a link between low birth weight and adult cardiovascular disease[59] is bound to initiate a search for developmental correlates that can explain why a poor intrauterine environment may have such far reaching consequences.

The evaluation of medical technology is another rapidly expanding area of perinatal research. Fetal heart rate monitoring in labor has become an integral part of obstetric practice, yet these recordings continue to pose major problems of interpretation for practising obstetricians.[89] New techniques such as Doppler ultrasonography, which has gained currency on the basis of empirical evidence, also need to be evaluated in an animal model. Thus indices derived from Doppler waveform analysis, and thought to reflect changes in placental vascular resistance during fetal hypoxemia, seem to depend more on alterations in fetal heart rate.[36] The full benefits of research in fetal physiology cannot be realized until refinement of these and other techniques, and of their application, leads to more reliable diagnosis.

REFERENCES

1. Barcroft, J., *Researches on Prenatal Life*, Blackwell Scientific Publications, Oxford, 1946.
2. Dawes, G. S., *Foetal and Neonatal Physiology*, Year Book Medical Publishers, Chicago, 1968.
3. Meschia, G., Cotter, J. R., Breathnach, C. S., and Barron, D. H., The hemoglobin, oxygen, carbon dioxide and hydrogen ion concentrations in the umbilical bloods of sheep and goats as sampled via indwelling plastic catheters, *Q. J. Exp. Physiol.*, 50, 185, 1965.
4. Rudolph, A. M., and Heymann, M. A., The circulation of the fetus in utero. Methods for studying distribution of blood flow, cardiac output and organ blood flow, *Circulation Res.*, 21, 163, 1967.
5. Makowski, E. L., Meschia, G., Droegemueller, W., and Battaglia, F. C., Measurement of umbilical arterial blood flow to the sheep placenta and fetus in utero, *Circulation Res.*, 23, 623, 1968.
6. Goodwin, D. H., *Sheep Management and Production*, London, Hutchinson, 1979.
7. Hecker, J. F., *The Sheep as an Experimental Animal*, Academic Press, London, 1983.
8. Mears, G. J., van Petten, G. R., Harris, W. H., Bell, J. U., and Lorscheider, F. L., Induction of oestrus and fertility in the anoestrous ewe with hormones and controlled lighting and temperature, *J. Rep. Fert.*, 57, 461, 1979.
9. van Petten, G. R., Mathison, H. J., Harris, W. H., and Mears, G. J., Chronic preparation of the pregnant ewe and fetus for pharmacological research: the placental transfer and fetal effects of bunitrolol, *J. Pharmacol. Meth.*, 1, 45, 1978.
10. Rudolph, C. D., Roman, C., and Rudolph, A. M., Effect of acute umbilical cord compression on hepatic carbohydrate metabolism in the fetal lamb, *Pediatric Res.*, 25, 228, 1989.
11. Noakes, D. E., and Young, M., Measurement of fetal tissue protein synthetic rate in the lamb in utero, *Res. Vet. Sci.*, 31, 336, 1981.
12. Mellor, D. J., and Slater, J. S., The use of chronic catheterization techniques in foetal sheep, *Br. Vet. J.*, 129, 260, 1973.
13. Kimberling, C. V., *Jensen and Swift's Diseases of Sheep*, 3rd edition, Lea & Febiger, Philadelphia, 1988.
14. Blood, D. C., Henderson, J.A., and Radostits, O.M., *Veterinary Medicine: A Textbook of the Diseases of Cattle, Sheep, Pigs and Horses*, 5th edition, Bailliere, London, 1979.
15. Fiset, P., and Woodward, T. E., Q fever, in *Bacterial Infections of Humans. Epidemiology and Control*, 2nd edition, Evans, A. S., and Brachman, P. S., Eds., Plenum Medical Book Company, New York, 1991.
16. Rankin, J. H. G., and Schneider, J. M., Effect of surgical stress on the distribution of placental blood flows, *Resp. Physiol.*, 24, 373, 1975.
17. Rudolph, A. M., and Heymann, M. A., Validation of the antipyrine method for measuring fetal umbilical blood flow, *Circulation Res.*, 21, 185, 1967.
18. Bristow, J., Rudolph, A. M., and Itskovitz, J., A preparation for studying liver blood flow, oxygen consumption, and metabolism in the fetal lamb *in utero*, *J. Dev. Physiol.*, 3, 255, 1981.
19. Ashwal, S., Majcher, J. S., Vain. N., and Longo, L. D., Patterns of fetal lamb regional cerebral blood flow during and after prolonged hypoxia, *Pediatric Res.*, 14, 1104, 1980.
20. Itskovitz, J., LaGamma, E. F., and Rudolph, A. M., The effect of reducing umbilical blood flow on fetal oxygenation, *Am. J. Obs. Gynecol.*, 145, 813, 1983.
21. Richardson, B. S., Patrick, J. E., Bousquet, J., Homan, J., and Brien, J. F., Cerebral metabolism in fetal lamb after maternal infusion of ethanol, *Am. J. Physiol.*, 249, R505, 1985.
22. Rudolph, A. M., and Heymann, M. A., Control of the foetal circulation, in *Foetal and Neonatal Physiology, Proc. of the Sir Joseph Barcroft Centenary Symp.*, Comline, K. S., Cross, K. W., Dawes, G. S., and Nathanielsz, P. W., Eds., Cambridge University Press, Cambridge, 1973, 89.
23. Morton, M. J., Pinson, C. W., and Thornburg, K. L., *In utero* ventilation with oxygen augments left ventricular stroke volume in lambs, *J. Physiol.*, 383, 413, 1987.

24. Reller, M. D., Morton, M. J., Geraud, G. D., Reid, D. L., and Thornburg, K. L., The effect of acute hypoxaemia on ventricular function during beta-adrenergic and cholinergic blockade in the fetal sheep, *J. Dev. Physiol.*, 11, 263, 1989.

25. Reuss, M. L., Rudolph, A. M., and Dae, M. W., Phasic blood flow patterns in the superior and inferior venae cavae and umbilical vein of fetal sheep, *Am. J. Obs. Gynecol.*, 145, 70, 1983.

26. Anderson, D. F., Parks, C. M., and Faber, J. J., Fetal O_2 consumption in sheep during controlled long-term reductions in umbilical blood flow. *Am. J. Physiol.*, 250, H1037, 1986.

27. Maulik, D., Yarlagadda, P., Nathanielsz, P. W., and Figueroa, J. P., Hemodynamic validation of Doppler assessment of fetoplacental circulation in a sheep model system, *J. Ultrasound Med.*, 8, 171, 1989.

28. Jensen, A., Roman, C., and Rudolph, A. M., Effects of reducing uterine blood flow on fetal blood flow distribution and oxygen delivery, *J. Dev. Physiol.*, 15, 309, 1991.

29. Fisher, D. J., Heymann, M. A., and Rudolph, A. M., Myocardial oxygen and carbohydrate consumption in fetal lambs in utero and in adult sheep, *Am. J. Physiol.*, 238, H399, 1980.

30. Makowski, E. L., Schneider, J. M., Tsoulos, N. G., Colwill, J. R., Battaglia, F. C., and Meschia, G., Cerebral blood flow, oxygen consumption, and glucose utilization of fetal lambs in utero, *Am. J. Obs. Gynecol.*, 114, 292, 1972.

31. Iwamoto, H. S., and Rudolph, A. M., Chronic renal venous catheterization in fetal sheep, *Am. J. Physiol.*, 245, H524, 1983.

32. Edelstone, D. I., Rudolph, A. M., and Heymann, M. A., Liver and ductus venosus blood flows in fetal lambs in utero, *Circulation Res.*, 42, 426, 1978.

33. Hanson, M. A., The importance of baro- and chemoreflexes in the control of the fetal cardio-vascular system, *J. Dev. Physiol.*, 10, 491, 1988.

34. Eik-Nes, S. H., Brubakk, A. O., and Ulstein, M. K., Measurement of human fetal blood flow. *Br. Med. J.*, ii, 283, 1980.

35. Gill, R. W., Trudinger, B. J., Garrett, W. J., Kossoff, G., and Warren, P. S., Fetal umbilical venous flow measured in utero by pulsed Doppler and B-mode ultrasound, *Am. J. Obs. Gynecol.*, 139, 720, 1981.

36. van Huisseling, H., Hasaart, T. H. M., Ruissen, C. J., Muijsers, G. J. J. M., and de Haan, J., Umbilical artery flow velocity waveforms during acute hypoxemia and the relationship with hemodynamic changes in the fetal lamb, *Am. J. Obs. Gynecol.*, 161, 1061, 1989.

37. Liggins, G. C., and Schellenberg, J.-C., Endocrine control of lung development, in *The Endocrine Control of the Fetus*, Künzel, W., and Jensen, A., Eds., Springer-Verlag, Berlin -Heidelberg, 1988, 236.

38. Pillai, M., and James, D., Hiccups and breathing in human fetuses, *Arch. Dis. Child.*, 65, 1072, 1990.

39. Gluckman, P. D., and Parsons, Y., Stereotaxic neurosurgery on the ovine fetus, in *Animal Models in Fetal Medicine III*, Nathanielsz, P. W., Ed., Perinatology Press, Ithaca, New York, 1984, 69.

40. Johnston, B. M., Bennet, L., and Gluckman, P. D., Inhibitory mechanisms in the control of breathing in the fetal lamb, in *Advances in Fetal Physiology: Reviews in Honor of G. C. Liggins*, Gluckman, P. D., Johnston, B. M., and Nathanielsz, P. W., Eds., Perinatology Press, Ithaca, New York, 1989, 177.

41. Richardson, B. S., Patrick, J. E., and Abduljabbar, H., Cerebral oxidative metabolism in the fetal lamb: relationship to electrocortical state, *Am. J. Obs. Gynecol.*, 153, 426, 1985.

42. Jensen, A., Bamford, O. S., Dawes, G. S., Hofmeyr, G., and Parkes, M. J., Changes in organ blood flow between high and low voltage electrocortical activity in fetal sheep, *J. Dev. Physiol.*, 8, 187, 1986.

43. Nijhuis, J. G., Prechtl, H. F. R., Martin, C. B., and Bots, R. S. G. M., Are there behavioural states in the human fetus? *Early Human Dev.*, 6, 177, 1982.

44. Stark, R. I., and Myers, M. M., Effect of electroencephalographic (EEG) state on fetal breathing activity (FBA) in the baboon, in *39th Annual Meeting, Society for Gynecologic Investigation*, 1992, Abstract No. 264.

45. Henderson-Smart, D. J., Pettigrew, A. G., and Campbell, D. J., Clinical apnoea and brainstem neural function in preterm infants, *New Eng. J. Med.*, 308, 353, 1983.

46. Gluckman, P. D., Cook, C., Williams, C., Bennet, L., and Johnston, B., Electrophysiological, neuromodulator and neurotransmitter development of the late gestation fetal brain, in *Fetal and Neonatal Development*, Jones, C. T., Ed., Perinatology Press, Ithaca, New York, 1988, 220.

47. Gluckman, P. D., Cook, C. J., Williams, C. E., Gunn, A. J., and Johnston, B. M., Electrophysiological and neurochemical response to asphyxia in the ovine fetus, in *The Endocrine Control of the Fetus*, Künzel, W., and Jensen, A., Eds., Springer-Verlag, Berlin - Heidelberg, 1988, 265.

48. Carter, A. M., Factors affecting gas transfer across the placenta and the oxygen supply to the fetus, *J. Dev. Physiol.*, 12, 305, 1989.

49. Hay, W.W., and Sparks, J.W., Placental fetal and neonatal carbohydrate metabolism, *Clin. Obs. Gynecol.*, 28, 473, 1985.

50. Elphick, M. C., Hull, D., and Broughton Pipkin, F., The transfer of fatty acids across the sheep placenta, *J. Dev. Physiol.*, 1, 31, 1979.

51. Thomas, C. R., Placental transfer of non-esterified fatty acids in normal and diabetic pregnancy, *Biol. Neonate*, 51, 94, 1987.

52. Power, G. G., and Dale, P. S., Placental water transfer with uneven blood flows, *Placenta*, Suppl. 2, 215, 1981.

53. Wintour, E.M., Water metabolism in the fetal-placental unit, in *Principles of Perinatal-Neonatal Metabolism*, Cowett, R.M., Ed., Springer-Verlag, New York, 1991, 340.

54. Künzel, W., and Jensen, A., Eds., *The Endocrine Control of the Fetus*, Springer-Verlag, Berlin - Heidelberg, 1988.

55. Fowden, A. L., and Comline, R. S., The effects of pancreatectomy on the sheep fetus in utero, *Q. J. Exp. Physiol.*, 69, 319, 1984.

56. Cetin, I., Corbetta, C., Sereni, L. P., Marconi, A. M., Bozzetti, P., Pardi, G., and Battaglia, F. C., Umbilical amino acid concentrations in normal and growth-retarded fetuses sampled in utero by cordocentesis, *Am. J. Obs. Gynecol.*, 162, 253, 1990.

57. Marconi, A. M., Battaglia, F. C., Meschia, G., and Sparks, J. W., A comparison of amino acid arteriovenous differences across the liver and placenta of the fetal lamb, *Am. J. Physiol.*, 257, E909, 1989.

58. Dunn, H. G., *Sequelae of Low Birthweight: The Vancouver Study*, Blackwell Scientific Publications, Oxford, 1986.

59. Barker, D. J. P., *Fetal and Infant Origins of Adult Disease*, British Medical Journal, London, 1992.

60. Carter, A. M., Placental blood flow and fetal oxygen supply in animal models of intra-uterine growth retardation, in *Placenta: Basic Research for Clinical Application*, Soma, H., Ed., Basel, Karger, 1991, 23.

61. Alexander, G., Studies on the placenta of the sheep (*Ovis aries* L.): effect of surgical reduction in the number of caruncles, *J. Rep. Fert.*, 7, 307, 1964.

62. Owens, J. A., Falconer, J., and Robinson, J. S., Effect of restriction of placental growth on fetal and utero-placental metabolism, *J. Dev. Physiol.*, 9, 225, 1987.

63. Giles, W. B., Trudinger, B. J., Stevens, D., Alexander, G., and Bradley, L., Umbilical artery flow velocity waveform analysis in normal ovine pregnancy and after carunculectomy, *J. Dev. Physiol.*, 11, 135, 1989.

64. Block, B. S., Schlafer, D. H., Wentworth, R. A., Kreitzer, L. A., and Nathanielsz, P. W., Regional blood flow distribution in fetal sheep with intrauterine growth retardation produced by decreased umbilical placental perfusion, *J. Dev. Physiol.*, 13, 81, 1990.

65. Trudinger, B. J., Stevens, D., Connelly, A., Hales, J. R. S., Alexander, G., Bradley, L., Fawcett, A., and Thompson, R. S., Umbilical artery flow velocity waveforms and placental resistance: the effects of embolization of the umbilical circulation, *Am. J. Obs. Gynecol.*, 157, 1443, 1987.

66. Liggins, G. C., The onset of labor: an historical review, in *Fetal and Neonatal Development*, Jones, C. T., Ed., Perinatology Press, Ithaca, New York, 1988, 381.

67. Challis, J. R. G., and Brooks, A. N., Maturation and activation of hypothalamic-pituitary-adrenal function in fetal sheep, *Endocrine Rev.*, 10, 182, 1989.

68. Liggins, G. C., Premature parturition after infusion of corticotrophin or cortisol into foetal lambs, *J. Endocrinol.*, 42, 323, 1969.

69. Ramsey, E. M., Corner, G. W., and Donner, M. W., Serial and cineradio-angiographic visualization of maternal circulation in the primate (hemochorial) placenta, *Am. J. Obs. Gynecol.*, 86, 213, 1963.

70. Novy, M. J., Piasecki, G. J., Hill, J. D., and Jackson, B. T., Cardio-respiratory measurements in fetal monkeys obtained by chronic catheters, *J. Appl. Physiol.*, 31, 788, 1971.

71. Paton, J. B., Fisher, D. E., Peterson, E. N., deLannoy, C. W., and Behrman, R. E., Cardiac output and organ blood flows in the baboon fetus, *Biol. Neonate*, 22, 50, 1973.

72. Jackson, B. T., Piasecki, G. J., and Novy, M. J., Fetal responses to altered maternal oxygenation in rhesus monkey, *Am. J. Physiol.*, 252, R94, 1987.

73. Stark, R. I., Daniel, S. S., James, L. S., MacCarter, G., Morishima, H. O., Niemann, W. H., Rey, H., Tropper, P. J., and Yeh, M.-N., Chronic instrumentation and longterm investigation in the fetal and maternal baboon: tether system, conditioning procedures and surgical techniques, *Lab. Anim. Sci.*, 39, 25, 1989.

74. Comline, R. S., and Silver, M., A comparative study of blood gas tensions, oxygen affinity and red cell 2,3 DPG concentrations in foetal and maternal blood in the mare, cow and sow, *J. Physiol.*, 242, 805, 1974.

75. Silver, M., and Fowden, A. L., Induction of labour in domestic animals: endocrine changes and neonatal viability, in *The Endocrine Control of the Fetus*, Künzel, W., and Jensen, A., Eds., Springer-Verlag, Berlin - Heidelberg, 1988, 401.

76. Benavides, C. E., Pérez, R., Espinoza, M., Cabello, G., Riquelme, R., Parer, J. T., and Llanos, A. J., Cardiorespiratory functions in the fetal llama, *Resp. Physiol.*, 75, 327, 1989.

77. Lemons, J. A., Perez, R., Schreiner, R. L., and Gresham, E. L., Acute small animal preparation — suitable for fetal metabolic studies? *J. Appl. Physiol.*, 49, 42, 1980.

78. Carter, A. M., The blood supply to the abdominal organs of the fetal guinea-pig, *J. Dev. Physiol.*, 6, 407, 1984.

79. Detmer, A., Gu, W., and Carter, A. M., The blood supply to the heart and brain in the growth retarded guinea pig fetus, *J. Dev. Physiol.*, 15, 153, 1991.

80. Umans, J. G., Cox, M. J., Hinman, D. J., Dogramajian, M. E., Senger, G., and Szeto, H. H., The development of electrocortical activity in the fetal and neonatal guinea pig, *Am. J. Obs. Gynecol.*, 153, 467, 1985.

81. Reynolds, M.L., and Young, M., The transfer of free α-amino nitrogen across the placental membrane in the guinea-pig, *J. Physiol.*, 214, 583, 1971.

82. Jansson, T., and Persson, E., Placental transfer of glucose and amino acids in intrauterine growth retardation: studies with substrate analogs in the awake guinea pig, *Pediatric Res.*, 28, 203, 1990.

83. Hagberg, B., and Hagberg, G., The changing panorama of infantile hydrocephalus and cerebral palsy over forty years — a Swedish survey, *Brain & Develop.*, 11, 368, 1989.

84. Bell, A. W., Kennaugh, J. M., Battaglia, F. C., Makowski, E. L., and Meschia, G., Metabolic and circulatory studies of fetal lamb at midgestation, *Am. J. Physiol.*, 250, E538, 1986.

85. Iwamoto, H. S., Kaufman, T., Keil, L. C., and Rudolph, A. M., Responses to acute hypoxemia in fetal sheep at 0.6-0.7 gestation, *Am. J. Physiol.*, 256, H613, 1989.

86. Akagi, K., and Challis, J. R. G., Hormonal and biophysical responses to acute hypoxemia in fetal sheep at 0.7-0.8 gestation, *Can. J. Physiol. Pharmacol.*, 68, 1527, 1990.

87. Gleason, C. A., Hamm, C., and Jones, M. D., Cerebral blood flow, oxygenation, and carbohydrate metabolism in immature fetal sheep in utero, *Am. J. Physiol.*, 256, R1264, 1989.

88. Blair, E., and Stanley, F., Intrauterine growth and spastic cerebral palsy, *Am. J. Obs. Gynecol.*, 162, 229, 1990.

89. Murphy, K. W., Johnson, P., Moorcraft, J., Pattinson, R., Russell, V., and Turnbull, A., Birth asphyxia and the intrapartum cardiotocograph, *Br. J. Obs. Gynecol.*, 97, 470, 1990.

90. Rudolph, A.M., personal communication.

91. Kaufmann, P., personal communication.

Chapter 9

Animal Models in Nephrological Research

H. Dieperink, S.T. Lillevang, and E. Kemp

CONTENTS

INTRODUCTION

In nephrological research, many animal models have been elaborated. This has resulted in fast progress in the understanding of renal disease and may eventually result in better treatment. In this chapter, three major fields of experimental nephrological research will be described:

1. renal physiology and pathophysiology
2. glomerulonephritis
3. renal transplantation

ANIMAL MODELS IN RENAL PHYSIOLOGY AND PATHOPHYSIOLOGY

The kidney is the central regulatory organ governing the maintenance of body fluid volume and composition. This has motivated the development of a formidable number of experimental models in both animal and human subjects. Because the kidneys are constructed from a large number of small, independently functioning units (nephrons) not directly accessible from the body surface, the current understanding of renal function in health and disease is critically dependent on invasive experiments only possible in animal laboratory models. Certainly, there is a long step from single nephron function in series of micropuncture experiments in

0-8493-4390-9/94/$0.00+$.50
© 1994 by CRC Press Inc.

anesthetized, laparectomized, and ventilated rats to whole-kidney function in humans. But data obtained with invasive and non-invasive techniques in animal models can been correlated, making it possible in the second line to compare data from non-invasive animal and non-invasive human models. When the relative influence of anesthesia, surgery, and species difference has been elucidated, the conclusions drawn from single nephron function in animals can sometimes be generalized to cover aspects of whole kidney function in human subjects.

It can be even more intricate to interpret data from kidney cell culture, microdissection preparations, isolated nephron segments, or isolated perfused whole kidneys, since the bias introduced by such preparations necessitates further comparative investigations. On the other hand, these methods in general either reduce the bias induced by the heterogeneity of the studied material, or give access to structures not otherwise accessible.

Among the many models used to elucidate kidney physiology in a variety of animal species, space permits only two models to be introduced in this chapter. Arguments for choice of model and species are presented, but the chapter does not pretend to give more than a short description of the selected models, aimed at the novice reader. Any major textbook on kidney physiology will describe these models in more detail. In general, the choice of model for a specific project is an expert question, and the non-expert reader is advised to consult a laboratory working with kidney physiology before embarking on a project.

MICROPUNCTURE METHODS

Micropuncture methods are the most powerful tools in renal physiology, because they give direct measurements of glomerular and periglomerular vascular hemodynamics, and allow assessment of reabsorption or secretion rates at different sites in the nephron.[1] Micropuncture experiments are indispensable for examining details in renal function, and they represent the gold standard to which new methods are correlated. The pros of the micropuncture models are that some of the data obtained with micropuncture are not available from any other method, and they give detailed data from single nephrons while other methods, for instance clearance measurements, yield results expressive of mean nephron function. However, the cons of micropuncture experiments are many. Only the very experienced researcher can perform a reliable micropuncture. A specially equipped laboratory is mandatory. The methods are laborious and because they give data from a number of single nephrons in animals prepared for micropuncture with anesthesia and laparatomy, they demand several series of other experiments if the bearings of the conclusions based on micropuncture are to be extended to whole kidney function in conscious not-operated animal or human subjects.

Glomerular micropuncture is difficult and most animal strains have only few glomeruli accessible on the kidney surface. But a mutant of the Wistar rat strain, the Münich-Wistar, has a substantial number of glomeruli on the kidney surface. This allows systematical studies on glomerular hemodynamics, but introduces the perplexing situation that data on glomerular function are obtained in a rat strain that is abnormal when it comes to the glomeruli. However, experiments have verified that the function of these surface glomeruli is similiar to that of the other glomeruli in the outer cortex.

Since micropuncture experiments in the Münich-Wistar rats have formed the backbone in our current knowledge of glomerular hemodynamics, most other renal physiological investigations are performed in the rat species. Also, the effects of surgery and anesthesia are best elucidated in various rat strains.

The proximal tubules are technically the most simple to puncture. Tubular hydrostatic pressure and transepithelial electrical potential difference can be measured directly. When a dye is injected intravenously and the kidney surface is observed, the convolutions of the proximal tubule are easily identified as the dye is ultrafiltrated and follows the flow of the tubular fluid. Provided inulin is given and plasma inulin is measured, single nephron glomerular filtration rate can be determined from tubular fluid inulin concentration and tubular flow rate, and furthermore the fractional fluid reabsorption in the segment of the proximal tubule proximal to the puncture site can be estimated from the ratio between tubular fluid and plasma inulin.

The superficial convolutions of the distal convoluted tubules are also accessible in the rat, while the renal papilla and hence the thin loop of Henle and the papillary collecting duct are only accessible in other rodents, the hamster for instance, and very young rats (body weight below 100g).

CLEARANCE METHODS

Clearance methods have a number of advantages. First, they can be used in almost all species and do not demand anesthesia or surgery, maneuvers that may markedly alter renal function. Therefore, they can make apparent some of the potential errors when extrapolating data from micropuncture to whole organ function in conscious animals. Secondly, they represent the single most efficacious means of studying human renal physiology, and thus they represent a link between animal and human experiments. Combined with surface micropuncture, they allow the calculation of data about deep nephrons, which is of interest if differential changes in superficial and deep nephrons are suspected in animal experiments. The disadvantages are that clearance methods cannot distinquish internephron variation, and that they present problems when it comes to localizing the specific nephron site of reabsorption or secretion. The gold standard for measurement of glomerular filtration rate (GFR) is inulin clearance, because inulin is completely filterable at the glomerulus, and is not reabsorbed or secreted by tubules. The actual rate of fluid filtration is approximately 92% of inulin clearance (C_{in}) because 8% of plasma volume consists of unfilterable protein, but only few studies need this correction. Creatinine clearance (C_{crea}) has the advantage that creatinine is endogenously produced, and therefore C_{crea} only requires collection of urine and blood samples. However, creatinine production is not constant in disease or stress states with inconstant food intake. Creatinine undergoes tubular secretion, and at low tubular flow rates studies in dogs have shown tubular reabsorption.[3] Measurements of creatinine are not straightforward, and the autoanalyzer methods owe their relative accuracy to the combined effects of analytical overestimation of creatinine in the blood and physiological overestimation of filtered creatinine due to creatinine secretion. Therefore, C_{crea} cannot be recommended for assessment of GFR in most animal experimental settings. As an unfortunate example, the manifest nephrotoxic effects of the currently most used immunosuppressive drug, cyclosporine A, was missed in the preclinical animal investigations using C_{crea}. As a method less laborious than standard C_{in} the single-bolus injection ^{57}Co-EDTA method has been evaluated in the rat, and can be recommended.[4] The glomerular pore size and charge selectivity can be estimated with differential clearance measurements.[2] Neutral dextran molecules of varying sizes are neither secreted nor reabsorbed by the renal tubules, and therefore their clearances are equal to their glomerular filtration. If dextran of a known size is filtered freely as is inulin, then the glomerular pores are greater than this specific dextran molecule. Thus, by studying the clearances of dextrans of various sizes, the size of the glomerular pores can be estimated noninvasively in animal and human subjects. However, also the charge of the glomerular capillary wall is interesting, since this charge may change in various disease or intoxication states. In normal subjects the glomerular sieving of small molecules of dextran sulfate is significantly lower than expected from the molecular size, due to the anionic charge of the glomerular membrane. In contrast, the transport of cationic diethylamino-ethyl dextrans are facilitated. But when the glomerular membrane is damaged, the sieving characteristics of the neutral and the charged dextrans of a certain size are almost identical, indicating that the damaged membrane has lost its charge. Renal blood and plasma flow can be accurately measured by dye or gas-dilution methods, or by methods using the renal excretion rates of substances undergoing tubular secretion, for instance paraaminohippurate (PAH). The latter is only precise if renal vein catheterization is carried out, but the clearance of PAH (C_{pah}) approximates renal plasma flow and can therefore be used in not-operated and conscious animals provided the PAH extraction fraction is known.

Tubular transport functions of various substances actively or passively transported across tubular membranes have added substantially to current understanding of many physiological and pathophysiological states. Clearance techniques may approach localization of transport to various nephron segments by several methods. Of these, the free-water clearance (C_{H_2O}) and lithium clearance will be presented. C_{H_2O} is defined as urine volume minus the clearance value of osmolar particles (often denoted $\tilde{C}_{osm}$). C_{H_2O} can be explained as follows: if solute-free water is extracted from hyposmolar urine until the remaining urine is isoosmolar, then the volume of solute-free water removed per time unit is C_{H_2O}. Because this free water is generated by the cortical thick ascending limb of Henle, C_{H_2O} is proportional to NaCl transport in that nephron segment. However, C_{H_2O} overestimates thick limb NaCl transport because urine may also be diluted in the distal convoluted tubule, and in general there are so many conditions or circumstances where free-water back-diffusion is modified that the method yields more questions than answers. The lithium-clearance (C_{Li}) method utilizes the observation, confirmed by micropuncture[5] that lithium is ultrafiltrated and reabsorbed in the proximal tubule in parallel with sodium and water, while in the nephron segment distal to the end of the proximal tubule lithium is not reabsorbed, in contrast to sodium. Thus, C_{Li} is claimed to represent end proximal delivery. While significant post-proximal lithium reabsorption may occur if sodium reabsorption is enhanced, at least in the rat, it will in most experimental settings be possible to eliminate this bias by adding to the diet a suitable amount of sodium. When GFR, C_{Li} and C_{Na} are known, the absolute reabsorption of tubular fluid in the proximal tubule can be calculated (GFR-C_{Li}), and so can the sodium reabsorption in the post-proximal nephron segment ((C_{Li}-C_{Na})*P_{Na}). Thus, if trace amounts of lithium are administered, data on segmental nephron reabsorptive activity can be obtained in animal or human subjects with a minimum of preparation.

ANIMAL MODELS OF HUMAN GLOMERULONEPHRITIS

Since the first half of the 19th century, symptoms of renal disease — proteinuria, hematuria, edema, hypertension, anemia, etc. — have been associated with structural changes in the kidney. The traditional means of studying the natural history of a disease and hypothesizing about its pathogenesis by morphological studies on autopsy material did not yield much to the understanding of kidney disease, since most cases had already progressed to an end stage (glomerulosclerosis) when the patients died. Therefore, great interest was aimed at the development of animal models of human glomerulonephritis. Numerous such models gave and continue to give insight into the natural history of kidney diseases, enabling us to study their pathogenesis, and providing means to study the effect of therapeutic intervention.

GENERAL CONSIDERATIONS

It should be emphasized that none of the many existing experimental models of glomerulonephritis present a picture identical to any of the human forms of glomerulonephritis. A useful point to bear in mind is the fact that no model seems to be identical in both etiology and pathogenesis to its human counterpart. Hence, we cannot without caution extrapolate results from experimental studies to human disease. On the other hand, the whole picture of human glomerulonephritis is reasonably well represented by all experimental models taken together, with each model contributing its own details to the mosaic. A major problem in the comparison of human glomerulonephritis with an experimental model is that the natural history of the human disease *before* onset of clinical symptoms is rarely known. This means that the starting point of morphological observations in the clinical setting is often represented by a kidney biopsy at the time of diagnosis, whereas in the experimental situation time is set by the scientist, and the natural history of the model disease can be elucidated in detail from day 0. This is indeed the case for most experimental models and, as a consequence, a great deal is known about preventive measures or treatment modalities in the early stages of most experimental models. Because of the diagnostic delay in the human situation, the very early stages in human glomerulonephritis are seldom accessible to treatment and extrapolating results from experimental treatment may be disappointing. Another problem of this delay is that autoantibodies, presumably present at the onset of disease, may no longer be present in serum at the time of diagnosis, making the search for pathogenic antigens unrewarding. Different models of glomerulonephritis induced by injection of antibody (Nephrotoxic Serum Nephritis, NTSN) or non-physiological antigen (serum sickness nephritis) provide excellent tools to gain insight into the pathogenesis of glomerulonephritis. These models are complicated by the fact that they involve excessive amounts of heterologous antigen, leading in the case of NTSN to an immune response against the disease-inducing antibody. In their etiology, these models are therefore quite different from any human situation. More promising in respect to parallelling the etiology of human disease are autoimmune models based on polyclonal activation of B lymphocytes and/or proliferation of autoreactive T lymphocytes as a common mechanism. These models are either spontaneously occurring like the SLE-like disease of certain mice strains or induced by drugs or heavy metals (penicillamine-, gold salt-, and $HgCl_2$-induced glomerulonephritis in the Brown Norway rat), by allogeneic lymphocytes in graft-vs.-host (GVH) reactions, or by stimulatory agents like LPS (T-cell superantigen). Contrary to human autoimmune diseases, in general, the induced autoimmune phenomena in rodents are down-regulated and the animals recover, hindering the study of chronic autoimmune glomerulonephritis. In spite of these objections, it seems fair to conclude that the use of experimental models of human glomerulonephritis is justified. Examination of different details of a given human disease entity — the cell-type mediating inflammation, the involvement of hormones, the mechanism of mesangial deposition etc. — may well have to be studied in more than one model to get the whole picture.

CHOICE OF ANIMALS

The animals used in models of glomerulonephritis are almost exclusively rodents, with rats and mice being by far the most frequently employed. Rabbits are used especially in models of NTSN, but a number of considerations regarding the use of rabbits in experimental models of kidney disease are pertinent: first of all, inbred rabbit strains are (practically) not available, making immunological studies difficult to carry out. Secondly, rabbits are immunologically less well-characterized than rats and mice, and monoclonal antibodies similar to the vast array of monoclonal antibodies against rat and mouse leukocyte antigens and differentiation markers are not yet available for rabbits. For studies of chronic disease, it is also important to note that uremia induces changes in rabbit calcium metabolism quite different from what is seen in humans — leading to massive alterations in bone morphology. Lastly, rabbits are usually more expensive and require more room in the animal facility than do smaller rodents. Mice and rats, on the other hand, are used extensively due to their convenient size, the availability of literally hundreds of inbred strains — facilitating design and interpretation of immunological studies — and the fact that the immune systems, including major histocompatibility complex (MHC) genes and antigens, of rats and mice are fairly well characterized. A note of caution concerning animal age: unlike humans, rodents are not born with a fully developed cellular immune system (as demonstrated by the ability to induce tolerance neonatally). Consequently, quite different results may be obtained in the same model using newborn or mature animals. On the other hand, some mice and most rats — especially male rats —are prone to develop progressive glomerulosclerosis with age, often resulting in proteinuria and of course interfering with the interpretation of glomerulonephritis study results. In the following, brief descriptions are given of some commonly used experimental models. By no means is this intended to be an exhaustive review of available glomerulonephritis models but merely to serve as an illustration of the general points made above.

Heymann Nephritis

As originally described by Heymann, a form of nephritis can be induced in rats by immunization with kidney cortex homogenate.[6,7] Outbred Sprague-Dawley rats were used when the model was developed but nowadays inbred strains like LEW are more often used. This experimental autologous immune complex glomerulonephritis morphologically closely resembles idiopathic membraneous glomerulopathy in humans, and because of the associated nephrotic syndrome Heymann nephritis is regarded as the model of choice of human membraneous glomerulopathy. In both conditions, immune deposits are confined to the subepithelial space and the basement membrane changes including the characteristic "spikes" occur in both. The importance of this model lies in its contribution to the understanding of the formation and disappearance of glomerular immune aggregates and the mechanisms of glomerular injury leading to proteinuria. Studies of the cellular events leading to induction and maintenance of the autoimmune response in Heymann nephritis have failed to demonstrate alterations in T-lymphocyte subsets — in contrast to the T-lymphocyte subset changes described in human membraneous glomerulopathy.

HgCl$_2$-Induced Autoimmune Disease

Repeated low-dose injections of mercuric chloride in Brown Norway rats result in the induction of a generalized autoimmune disease characterized by polyclonal activation of B-lymphocytes, proliferation of autoreactive CD4$^+$ self-MHC class II-restricted T-lymphocytes, very high levels of IgE in serum, and the production of antibodies against a wide array of self and non-self antigens.[8] Autoantibodies to different components of the glomerular basement membrane such as laminin, type IV collagen, and fibronectin lead to the development of glomerulonephritis accompanied by severe proteinuria, clinically the most prominent feature of the model. The susceptibility to disease is under genetic control and other rat strains (e.g., Lewis) will develop unspecific suppression phenomena upon HgCl$_2$ challenge. Interestingly, similar autoimmune pathology can be induced in susceptible strains by gold salts, penicillamine, and allogeneic disease induced by transfer of parental lymphocytes to an F$_1$ hybrid (e.g., BN $\rightarrow$ (BNxLEW)F$_1$). A human parallel to these phenomena is the nephrotic syndrome developed in some patients under treatment with gold salts or penicillamine, the susceptibility of patients to develop disease again believed to be MHC-associated. The strength of the experimental models lie in the elucidation of the cellular events leading to autoimmunity. There is increasing focus on the interaction between different T-lymphocyte subsets, and in particular there is growing evidence of the significance of the subdivision of CD4$^+$ T-helper lymphocytes into T$_H$1 and T$_H$2 phenotypes.[9] The major drawback to this and other models of induced polyclonal B lymphocyte activation is the spontaneous downregulation of disease, which generally does not occur in human autoimmune disease with renal pathology.

Murine Lupus Nephritis

Spontaneously occurring SLE-like disease associated with glomerulonephritis in certain lupus-prone mouse strains has been used as a model of human SLE glomerulonephritis.[10] Many of the features described for the mercuric chloride-induced autoimmune disease including polyclonal B lymphocyte activation and CD4$^+$ T-lymphocyte mediated regulation hereof are true for this model as well, but in contrast the spontaneously occurring disease most often takes a chronic course. A large number of (NZBxNZW)F$_1$ female mice, BxSD mice, and

MRL-lpr/lpr mice develop the lupus-like syndrome accompanied by renal injury. The model has provided different hypotheses of pathogenesis, many with a focus on the importance of DNA/anti-DNA immune complex deposition in glomeruli, but others question this notion and ascribe the development of glomerulonephritis to the presence of gp70/anti-gp70 immune complexes (gp70 is a serum glycoprotein with structural resemblance to the murine leukemia virus envelope glycoprotein). Because of the chronic course of this model, it has been extensively used in studies of treatment modalities in both early and late stages of disease, often forming the basis of working hypotheses used for the study of its human counterpart or the introduction of tentative preventive/therapeutic measures in the human situation. The importance of prostaglandins in this model has been established by improvement in renal pathology and proteinuria by the administration of PGE_1 and PGE_2 or the synthetic prostacycline analogue Iloprost. Similar effect has been seen after treatment with a diet rich in ω-3 fatty acids. The importance of T-lymphocyte involvement in the model is demonstrated by protection from renal injury by treatment with anti-CD4 mAb or anti-IL2R mAb.

Nephrotoxic Serum Nephritis

NTSN (or the synonymous Masugi nephritis, experimental crescentic glomerulonephritis, or anti-glomerular basement membrane [-GBM] glomerulonephritis) is induced by the injection of a heterologous antibody against GBM antigens (nephrotoxic serum), most commonly studied in rabbits. After initial binding of the antibody to the glomerular basement membrane, resulting in linear immunofluorescence, the animals develop a proliferative glomerulonephritis with crescent formation, which eventually leads to renal failure. This resembles rapidly progressive crescentic glomerulonephritis in humans in morphology, albeit not in etiology. The development of tissue injury in the model is dependent on the influx of polymorphonuclear leukocytes, T-lymphocytes, and monocytes with procoagulant activity giving rise to fibrin deposition and further inflammation.[11] The importance of T-lymphocytes in the induction of NTSN is supported by the fact that bursectomy does not influence the occurrence of disease in a chicken model of NTSN whereas T lymphocytes can transfer the disease to native animals. NTSN has, in the past, been a valuable tool in the study of events causing glomerular damage, including the relative importance of antibodies, T-lymphocytes, and inflammatory cells and mediators released by these cells. Isolation of glomeruli and elution of bound antibody or characterization of the cellular outgrowth from cultured glomeruli has been extensively used in this model and has paved the way for similar studies in human glomerulonephritis.

ANIMAL MODELS IN RENAL TRANSPLANTATION

Transplantation research has always been based on animal experiments. Kidney transplantation was the first and leading organ transplantation and is now widely used all over the world as routine treatment. Many human lives are saved due to the treatment and due to basic experimental animal work. In this section renal allo- and xenotransplantation will be dealt with.

ALLOTRANSPLANTATION

In the early days of renal allotransplantation, animals were used for surgical training. Today, this is rarely necessary as young surgeons can learn the technique in the operating theater. Today, experimental renal allotransplantation is used for at least three important purposes:

1. investigation of the natural history of the fate of the transplanted kidney
2. renal preservation
3. treatment experiments with various immunosuppressive substances

The Fate of the Transplanted Kidney

Experiments have elucidated the rejection mechanism in allografting. In the past, surgeons usually used larger animals such as dogs and pigs for the purpose, but nowadays most experiments are performed with smaller animals, especially rats. In spite of the existing differences between humans and rats, many of the findings in the rat can be seen occurring in humans.

Transplantation immunology has gained much knowledge from experimental renal allotransplantation. Here larger animals, for instance monkeys, often have to be used in order to study animals close to humans regarding tissue typing, blood groups, etc. The whole concept of allograft rejection is based on animal experiments. The rejection phenomenon is very similar in humans and the above-mentioned animals.[12]

Another branch of experimental immunological animal research is attempts to make so-called rescue treatment. Animal research has contributed a great deal here.

Renal Preservation

Renal preservation has made great progress since the beginning of renal transplantation. In this almost "mechanical" business, it is very helpful to do animal research before clinical treatment. Rabbits and dogs are very convenient for preservation studies. Nowadays preservation times of 24 to 48 hours are acceptable provided there is a short warm ischaemia time.

Preservation studies are performed with both (and most often) flush experiments and machine perfusion. With machine perfusion, good graft function can be obtained even after several days of preservation. The composition of the perfusion fluid undergoes alterations all the time and is of course developed according to the experimental results.

Last but not least, the experience gained from renal preservation has been used and adapted to the preservation of heart, lung, liver, etc.

Immunosuppressive Substances

Animal research into rejection of transplants leads to a rational investigation of a means to avoid rejection. Nearly all new immunosuppressive substances have been tested in transplanted animals before clinical use. Administration rules and dosage of the substances are empirically ruled out. Concerning dosage, one often finds greater differences from species to species and here it can be difficult to know how to start treatment in the clinic. The rat and the pig often seem to be like the human but there are many exceptions.

Even more difficult and at the same time very important are studies of side effects. Many side effects have been observed in animal research, and unexpected side effects may appear when introducing a new immunosuppressant in humans. For instance, Cyclosporin A — one of the best immunosuppressants in kidney transplantation — was not known to be nephrotoxic when introduced for use in the clinic.

Work on immunosuppression is in a prolific phase. New immunosuppressive substances and treatment schemes for these substances have been developed. Many new drugs have appeared and are either undergoing tests *in vitro*, in animal research, or in trials in patients receiving renal transplants.

Conventional therapy with Azathioprine and steroids has in many places been changed to Cyclosporine, prospectively, with addition of newer drugs such as FK-506, Deoxyspergualin or Rapamycin — just to mention a few. In addition, many centers see possibilities in both rejection therapy and rescue therapy with monoclonal antibodies in conjunction with conventional therapy.

Innumerable combinations of substances and schemes for treatment now exist. Only animal experiments with well-defined models can bring at least some order in this almost chaotic situation. The future is promising but demands a very great deal of experimental work.

The final goal in all transplantation research is creating transplantation tolerance. New and exciting experiments have been made recently in this field. For instance, injection of donor renal tissue from one kidney into the thymus of the recipient creates tolerance for the other kidney when transplanted in rat experiments. Also, monoclonal antibodies can introduce tolerance.

When such experiments can be translated and performed in humans, we will have a brave new future with patients receiving renal transplants and no long-lasting immunosuppressive treatment.

XENOTRANSPLANTATION

As xenotransplantation definitely is not a clinical procedure today, all renal xenotransplantation research is bound to be experimental work. As in the case with allotransplantation, we have at least two purposes here:

1. Investigation of the natural histology of the fate of the transplanted kidney
2. Treatment experiments with various immunosuppressive substances (Renal preservation is better studied in allotransplants)

Fate of the Transplanted Kidney

At the beginning, many xenotransplants were performed in models using larger animals such as dogs and sheep. As time has passed, smaller animals have been more widely used. Rabbits, cats, baby pigs, hamsters, guinea pigs, and rats have been used for the purpose. The rat is an excellent animal to study as a recipient. It is easy to breed and there are well-defined strains, so experiments can easily be reproduced. The drawback of using smaller animals for renal transplantation is, of course, that microvascular surgery is necessary and must be learned.

In xenotransplantation, a distinction is made between the very fast rejection occurring from minutes to a few hours after transplantation, after so-called discordant xenografting, and concordant rejection. The mechanism of discordant rejection is activation of the complement system (often by natural antibodies) and complement-dependent destruction of the endothelium in renal vessels followed by thrombocyte aggregation and, finally, complete obstruction of the renal vessels. Especially histology, immunofluorescence microscopy, and electron microscopy have helped to describe this rejection form.

In concordant species combinations (usually more closely related species), another rejection pattern is seen starting with activation of macrophages but few lymphocytes, and the destructive process continues for several days. Eventually, necrosis of the renal tissue and destruction of the renal vessels will occur. While the rejection pattern in allografting is T-lymphocyte dependent, the xenograft rejection seems to be much more of a humoral type with macrophages and probably B-lymphocytes as the "main acteurs".

Further studies of the responsible immunocytes and the influence of various cytokines and adhesion molecules must also be performed.

Immunosuppressive Substances

In xenotransplantation, experiments were previously almost exclusively conducted with immunosuppressive substances known to be good in allotransplantation. Up to a certain limit, this has been all right, but as more and more is understood about the differences between the rejection mechanisms in allo- and xenotransplantation, other ways of immunosuppression are being tried, for instance, the use of monoclonal antibodies against macrophages and against B-lymphocytes or, immunosuppressive drugs with greater power against these cells than against T-lymphocytes.[13]

Concerning discordant xenografts, the best result obtained thus far has been the removal of the complement. For instance, in our laboratory, a rabbit kidney transplant in a cat is usually rejected in 10 minutes. After decomplementation, the graft has survived for up to a week. At the moment, work is being done on antibodies against complement C3, aiming at further prolongation of survival time.

One of the best possibilities to a successful survival of discordant xenografts is production of transgeneic animals. Some very exciting experiments are in development especially from the xenotransplantation group in Cambridge. The group has created a pig with human complement decay factor "spliced in". Also, xenotolerance is a hope for the future. This has been done to some extent with pancreatic islets and now also with kidneys (rats→mice).[14]

Animal research is essential to renal transplantation. In allotransplantation, as well as in xenotransplantation, there is a vast experience in elucidating the natural history of rejection and attempts to prevent rejection. Future research will also include many animal experiments. This is mandatory in testing all new immunosuppressive substances and combinations of these in evaluating treatment schemes.

Hope for the future is, first of all, a creation of immunologic tolerance. Perhaps it can be found in xenotransplantation with the use of transgenic animals.

REFERENCES

1. Andreucci, V. E., (Ed.), *Manual of Renal Micropuncture,* Idelson Publishers, Naples, Italy, 1978.
2. Ladd, M., Liddle, L. and Gagnon, J. A., Renal excretion of inulin, creatinine, and ferrocyanide at normal and reduced clearance levels in the dog, *Am. J. Physiol.,* 184, 505, 1956.
3. Ido, Y., Tilton, R. G., Chang, K., Pugliese, G. and Williamson, J. R., Rapid measurement of glomerular filtration rate in small animals, *Kidney Int.,* 41, 435, 1992.
4. Chang, R. L. S, Deen, W. M., Robertson, C. R. and Brenner, B. M., Permselectivity of the glomerular capillary wall. III, *Kidney Int.,* 8, 212, 1975.
5. Thomsen, K., Holstein-Rathlou, N. H, Leyssac, P. P., Comparison of three measures of proximal tubular reabsorption: Lithium clearance, occlusion time, and micropuncture, *Am. J. Physiol.,* 241, F348, 1981.
6. Heymann, W., Hackle D. B., Harwood, J., Wilson, S. G. F. and Hunter, J. L. P., Production of nephrotic syndrome in rats by Freund´s adjuvant and rat kidney suspensions, *Proc. Soc. Exp. Biol. Med.,* 100, 660, 1959.
7. Salant, D. J., Quigg, R. J. and Cybulsky, A. V., Heymann nephritis: Mechanisms of renal injury, *Kidney Int.,* 35, 976, 1989.
8. Sapin, C., Druet, E. and Druet, P., Induction of anti-glomerular basement membrane antibodies in the Brown Norway rat by mercuric chloride, *Clin. Exp. Immunol.,* 28, 173, 1977.
9. Powrie, F., Fowell, D., McKnight, A. J. and Mason, D., Lineage relationships and functions of CD4[+] T-cell subsets in the rat, *Res. Immunol.,* 142, 54, 1991.
10. Theofilopoulus, A. N. and Dixon, F. J., Etiopathogenesis of murine systemic lupus erythematosus, *Immunol. Rev.,* 55, 179, 1981.
11. Holdsworth, S. R, Thomson, N. M., Glasgow, E. F, Dowling, J. P. and Atkins, R. C., Tissue culture of isolated glomeruli in experimental crescentic glomerulonephritis, *J. Exp. Med.,* 147, 98, 1978.
12. Williams, G. M., Burdick, J. F. and Solez, K., *Kidney Transplant Rejection. Diagnosis and Treatment,* Marcel Dekker, Inc., New York, 1986.
13. Cooper, D. K. C., Kemp, E., Reemtsma, K. and White, D. J. G., *Xenotransplantation. The Transplantation of Organs and Tissues Between Species,* Springer Verlag, Berlin Heidelberg, 1991.
14. Chen, Z., Cobbold, S., Metcalfe, S. and Waldmann, H., Tolerance in the mouse to major histocompatibility complex -mismatched heart allografts, and to rat heart xenografts, using monoclonal antibodies to CD4 and CD8, *Eur. J.Immunol.,* 22, 805, 1992.

Chapter 10

Diabetic Animal Models

Ida Hageman and Karsten Buschard

CONTENTS

INTRODUCTION

Insulin-dependent (type I) diabetes mellitus (IDDM) is a relatively common disease; among caucasians about 1/2% of the population are affected and the incidence is increasing. The disease is characterized by a rather sudden onset of hypoinsulinemia, high blood glucose levels, and excessive amounts of ketone bodies in the blood. At onset, maybe only 10% of the beta cells of the pancreas, which synthesize and secrete insulin, remain.[1] For survival, the patient is therefore dependent on lifelong exogenous insulin treatment. However, the possibility of this insulin admission also allows the patient to live long enough for the chronic complications to become manifest, with the result that diabetes is now the most common cause of acquired blindness, the third most common cause of renal failure, and about the fifth most common cause of death in many countries.

0-8493-4390-9/94/$0.00+$.50

IDDM perhaps is the human disease having the very best animal models. These models provide an excellent opportunity for studying the multitude of interacting factors contributing to the syndrome, which is not feasible in the afflicted humans. A desirable feature of a model syndrome is, of course, that it approximates the phenotypes of human disease thereby leading to a more complete understanding of etiology, pathogenesis, and treatment in humans. Especially, the animal models provide material for examining the very earliest steps in the pathological process (before overt IDDM), since such investigations cannot be conducted in humans as the manifest disease covers up a long preceding process. This review will deal with the spontaneously diabetic BB rat, the NOD (Non-Obese Diabetic) mouse, and the low-dose streptozotocin and the virus-induced diabetic models in mice.

THE BB RAT

The BB-rat syndrome was recognized initially in 1974 by Clifford Chappel at the BioBreeding Laboratories, Ottawa, Canada.[2] Overt IDDM, associated with hypoinsulinemia, occurred sporadically in this commercial breeding colony of non-inbred Wistar derived laboratory rats kept under strict gnotobiotic conditions. A breeding program was established, and it was decided to name the syndrome "BB" after the initials of the breeding laboratory.

All BB rats are descendants of the original Ottawa litters, but rats in different colonies now vary in frequency of diabetes. To identify the specific strain, all animals are named after the city or institution where they are bred, e.g., BB/W for Worcester.[3]

CLINICAL COURSE OF THE DIABETIC SYNDROME

Diabetes in the BB rat typically has an abrupt onset with glucosuria, hyperglycemia, hyperketonemia, ketonuria, and hypoinsulinemia. The age at which diabetes is diagnosed is generally between 60 and 120 days of age.[4] The mean is about 90 days in most reported data. This age distribution at the diagnosis of IDDM is analogous to that observed in humans: a preponderance of cases among the juvenile and adolescent population. The incidence of diabetes varies in the different rat colonies from 10 to 80%. The animals are not obese and diabetes occurs with almost equal frequency in both sexes.

Acutely diabetic animals die from ketoacidosis within 2 weeks of onset unless insulin is given. Morphological studies show infiltration of mainly mononuclear cells in the islets of Langerhans, a condition called insulitis. The most severe form of insulitis is found in rats with overt IDDM. Insulitis is present before the disease is manifest, but insulitis is not tantamount to the development of diabetes. The pancreas of rats with overt IDDM shows less than 0.1% of normal insulin content.[5,6] The progression from normal to seriously decompensated can be counted in days. The hyperglycemia is associated with hypoinsulinemia and hyperglucagonemia. Until glucosuria begins, absolute values and rates of gain in body weight in the majority of rats are indistinguishable from those of litter mates.

Despite hyperphagia and polydipsia, weight loss is rapid and a good indicator of diabetes development. Physical activity is clearly decreased and tachypnea can be seen. In contrast to humans, the BB rat (diabetic as well as non-diabetic) has an unusual predisposition to lymphopoietic malignancy and to infection, especially with Mycoplasma pneumoniae which is often fatal. The animals exhibit a pronounced decrease in the population of T-lymphocytes and thereby a functional deficiency of a variety of lymphocyte-mediated immune reactions, that is a marked immunoregulatory defect. A line of "nonlymphopenic diabetic" (NLD)-BB rats has, however, been developed.[7]

GENETICS

Human IDDM as well as the BB-diabetic syndrome is a heritable disorder. In humans, there is a 30% concordance for IDDM among monozygotic twins and in the BB-rat model about

70% of the animals develop diabetes in colonies that have been inbred for many generations, indicating that factors other than genetics must play a role. It is most likely that the mode of inheritance of BB-rat diabetes involves an autosomal recessive gene or gene cluster with incomplete penetrance (approximately 50%),[8,9] leaving room for environmental factors to influence the expression of the gene(s) or its (their) product. Furthermore, diabetes in the BB rat also shows a major histocompatibility complex association.

DISEASE MECHANISMS

As in humans, diabetes in the BB rat is believed to be an autoimmune disease. Three main causes contribute to this conviction: (1) involvement of the humoral immune system, (2) involvement of the cellular immune system, and as discussed before (3) involvement of a genetic factor, i.e., the association with the major histocompatibility complex. The exact series of events that may initiate the diabetes is still hypothetical.

Role of the Humoral Immune System

A phenotypic feature of diabetic and diabetes-prone (DP) BB rats is the presence of autoantibodies, of the IgG class, which bind to smooth muscle, thyroid colloid, and gastric parietal cell antigens.[10,11] Although there is high concordance between the presence of diabetes, thyroiditis, and autoantibodies, 50% of animals without thyroiditis evidence antithyroid colloid antibodies. Perhaps more important is that beta islet cell surface antibodies (ICSA) have been detected as early as 40 days of age. Complement-fixing islet cell antibodies (CF-ICA) have also been detected and may be present 2 weeks before the onset of diabetes. Thus, these two autoantibodies actually antedate the manifest disease. Antilymphocyte antibodies are also prevalent in diabetic animals.[12, 13]

It is not probable that the B-lymphocyte abnormality alone is responsible for the development of diabetes, but certainly it has a place in the pathogenesis — most likely in an intimate interplay with the cellular immune system. In addition, direct testing of the ability of the BB rat to mount an antibody response to various injected immunogens has also suggested that responses to T-independent antigens are normal, whereas responses to T-dependent antigens are subnormal.

Role of the Cellular Immune System

As mentioned, the BB rat is lymphopenic, and this can be recognized before the clinical onset of diabetes.[14] The lymphopenia is characterized by a marked decrease in the number of T-lymphocytes in the peripheral blood, lymph nodes, and spleen.[15] While all T-cell subsets are diminished, the CD8+ T-cell subset (cytotoxic/suppressor) is the most diminished.[16] In addition, the RT6 differentiation alloantigen, which is normally expressed on about half the peripheral T-cells (but absent in bone marrow and thymocytes), is absent in rats with lymphopenia.[17] The RT6+ peripheral T-cell subset includes members of both the helper/inducer (W3/25) and suppressor/cytotoxic (OX8) antigenic phenotypes.

Though the BB rats are lymphopenic, cell-mediated immune processes are implicated in the destruction of the islet cells; pancreatic lymphocytic insulitis is observed in young asymptomatic BB rats with normal levels of blood glucose and insulin so insulitis actually precedes overt diabetes. Studies have shown the lymphocytic infiltrate to consist of cytotoxic effector cells, T-lymphocytes (they are Ia+, which express activation and also in the possession of interleukin 2 receptor expression) and/or natural killer (NK) cells. Macrophages are believed to be the first cells invading the islets, an important cell type both for cytokine production and antigen presentation.[18] Additionally, it has been demonstrated that NK-cell activity is increased in acutely diabetic as well as DP BB rats and that islet cells can serve as target cells for these large granular lymphocytes *in vitro*, NK-cells being capable of lysing islet cells.[19] The exact role of the various cell types is not clarified.

Within a very short time after the detection of hyperglycemia, insulitis rapidly decreases and finally disappears with the appearance of the so-called "end-stage islets". These structures are much smaller than normal islets and can be very difficult to detect in hematoxylin-eocin (HE) stained pancreatic sections. With immunocytochemical stains, it is apparent that the end stage islet consists almost exclusively of glucagon, somatostatin, and pancreatic polypeptide-synthesizing islet cells.

The presence of lymphocytic thyroiditis in a large proportion of BB rats suggests that this organ is the target of a cell mediated autoimmune attack. Lymphocytic thyroiditis occurs in diabetic and normoglycemic BB/W rats, but is more frequent among diabetic animals. However, the thyroiditis is not followed by clinical thyroidea disease.

Further evidence for the involvement of cellular immunity in the pathogenesis of diabetes in the BB rat is found in the fact that DP rats have been protected from developing diabetes by neonatal thymectomy. Another study has shown incomplete thymectomy to influence the incidence, indicating that the mass of functional thymic tissue is a factor in the pathogenesis.[20] Neonatal bone marrow allografts,[21] sublethal whole body irradiation,[22] and total lymphoid irradiation[23] also have been shown to protect DP rats from diabetes. Administration of antilymphocyte globulin alone prevents diabetes when given to prediabetic animals and will cure diabetes in approximately one third of BB rats treated on the day diabetes is detected. Also, transfusions of whole blood[24] or peripheral T-lymphocytes[25] from the diabetes resistant (DR) subline of BB rats (so-called immune "enhancement") have been reported to prevent the appearance of diabetes in the DP rat. Conversely, Concanavalin A (ConA) activated spleenic lymphocytes have been shown to adoptively transfer insulitis and diabetes upon injection into young DP BB/W-rats[26] or into otherwise DR BB rats[27] and Wistar-Furth rats[28] that have been pretreated with cyclophosphamide. Administration of cyclosporin A will effectively reduce the frequency of diabetes but does not cure the disease.[29,30] Cyclosporin A itself is not cytotoxic, but is believed to act by inhibiting T-lymphocyte proliferation in response to antigenic stimulation. Cyclosporin A is able to protect the beta cell from injury caused by the cytotoxic effect of interleukin 1 and probably also interleukin 6, which functionally and structurally has been shown to modify beta cells *in vitro*. Cyclosporin A is used to treat prediabetic rats when needed for breeding, but cannot be used in humans as side effects (especially nefrotoxicity) are too serious. On the other hand, Freund's Adjuvant, which causes immunostimulation, lowers the diabetes incidence, maybe because of an influence on the suppressor T-cells, in accordance with the fact that elimination of infectious agents from the environment actually increases the frequency and accelerates the tempo of spontaneous diabetes among DP rats.[31]

THE QUESTION OF SELF-TOLERANCE

As mentioned, diabetes is believed to be an autoimmune disease. Failure to induce islet tolerance may be caused by (1) thymic antigen-presenting cells in DP animals being defective in their ability to present beta cells to establish islet tolerance,[32] or (2) the fact that islets from rats of the age when self-tolerance is normally induced, neonates, lack certain antigenic determinants that develop later, leaving them susceptible to destruction by their own immune system. A study has shown that diabetes in BB rats can be prevented by neonatal stimulation of beta cells; a procedure that is thought to induce or enhance antigen expression on the beta cells, which facilitates the ability of the immune system to develop self-tolerance.[33,34] The neonates were stimulated for the first 6 days after birth by glucose accompanied by glucagon or arginin, the immature beta cells producing only a basal amount of insulin and being unresponsive to glucose alone in order to accelerate beta cell maturation and possibly to induce antigen expression and tolerance. Over the first 200 days of life, only about 40% of the treated rats developed diabetes compared with 65% of untreated controls. This may explain the observation that children of mothers who have type I diabetes are three times less likely to develop the disease than children of fathers with IDDM. Earlier maturation of the beta cells during the diabetic pregnancy may thus protect against diabetes in later life.

Also intrathymic injections have been carried out.[35] This was done thinking that the introduction of islet cells into the thymus might directly induce islet tolerance — a mechanism for the establisment of self-tolerance might then be an enhancement of the activity of the above-mentioned antigen-presenting cells. The islets needed for injection were isolated from DR rats. In fact, only 35% of the rats that had had an intrathymic injection of islets developed diabetes compared to 88% of the control sham-operated rats. Thus, it seems that exposing the cells of the thymus directly to islet antigen can prevent an autoimmune attack, induce tolerance, and significantly reduce the incidence of the disease.

ENVIRONMENTAL FACTORS

The concordance of only about 30% in human monozygotic twins and the fact that the incidence of diabetes varies from 50 to 80% in highly inbred BB rat colonies, can be considered as very strong arguments for the involvement of environmental factors. They may either trigger the autoimmune process or modify its course.

An environmental influence operating on a basis of genetic susceptibility may be the diet.[36] Diet has clearly been shown to modify the frequency of diabetes among BB rats; substitution of a defined diet for rat chow lowers the frequency to about half of that seen for normal rat chow, and feeding a diet containing only a casein hydrolysate further decreases the frequency of disease. Wheat gluten and cow's milk also decreases incidence but less than the casein hydrolysate. It is unknown whether the lower incidence is secondary to removal of a specific dietary protein or whether it is caused by the removal of many components (e.g., fibers, lectins, viral, and bacterial toxins) which may be present in chow and thus affect the gut of the young weanlings. Other environmental factors have been evaluated: castration, vagotomy, hypophysectomy, and stress produced by ultrasound, for instance, could not prevent diabetes.[37]

Administration of nicotinamide,[38,39] a precursor for the synthesis of nicotinamide adenin dinucleotide (NAD), has proven to be able to delay the onset of diabetes. Histological examinations of pancreata collected from treated animals showed a reduction of insulitis and preservation of the number of beta cells and the overall islet architecture. Moreover, treatment with large doses of nicotinamide from the first day of glucosuria precipitated the disappearance of glucosuria and an improvement of glucose tolerance during the treatment period.

Exogenous insulin treatment is another way of trying to influence the incidence through environmental factors: reduction of the diabetes incidence of BB rats has been seen with early prophylactic insulin treatment of DP animals. In a specific study, BB rats were given insulin from day 50 to day 142 of age.[40] At withdrawal, this group was compared to a control group of rats given insulin only from the first day of glucosuria. The incidence in the prophylactically treated group was 22% compared to 44% among the controls. The findings of this study suggest that administration of exogenous insulin to BB rats during the prediabetic period could render the beta cells, characterized by a low rate of insulin synthesis, less vulnerable to immune aggression. Specifically, a reduction of endogenous insulin secretion might reduce the amount of antigens on the beta-cell surface, which are recognized by the immune system, to such a level that the autoimmune cascade is either not initiated or alleviated.[41] In another study, when insulin treatment was started earlier in life (day 35), the diabetes incidence was reduced from 56 to 2%.[42]

Another study concerning prophylactic insulin treatment has been carried out using the DR BB rat, in which diabetes and thyroiditis occur in less than 1% of the animals and the RT6 alloantigen is present on about 60% of the T-cells. Thirty-day-old DR rats were treated with anti RT6 monoclonal antibody, exogenous insulin, or both until the age of 60 days.[43] *In vivo* depletion of RT6-T-cells by giving cytotoxic monoclonal antibodies induced diabetes and thyroiditis in more than 50% of treated animals by 60 days of age. Co-administration of insulin during this prediabetic period prevented nearly all cases of diabetes, but not thyroiditis. Spleen cells from these insulin-treated and RT6-depleted non-diabetic DR rats were still capable of adoptive transfer of diabetes.

The precise mechanism of insulin action is unproven, but the possibility exists that the action could take place either at the beta-cell level or at the T-cell level. In favor of the T-cell level is the fact that insulin is known to be immunosuppressive.[44] On the other hand, as is obvious from, e.g., prophylactic insulin treatment not being able to prevent thyroiditis, a great deal of evidence exists that insulin treatment acts on the beta-cell level, where it suppresses insulin secretion: prolonged insulin treatment means prolonged hypoglycemia, which again causes reduced beta-cell mitotic activity and suppressed endogenous insulin production, secretion, and stores. Such depression of beta-cell metabolic activity might very well render them resistant to the cytotoxic effect of cytokines such as interleukin 1 released in the course of the autoimmune process. On the basis of *in vitro,* cytokines have been hypothesized to participate directly in beta-cell destruction, although this theory still needs to receive experimental support *in vivo.*

As already partly discussed, alteration of antigens that are targets of the autoimmune process could also occur in response to exogenous insulin keeping the blood glucose low. Studies have been carried out demonstrating that islet cells incubated at different glucose concentrations showed different labeling with specific autoantibodies.[41] Labeling was found to be more frequent and more pronounced in islet cells incubated at high glucose concentrations. The labeling was of cell surface antigens that were detected by the beta-cell specific monoclonal antibody IC2 and A2B5, the latter directed against a gangliosid. Thus, beta-cell antigen expression very likely depends on the functional state of the cells.

THE NON-OBESE DIABETIC MOUSE

Like the BB-rat model, the non-obese diabetic (NOD) mouse model is a genetically determined model and the NOD mouse is in many ways the mouse equivalent to the BB rat. The ultimate effector mechanisms, however, are different.

The pedigree of the NOD mouse is as follows: In 1966, a cataract-prone mouse arose from outbred ICR mice and gave rise to the CTS strain. Since cataract is frequent in diabetic patients, the suspicion of a pathogenetic relationship to diabetes arose. Selective breeding was carried out and two sister strains, one euglycemic and the other slightly hyperglycemic, arose after 13 generations of breeding. The mouse that developed non-obese diabetic symptoms was obtained in the 20th generation and ironically in the euglycemic sister strain. The mouse was female and exhibited polyuria, severe glycosuria, and weight loss. The strain was established in 1974 by Makino et al. in Osaka, Japan. Breeding was continued using offspring selected for both spontaneous diabetes and reproductive ability, leading after the 6th generation to the NOD mouse, which is not cataract-prone.[45,46]

In 1980, the original NOD strain had a cumulative diabetes incidence by 30 weeks of age of 60 to 80% in females vs. only about 10% in males.[45] The main period of diabetes manifestation was between 80 and 200 days.[47] A corresponding non-diabetic substrain was also maintained, to serve as a control strain and termed non-obese normal (NON).

CLINICAL COURSE OF THE NOD DIABETIC SYNDROME

Many NOD lines have been established around the world and they differ significantly in diabetes incidence, time of onset, and degree of female preponderance. Apart from a higher frequency, NOD females also exhibit permanent hyperglycemia at an earlier age than males: peak onset between 16 and 20 weeks as compared to between 21 and 28 weeks in males.[48] Gonadal sex steroids are important modulators of pathogenesis: castrated males show a higher incidence of diabetes and oophorectomized females show a lower incidence.[49] Castration of mice up to the age of 7 weeks results in an increase in males and a decrease in females.[50]

The clinical features of the diabetes syndrome in NOD mice are quite similar to human IDDM and characterized by hypoinsulinemia, hyperglycemia, glycosuria, hypercholesteromia, ketonuria, polydipsia, polyuria, and polyphagia. The blood glucose rises from a normal level of approximately 7 to 9 mM to permanent hyperglycemia, i.e., a blood glucose level >25 mM over a period of 3 to 4 weeks and, in contrast to the BB rat, the NOD mouse can survive quite long without insulin treatment, i.e. 1 to 12 weeks. [47,48]

HISTOPATHOLOGY

Despite sex difference in incidence almost all animals (>95%) display mononuclear cellular infiltration, insulitis.[52,52] In fact, 80% of males and 30% of females show insulitis without developing diabetes up to the 30th week of age. So, somehow a much higher frequency of male NOD mice avoid pancreatic lesions severe enough to cause overt glycosuria.

The pathological features of lymphocytic infiltration become evident at about 4 to 5 weeks of age;[51,53] by week 6, initial insulitis is seen in >50% of NOD mice; at 8 weeks the lymphocytes begin to invade the islets,[54] and the insulitis process is virtually completed as the animals approach 12 weeks of age. Overt glycosuria, i.e., manifest disease, appears several weeks after the completion of insulitis.

The earliest change is periinsulitis adjacent to the pancreatic ducts, followed by invasion of the islet capsule by small lymphocytes that penetrate the islets. The final stage is characterized by small islets from which beta cells have disappeared, with resolution of insulitis.[50] The different stages of the process can, however, be found within the same pancreas at any time, so intact islets may be seen not far from severely affected ones. Phenotyping of lymphocyte subsets involved in insulitis has produced conflicting results.[55-58] Some investigators report monocytes and B-lymphocytes (IgM+) to be the predominant cell populations; other reports claim L3T4 cells (mainly helper/ inducer) and MHC class II cells (B-lymphocytes and macrophages) to be predominant. NK-cells and Ia+ lymphocytes also seem to be present.

The NOD mice lymphocytic infiltration is not restricted to islets but also occurs in the submandibular glands, as well as in the lacrimal, thyroid, and adrenal glands, suggesting a wider disturbance of immune tolerance in this animal. Human type I diabetes has also been associated with other endocrine abnormalities; however, infiltration of salivary glands has not been described.

GENETICS

Basically, the genes involved are recessive since animals of the F1 generation from mating between the NOD and a non-diabetic strain do not develop diabetes or insulitis. From backcross experiments with, e.g., C57BL mice and the NON strain a minimum of three recessive genes have been suggested.[59,60] One is MHC (H-2)-linked and is not needed for insulitis to evolve but necessary for the development of diabetes. The dominant H-2 types are H-2K^d and H-2D^b.[61] A second recessive gene controls the development of severe insulitis and the third gene is involved in the progression to diabetes, perhaps via a lack of specific suppressor cells.

Since NOD mice can be considered genetically identical, but not all develop diabetes, it is susceptibility to diabetes that is inherited rather than the expressed disease, as is also the case in humans (identical twins) and the BB rat as mentioned.

DISEASE MECHANISMS

There is every indication that the spontaneous diabetic syndrome of the NOD mouse is an autoimmune disorder since there is (1) involvement of the humoral immune system, (2) involvement of the cellular immune system, and (3) involvement of a genetic factor.

Humorally Mediated Immunity

One of the immunological observations in the NOD mouse is the occurrence of autoantibodies. Islet cell antibodies (ICA) have been described in about 50% of NOD mice up to the 21st week of age. Islet cell surface antibodies (ICSA) appear at 3 to 6 weeks and reach peak incidence and titer at 12 to 18 weeks. The ICA as well as the ICSA tend to respectively disappear or decline later on.[62,63] The question is whether these autoantibodies are primarily involved in beta-cell destruction or are secondary to islet cell destruction/damage and massive leakage or expression of antigens. The last suggestion could be correlated with the time course of insulitis.

The presence of insulin autoantibodies (IAA) before development of diabetes has been reported.[64] A study showed that IAA were only found in sera from NOD mice with insulitis and not from those without insulitis. This study showed that the prevalence of IAA was 0% before the appearance of insulitis, 80% at 12 to 14 weeks of age, and 30% after 20 weeks of age in females. In males, IAA were found in 45% at 12 to 14 weeks of age and 20% after 20 weeks. The IAA were detected by the polyethylene glycol method.[65] Two different studies, however, report that IAA could be detected by an ELISA assay before insulitis developed.[62,63] Antilymphocyte antibodies also appear, most frequently at 3 weeks of age, and decrease thereafter.[58]

Cell-Mediated Immunity

Strong evidence for the involvement of the cellular immune system is found in the fact that neonatally thymectomized and nude NOD mice do not develop diabetes.[66] This means that T-lymphocytes are required for diabetes pathogenesis, but the T-lymphopenia characteristic of the BB rat is not found in the NOD mouse or for that matter in human diabetics. On the contrary, a markedly increased concentration of T-lymphocytes in spleen and peripheral blood is found in NOD, but not in NON mice.[67] This is reflected in an enlargement of thymic cortex and lymph nodes. The increase in T-cell number appears to include both $Lyt1^+$ and $Lyt2^+$ phenotypes. This lymphoproliferation is very likely the result of an underlying immunoregulatory defect.

If the insulitis and overt diabetes observed in the NOD mouse is based on cellular mechanisms, the disease should be transferable with lymphocytes. Direct demonstration of the involvement of the cellular immune system was actually made in a study concerning transfer of splenocytes from overtly diabetic NOD to non-diabetic NOD mice.[55] Splenocytes from overtly diabetic NOD mice were unable to transfer diabetes to very young (<7 weeks) irradiated NOD mice, but effectively transferred the disease to irradiated mice >6 weeks of age; overt diabetes was induced within 12 to 22 days in more then 95% of the recipients. This transfer to young mice induces them to become diabetic at a higher frequency and at a younger age than their untreated littermates. An explanation of the failure to induce diabetes in the very young mice could be that the immune or hormonal system of the recipient must reach a certain degree of maturation before the transfer can be accomplished. Another very likely possibility is that the beta cells of the very young mice may not express the critical antigenic determinants for which the transferred splenocytes are specific until about 6 to 7 weeks after birth.[54]

Not only the age of the recipient seems important, since spleen cells obtained from 7-week-old non-diabetic mice were unable to transfer diabetes, presumably reflecting that an insufficient number of effector cells are present in the spleen at this age. On the other hand, non-diabetic mice donors >15 weeks of age have high levels of intraislet insulitis but their ability to transfer diabetes is variable, suggesting that in at least some older non-diabetic NOD mice, either an insufficient number of effectors are present in the spleen or suppressor cells can interrupt effector cell function. NOD mice that have been insulin-dependent for 2 months presumably lack beta cells and fail to express the antigenic stimulus for the autoimmune response. A spleenic transfusion from these animals, however, showed retained ability to transfer diabetes, indicating that long-lived memory cells are present for at least several months after the destruction of beta cells.

It is noteworthy that transfer of diabetes as mentioned above was not limited to female donors and recipients; splenocytes from diabetic males consistently induced diabetes in non-diabetic NOD males. This is of interest as male mice display a lower spontaneous incidence of diabetes than females, as already mentioned. All the transfers were carried out with as few as 5×10^6 spleen cells, which did not have to be stimulated by ConA in advance, as is necessary in similar spleen transfusion experiments performed in BB rats.

Notable is also the fact that treatment with anti-Thy 1.2 mAb (T-cells) prevents diabetes but does not influence the progression of insulitis.[68] Prevention of diabetes as well as insulitis is obtained by administration of L3T4 (helper/inducer) mAb. The necessity of the presence of suppressor/cytotoxic cells and macrophages for the development of insulitis was proved by admission of anti-Lyt2 antibodies and silica particles, thereby preventing beta cell destruction.[69]

Other cytotoxicity systems also show abnormalities, i.e., NK-cell and monocyte activity is depressed[70] and antibody-dependent cell-mediated cytotoxicity (ADCC) is elevated in diabetic NOD mice compared to ICR mice.[71] IL-1 production from NOD macrophages is low, and it has been suggested that it may be defective communication between macrophages and T-helper cells that causes the hyperplasia of T-lymphocytes in lymphoid tissue by way of a defective suppression mechanism.[48] A lack of suppressor cells may be a result of decreased endogenous production of IL-2, since ConA stimulated splenocytes supplemented with IL-2 allow generation of T-suppressor/inducer cells.[72]

Finally, irradiation followed by reconstitution with bone marrow cells from young BALB/c nu/nu mice, leading to full T-cell reconstitution, reverses insulitis and prevents the onset of diabetes.

IMMUNOTHERAPY AND OTHER ENVIRONMENTAL FACTORS

Cyclosporin A can prevent the onset of diabetes and reduce insulitis in the NOD mouse.[73,74] On the contrary, cyclophosphamide strikingly enhances diabetes development especially in males, perhaps via depression effects on suppressor cells or enhancement of ADCC.[75] The effect of cyclophosphamide can be prevented by admission of nicotinamide.[76] Nicotinamide and cyclosporin A are more closely discussed in the BB-rat section. Nicotinamide itself reduces the incidence of insulitis and diabetes in NOD mice and the blocking of the cyclophosphamide effect is probably brought about by inhibition of ADCC.[76] Nicotinamide seems to be of some benefit in newly diagnosed type I diabetic patients and increases C-peptide secretion in the first year after detection.[77,78]

Monosodium glutamate is another drug capable of substantially decreasing incidence of diabetes and severe insulitis.[79,80] Perhaps this immunomodulation of glutamate is due to elevated corticosterone levels since delayed type hypersensitivity after treatment with the drug has been observed.

As was the case with the BB rat, prophylactic insulin treatment of NOD mice during the prediabetic phase has been shown to prevent and/or delay the clinical onset of the disease.[81] Insulin therapy has also proven to be able to protect non-diabetic NOD mice from the effects of transferred splenocytes.[82] In this last study, the maximum tolerable dosage of fast-acting insulin was given until 30 days after the cell transfer. The diabetes incidence of the insulin-treated group was about 27% compared to 83% in a control group.

Diet can also influence the incidence, especially the amount of fat seems to be important for the development of the syndrome in the male NOD mouse, i.e., a diet reduced in fat can strongly increase incidence.[76] The admission of gamma interferon to NOD mice did not alter diabetes development and treatment with interleukin-2 could only reduce blood glucose values slightly.[83] A preparation of group A streptococcus pyogenes, however, protects mice

112

from diabetes and insulitis.[84] The preparation is known to enhance interferon and Il-2 production, and normalized lymphokine levels could result in normal suppressor cell activity in NOD mice.

LOW-DOSE STREPTOZOTOCIN-INDUCED DIABETES

Streptozotocin (SZ) is a naturally occurring broad spectrum antibiotic produced by Streptomyces acromogenes.[85] The drug possesses oncolytic, oncogenic, as well as diabetogenic properties, diabetogenesis being mediated by pancreatic beta-cell destruction, and is widely used as a method for induction of diabetes in experimental animals.

SZ consists of a nitrosamine group linked to a glucose molecule. The glucose moiety is apparently the essential component that specifically leads SZ into the beta cell. SZ is rapidly cleared from the bloodstream with a serum half-life of 15 minutes.

From 1963, SZ was conventionally administered as a single dose (200 mg/kg body weight), causing complete beta-cell necrosis and diabetes within 24 hours.[86] The islets, however, were virtually inflammation-free. In 1976, Like and Rossini presented a new model where multiple subdiabetogenic doses to mice were applied.[87] The result was a delayed onset of hyperglycemia, which for reasons of kinetics could not be due to the direct and rapid toxic activity of the drug. Fortunately, this new model also showed islets with insulitis and until the discovery of the two spontaneously occurring models (the BB rat and the NOD mouse), this model provided one of the few experimental ways to study insulitis.

The mouse strain used by Like and Rossini was outbred CD-1 mice. The dosage used was 40 mg/kg body weight and was administered for 5 consecutive days, i.e., a total dose equal to the single dosage used previously. Seven days after the completion of injections, the animal evidenced mild hyperglycemia, and plasma glucose elevation became progressively more pronounced 10 to 25 days after the last injection, i.e., long after SZ was cleared from the bloodstream and the shortlived SZ beta cytotoxic activity was completed. Severe insulitis and disruption of islet cytoarchitecture was noted by experimental day 11. Light microscope examination revealed large numbers of lymphocytes, moderate numbers of macrophages, and few neutrophiles surrounding and permeating the islets of Langerhans. Ultrastructural studies unexpectedly showed the presence of large numbers of type C virus particles within the many partially degranulated beta cells, a discovery that was not made in usually well-granulated beta cells, nor in alpha, delta, or inflammatory cells. Obviously SZ was somehow responsible for the activation of virus replication.

Sex seemed to be an important modifier of the diabetogenic action of SZ, since only males were susceptible. Later investigations confirmed this by showing that orchiectomy of CD-1 males depressed the level of hyperglycemia induced by SZ, whereas testosterone treatment restored full sensitivity. Testosterone treatment of both ovariectomized and normal CD-1 females also increased hyperglycemic responsiveness to levels comparable with those observed in intact males.[88]

MECHANISMS OF ACTION
There seem be two ways by which the low-dose streptozotocin model can produce diabetes, the one not excluding the other: (1) by direct cytotoxic effect of SZ, and (2) by immune mechanisms (possibly autoimmune).

Direct Cytotoxic Action of Streptozotocin
The very specific toxicity of SZ within islets for beta cells is linked to the capacity of the drug to accumulate rapidly in these cells. It seems probable, though not proved in *vitro*, that SZ binds with a glucose recognition site on beta cells, since 3-O methylglucose and at a higher dose D-glucose (partially) protect against streptozotocin.[89] Once inside the cell, SZ decom-

poses to other components, one of which is a highly reactive carbonium ion, which is able to alkylate various cellular components such as DNA or protein. Lesions in DNA of this type are removed by excision repair. Part of this excision repair process is the activation of the enzyme poly(ADP-ribose) synthetase to form poly (ADP-ribose) using nicotinamide adenin dinucleotide (NAD) as a substrate. It is probable that the enzyme becomes activated to such an extent in the beta cells that NAD becomes critically depleted, resulting in a cessation of cellular function and ultimately cell death.[90] Perhaps SZ, on entering the cell, alkylates not only DNA but also important components necessary for generation of ATP, e.g. glycolytic and mitochondrial enzymes. A drop in ATP generation would further impair the resynthesis of NAD, causing this key component to drop below critical levels.[91]

Immune Mechanisms

There is also the possibility of SZ causing point mutation. This type of lesion could cause the expression of a repressed gene that codes for a protein or other hapten not normally recognized by the immune system, e.g., a fetal protein or a retrovirus.[91] In support of the latter is the finding of the low-dose SZ model inducing the expression of type C retrovirus (or type A in the C57BL/KsJ strain). Although there seems to be little cytotoxic activity of these vira, they may increase islet cell antigenicity. Alkylation of DNA bases or the phosphate backbone could, if not repaired, cause conformational changes in DNA. These conformational lesions could alter the binding of a repressor protein and lead to the expression of a normally silent gene, which could elicit an immune reaction. SZ could also cause the expression of neoantigens by simply altering surface proteins on the beta cell surface directly. These altered surface proteins are very likely to be immunogenic.

The involvement of the immune system is supported by the fact that (1) T-cell deficient mice do not develop hyperglycemia,[92-95] and that (2) conventional immunosuppression protects from diabetes: irradiation, prednisolon, cyclophosphamide, anti-lymphocyte serum, and antibodies to T-cells.[96-102] Cyclosporin A, however, is not able to inhibit diabetes development, probably because it is also beta-cell cytotoxic in mice and might thereby amplify the effects of streptozotocin.[103]

Involvement of immune processes normally leads to an immunological "memory", i.e., transfer of diabetes from diabetic SZ-treated mice to normal mice should be possible. However, permanent hyperglycemia has not been convincingly transferred into normal mice receiving splenocytes from SZ-treated donors.[91] This is explainable if one considers that the memory cells are specific for beta cells only when the beta cells have been modified by streptozotocin. This is not an autoimmune mechanism in the classical sense since the organism has not lost tolerance to normal cells, but immune mechanisms have been induced by altered cells. A normal mouse not treated with SZ does not, of course, possess these altered cells.

Several investigations have examined the susceptibility to SZ in different mice strains. Studies have shown "BALB/cBOM-nu/+" males to be susceptible and nu/nu males to be resistant unless reconstituted with T-lymphocyte-enriched splenocytes from euthymic donors,[92-94] clear demonstrations of the diabetogenic potential of T-lymphocytes. On the other hand, studies have also shown BALB/cBOM-nu/nu males to be as sensitive to SZ as euthymic littermates, using 60 mg/kg for 5 consecutive days.[104] Yet another study of low-dose streptozotocin showed nude mice of the C57BL/KsJ background to develop blood glucose levels not significantly lower than their thymus-intact littermates.[105] Possible explanations for this variety include different dosage regimes (as already mentioned), different contents of the alpha and beta isomers of SZ, alpha having the highest beta cell cytotoxicity, and (genetically) different sensitivity among different mouse strains — there even seem to be considerable variations among certain well-characterized BALB/c-substrains, e.g., the BALB/cBOM stock itself is genetically heterogenous and thus should not be considered as an inbred BALB/c-substrain.[106] The specific pathogen free status of a colony may also be one of the major variables controlling multiple low-dose SZ sensitivity, i.e., mice whose immune system has been stimulated by environmental vira may respond to SZ more strongly than mice kept under strict gnotobiotic conditions: a stressed (recently stimulated) immune system is more susceptible than one "resting" from provocation.

INSULITIS

Though well described in the CD-1 mouse strain, insulitis is not a consistent finding in the low-dose SZ model: some strains such as BALB/cByJ develop hyperglycemia without insulitis.[107] On the contrary, DR C57BL/KsJ females develop severe insulitis, but not hyperglycemia, presumably because of the protective effect of estrogens.[108]

The insulitis of the low-dose streptozotocin model may be due to autoimmune mechanisms, but may also simply constitute a normal response to either tissue damage or beta-cells that have been structurally modified by SZ. Macrophages and neutrophiles are probably the earliest infiltrating cells. Interleukin I, a cytokine secreted by macrophages, has been shown to inhibit insulin secretion of mouse islet monolayers, but is not cytotoxic itself.[101] A strong cytolytic action is, however, obtained in combination with gamma interferon, a lymphokine secreted by T-cells.[109] On the basis of these findings, a new pathogenetic model for IDDM has been proposed, involving local accumulation around beta cells of toxic cytokines from macrophages and activated T-helper cells rather than "classical" MHC-restricted action of T-lymphocytes.[110]

VIRUS-INDUCED DIABETES

A viral agent has been suggested as a trigger of diabetes. This is based on the seasonal trend, the presence of viral antibodies with rising titers in paired sera from newly diagnosed IDDM patients,[111] the presence of inflammatory cells in the islets of Langerhans, the decrease in number of beta cells, and the concordance of only about 30% between monozygotic twins, which speaks in favor of an ethiological importance of the environment — this might very well be viral.

THE EMC VIRUS

Evidence that viruses may be involved in beta-cell destruction comes from experiments in animals. The experimental model most extensively studied has been the diabetogenic encephalomyocarditis (EMC) virus introduced by Craighead and McLane in 1968.[112] The EMC virus is a small RNA-virus belonging to the family of picornavirus and is categorized as an enterovirus. It is a pantropic virus, which can attack all organs, but only the laboratory-selected M-variant of the virus has a specific tropism for beta cells. When inoculated into mice, the virus attacks and destroys the beta cells, and a diabetes-like syndrome evolves. However, the development of diabetes by EMC-M virus varied with different virus pools and passage history of the virus: plaque-purification of the EMC-M virus resulted in the isolation of two stable variants, the highly diabetogenic EMC-D and the non-diabetogenic EMC-B.[113,114] A new variant, EMC-DV$_1$, which is non-diabetogenic, was, however, recently obtained by plaque purification of the EMC-D variant stock pool and comparison between nucleotide sequence and biological characteristics of the three variants made it likely that only two amino acids, one on the leader peptide, the other on the capsid protein, are responsible for the diabetogenicity of the EMC-virus.[115]

Tissue culture experiments showed that EMC-D induced little, if any, interferon whereas substantial amounts of interferon were produced by EMC-B.[113,116] These results suggested that the interferon system might be one of the factors limiting the number of beta cells that become infected and thereby might inhibit the induction of diabetes. In support of this, studies have shown that repeated administration of interferon or an interferon inducer reduces the development of diabetes in mice infected with the D-variant.[117] Mice treated with the interferon inducer had less virus, fewer pathological changes and higher concentrations of immunoreactive insulin in the islets of Langerhans in comparison with untreated mice. In this study, the normally non-diabetogenic EMC-B variant was also inoculated into mice given antibody to interferon. The result was an increased content of EMC-B virus in islets and other tissues, which resulted in diabetes in about 40% of the surviving animals. This result demonstrates that EMC-B is in fact able to infect islet cells, which therefore probably have receptors for both the EMC-B and EMC-D variants.

Even though interferon clearly influences diabetes incidence, the importance of the cytokine has been seriously questioned by the fact that the EMC-DV$_1$ variant is neither diabetogenic nor interferon inducing.[115] Actually, it has been proposed that the protection against diabetes by interferon is merely strain-dependent and not the cause of the different diabetogenecity of the B and D variants. The difference in diabetogenic properties of the D and B variants might, however, be related to the affinity of the vira for beta-cell receptors. Thus, a study has shown that up to six times more EMC-D than EMC-B virus attaches to primary beta cells extracted from male ICR-Swiss mice.[118] As mentioned, two amino acid changements between the B and D variants might be responsible for the diabetogenicity and one of the changements, a change from Thr (EMC-B) to Ala (EMC-D), has been shown to reduce the hydrophilicity of the region by 37%. Thus, this change unique to EMC-D may be responsible for the diabetogenicity of EMC-D virus by increasing the efficiency of viral attachment to the beta cells of mice. The resistance of certain mouse strains to the diabetogenic effects of EMC-D virus could be due to genetically determined modifications in virus receptors on the surface of beta cells.

Clinical Course of the Diabetes-Like Syndrome

After subcutaneous inoculation, the virus multiplies under the skin and disseminates in the blood, but viremia is transient (48 to 72 h). The infected mice develop necrotizing lesions of the beta cells and immunofluorescence studies have demonstrated viral antigens exclusively in the islets of Langerhans. During the acute stages of infection, virus multiplication is associated with degranulation of the beta cells and the release of insulin into the circulation. Promptly thereafter, blood levels of insulin fall and hyperglycemia develops.

The number of animals who survive the infection and mortality during the acute stages varies with animal age, dosage, and strain.[119] Surviving animals either recover, exhibit abnormal glucose tolerance, or develop chronic hyperglycemia and a frank diabetes-like syndrome.[120] Metabolically, many appear normal, even though they were hyperglycemic at some time during the first two weeks after virus inoculation.

Histological changes of the pancreatic islets become evident after about 4 days. At this time, disruption of the overall architecture of the islets can be found. Mononuclear cells appear around the islets; especially macrophages are present in the tissue early in the course of infection. The inflammatory response varies from islet to islet and is relatively transient, since foreign mononuclear cells are rarely found after the second week of infection.[119] Other things being equal, the insulitis in the EMC virus model is more moderate than described in the other animal models of diabetes.

Genetic Susceptibility and Environmental Factors

When mice are infected with EMC virus (D or M variants), only certain inbred strains such as C3H/J, SJL/J, SWR/J, DBA/1J, and DBA/2J are susceptible and develop diabetes, while other strains such as C57BL/6J, CBA/J and AKR/J remain unaffected.[121] As mentioned previously, there seem to be considerable genetic variations among certain well-characterized BALB/c substrains: the BALB/c/BOM mouse is susceptible to EMC-virus infection[122] while the BALB/cJ mouse is resistant.[123] Backcross studies have indicated that susceptibility is inherited as an autosomal recessive trait.

It appears that even though mice seem uniformly susceptible to EMC regarding diabetes development, the insular tissue of some strains is more readily damaged by the virus. The course of the infection in two susceptible strains, DBA/2J and C3H/J, has been compared: it was found that the amounts of virus in the pancreas of the two strains were similar, but the morphological changes in the islets of Langerhans, however, differed since the beta cells of the DBA/2J animals were strikingly degranulated and exhibited evidence of necrosis, whereas the insular cells of C3H mice were less severely affected. [119]

As it is only the susceptibility to EMC-induced diabetes that is inherited, it is not surprising that environmental factors also influence the expression of diabetes. Metabolic stress, for instance, has been shown to influence the severity of the disease: by inducing hyperphagia and thus obesity in mice by administration of gold-thio-glucose, which has a damaging effect on the satiation center of the hypothalamus, hyperglycemia occurred more often and was of greater severity than in infected non-obese controls. Corticosteroid hormones are able to increase the severity of the pancreatic lesions of the EMC virus; the islets often exhibit frank necrosis and significantly greater amounts of insulin are found in the blood than in controls.[119]

Immune Mechanisms

The importance of the immune system in this animal model is a highly interesting question: does the diabetic state occur predominately on the basis of direct islet-cell destruction by the beta tropic virus or are immune mechanisms, especially T-cells involved in the pathogenesis? Using the M-strain of EMC virus (originating from Craighead), Buschard et al. (in 1976) demonstrated the absence of a diabetogenic effect of EMC virus in nude mice of the C57/B16-strain.[124] These mice did not, like heterozygotic littermates and homozygotic mice, develop diabetes as shown by abnormal glucose tolerance. Diabetes in the latter developed 2 to 3 weeks after administration of the virus, at a time when the virus could no longer be isolated from the mice. Similar investigations in support of the role of an immune mechanism have been carried out using other mice strains.[122,125] Thymectomy[126] and irradiation[127] have also been shown to prevent the development of diabetes in DBA/2 mice after EMC-virus inoculation, while treatment of the same mice with antilymphocyte serum reduced both the degree and the duration of hyperglycemia.[128] Thymectomized and irradiated BALB/cBy mice also fail to develop diabetes when infected.[129,130] Interestingly enough, Buschard et al. observed that the thymus-intact BALB/c mice developed not only diabetes, but also paresis after administration of EMC-M virus, suggesting that neural and islet tissue have antigenic components in common.[122] Another study in which mice (BALB/cByJ) were treated with the anti-T-lymphocyte monoclonal anti-L3T4 and anti-Lyt 2.2 antibodies before virus inoculation showed that mice depleted of L3T4+ cells exhibited a reduced incidence and severity of diabetes compared with both untreated and anti-Lyt 2.2-treated animals. All mice sustained pancreatic infection, but islet lesion with beta-cell degranulation only occurred in immune intact and anti-Lyt 2.2 treated animals.[131] These data clearly support the involvement of the immune system, especially suggesting a pivotal role for helper/inducer T-lymphocytes in the pathogenesis of the disease.

On the basis of studies showing that depletion of lymphocytes failed to alter the incidence of diabetes,[132] and that athymic nude mice infected with EMC-D virus showed a response nearly identical to the diabetogenic response of heterozygous litter mates,[133] Yoon et al. did not find a primary role for the T-cells in pathogenesis using his strain of virus. What seems important in this connection is that the passage histories of the virus used by Buschard and Yoon are different: the virus used by Yoon is passaged in beta-cell cultures, a process known to increase direct beta-cell toxicity, whereas the virus used by Buschard is passaged in mouse fibroblast cultures. Using very beta-cell toxic vira, the direct action of the vira on the beta cells overrules a role of the T-immune system, which is obvious when less beta-cell toxic vira are used. The model using the very toxic EMC virus makes an interesting experimental model, but the T-cell dependent model is probably more relevant to human IDDM since the human disease very seldom has an acute onset, as would be expected from the actions of a toxic virus.

Recently, even Yoon demonstrated immune mechanisms to be involved in his experimental model.[133] It was determined by various MAbs against mouse immunocytes that Mac-2-positive macrophages were predominant at an early stage of viral infection, whereas helper/inducer T-cells and cytotoxic/suppressor T-cells were present at intermediate and late stages of viral infection. Since it has been reported that Mac-2 expression is induced only by strong inflammation stimuli and appears to be specific for mononuclear phagocyte subpopulations, it was examined whether macrophages truly play a role in destruction of beta cells. This was done by depleting mice of macrophages by administration of silica, and long term (but not short term) treatment with silica resulted in complete prevention of diabetes in animals given a low dose of the virus. Thus, macrophages are very likely to contribute to the development of the disease in this model, probably through the release of soluble factors such as cytokines (e.g., interleukin 1 and gamma-interferon) and free radicals (oxygen radicals), and it is suggested that the presence of Mac-2-positive macrophages at an early stage of the viral infection is merely due to scavengers present as a consequence of beta-cell damage by viral infection.

Since the lymphocytic infiltration in the islets of Langerhans is modest during virus infection, the possible role of humoral mechanisms has also been studied.[134] Using fluorescence microscopy, the presence of immunoglobulins in the islets of Langerhans could be shown 3 days after EMC-M-virus inoculation, gradually disappearing about day 14. The Igs deposit was scattered throughout the islets, but the precise target of Igs has not been detected. A possible functional significance of the immunoglobulin deposits is unknown, but it has been shown that human Ig containing islet cell surface antibody can affect insulin secretion in isolated cells *in vitro* without destroying the beta cells.[135] Thus, it may be that a reaction of this type as well as other immunoglobulin-dependent types of immunological reactions, may be involved in the pathogenesis of diabetes.

REFERENCES

1. Colle, E., Genetic susceptibility to the development of spontaneous Insulin-dependent Diabetes Mellitus in the rat, *Clin. Immunol. Immunopath.*, 57, 1, 1990.
2. Chappel, C. I., and Chappel, W. R., The discovery and development of the BB-rat colony: An animal model of spontaneous Diabetes Mellitus, *Metabolism*, 32, 7(1), 8, 1983.
3. Marliss, E. B., Recommended nomenclature for the spontaneously diabetic syndrome in the BB-rat, *Metabolism*, 32, 7(1), 6, 1983.
4. Mordes, J. P., Desemone, J., and Rossini, A. A., The BB-rat, Diabetes/ *Metabolism Rev.*, 3, 3, 725, 1987.
5. Nakhooda, A. F., Like, A. A., and Chappel, C. I., The spontaneously diabetic Wistar rat, *Diabetes*, 26, 100, 1977.
6. Marliss, E. B., Nakhooda, A. F., and Poussier, P., Clinical forms and natural history of the diabetic syndrome and insulin and glucagon secretion in the BB-rat, *Metabolism*, 32, 7(1), 11, 1983.
7. Like, A. A., Guberski, D. L., and Butler, L., Diabetic BioBreeding/ Worcester (BB/Wor) rats need not be lymphopenic, *J. Immunol.*, 136, 3254, 1986.
8. Butler, L., Guberski, D. L., and Like, A. A., Genetic analysis of the BB/W diabetic rat, *Can. J. Genet. Cytol.*, 25, 7, 1983.
9. Like, A. A., and Rossini, A. A., Spontaneous autoimmune Diabetes Mellitus in the BioBreeding/Worcester rat, *Surv. Synth. Path. Res.*, 3, 131, 1984.
10. Elder, M., Macloren, N., Riley, W., and McConnell, T., Gastric parietal and other antibodies in the BB-rat, *Diabetes*, 31, 816, 1982.
11. Like, A. A., Appel, M. C., and Rossini, A. A., Autoantibodies in the BB/W rat, *Diabetes*, 31, 816, 1982.

12. Rossini, A. A., Mordes, J. P., and Like, A. A., Immunology of Insulin-dependent Diabetes Mellitus, *Ann. Rev. Immunol,* 3, 291, 1985.
13. Dyrberg, T., Poussier, P., Nakhooda, A. F., Bækkeskov, S., Marliss, E. B., and Lernmark, A., Islet cell surface and lymphocyte antibodies often precede the spontaneous diabetes in the BB-rat, *Diabetologia,* 26, 159, 1984.
14. Poussier, P., Nakhooda, A. F., Falk, J. F., Lee, C., and Marliss, E. B., Lymphopenia and abnormal lymphocyte subsets in the "B" rat: Relationship to the diabetic syndrome, *Endocrinology,* 110, 1825, 1983.
15. Elder, M. E., and Maclaren, N. K., Identification of profound peripheral T Lymphocyte immunodeficiencies in the spontaneously diabetic BB-rat, *J. Immunol.,* 130, 1723, 1983.
16. Nakamura, N., Woda, B. A., Tafuri, A., Greiner, D. L., Reynolds, C. W., Ortaldo, J., Chick, W., Handler, E., Mordes, J. P., and Rossini, A. A., Intrinsic cytotoxicity of natural killer cells to pancreatic islets in vitro, *Diabetes,* 39, 836, 1990.
17. Greiner, D. L., Handler, E. S., Nakano, K., Mordes, J. P., and Rossini, A. A., Absence of the RT-6 cell subset in diabetes prone BB/W-rats, *Am. Ass. Immunol.,* 136, 1, 148, 1986.
18. Appel, S. B., Burkart, V., Kantwerk-Funke, G., Funda, J., Kolb-Bachaofen, V., and Kolb, H., Spontaneous cytotoxicity of macrophages against pancreatic islet cells, *J. Immunol.,* 142, 3803, 1989.
19. Mackay, P., Jacobsen, J., and Rabinovitch, A., Spontaneous Diabetes Mellitus in the BioBreeding/Worcester rat: Evidence in vitro for NK cell lysis of islet cells, *J. Clin. Invest.,* 77, 916, 1986.
20. Like, A. A., Kislauskis, E., Williams, R. M., and Rossini, A. A., Neonatal thymectomy prevents spontaneous diabetes mellitus in the BB/W rat, *Science,* 216, 644, 1982.
21. Naji, A., Silvers, W. K., Belgrau, D., Anderson, A. O., Plotkin, S., and Barker, C. F., Prevention of diabetes in rats by bone marrow transplantation, *Ann. Surg.,* 194, 328, 1981.
22. Like, A. A., Rossini, A. A., Appel, M. C., Guberski, I., and Williams, R, M., Spontaneous diabetes mellitus: reversal and prevention in the BB/W rat with antiserum to rat lymphocytes, *Science,* 206, 1421, 1983.
23. Rossini, A. A., Slavin, S., Woda, B. A., Geisberg, M., Like, A. A., and Mordes, J. P., Total lymphoid irradiation prevents diabetes in the Bio-Breeding/Worcester (BB/W) rat, *Diabetes,* 33, 543, 1984.
24. Rossini, A. A., Mordes, J. P., Pelletier, A. M., and Like, A. A., Transfusions of whole blood prevents spontaneous diabetes mellitus in the BB/W rat, *Science,* 210, 975, 1983.
25. Rossini, A. A., Faustman, D., Woda, A., Like, A. A., Szymanski, and Mordes, J. P., Lymphocyte transfusions prevent diabetes in the Bio-Breeding/Worcester rat, *J. Clin. Invest.,* 74: 39-46 1984.
26. Koevary, S., Rossini, A. A., Stoller, W., Chick, W., and Williams, R. M., Passive transfer of diabetes in BB/W rats, *Science,* 2, 220, 727, 1983.
27. Like, A. A., Weringer, E. J., Holdash, A., McGill, P., and Rossini, A. A., Adoptive transfer of autoimmune diabetes in BioBreeding Worcester (BB/W) inbred and hybrid rats, *J. Immunol.,* 134, 1583, 1985.
28. Koevary, S. B., Williams, D. E., Williams, R. M., and Chick, W., Passive transfer of diabetes from BB/W to Wistar-Furth rats, *J. Clin. Invest.,* 75, 1904, 1985.
29. Like, A. A., Anthony, M., Guberski, D. I., and Rossini, A. A., Spontaneous diabetes mellitus in the BB/W rat. Effects of glucocorticoids, cyclosporin-A, and antiserum to rat lymphocytes, *Diabetes,* 32, 326, 1983.
30. Laupacis, A., Stiller, C. R., Gardell, C., Keown, P., Dupre, J., Wallace, A. C., and Thibert, P., Cyclosporin prevents diabetes in BB Wistar rats, *Lancet,* 1, 10, 1983.
31. Like, A. A., Guberski, D. L., and Butler, L., Influence of environmental viral agents on frequency and tempo of diabetes mellitus in BB/Wor rats, *Diabetes,* 40 (2), 259, 1991.
32. Georgiou, H. M., Lagarde, A. C., and Bellgrau, D., T cell dysfunction in the diabetes-prone BB-rat: a role of thymic migrants that are not T cell precursors, *J. Exp. Med.,* 167, 132, 1988.
33. Buschard, K., Jørgensen, M., Aaen, K., Bock, T., and Josefsen, K., Prevention of diabetes mellitus in the BB rats by neonatal stimulation of B cells, *Lancet,* 335, 134, 1990.

34. Ihm, S. H., Lee, K. H., and Yoon, J. W., Studies on autoimmunity for initiation of beta cell destruction, VII, Evidence for antigenic changes on beta cells leading to autoimmune destruction of beta cells in BB rats, *Diabetes*, 40, 269, 1991.
35. Koevary, S. B., and Blomberg, M., Prevention of diabetes in the BB/W rat by intrathymic islet injection, *J. Clin. Invest.*, 89, 512, 1992.
36. Scott, F. W., Dietary initiators and modifiers of BB-rat diabetes, in *Lessons from Animal Diabetes II*, Shafrir, E., and Remold, A. E., Eds., Libbey, London, 1988.
37. Rossini, A. A., Mordes, J. P., Gallina, D. L., and Like, A. A., Hormonal and environmental factors in the pathogenesis of BB rat diabetes, *Metabolism*, 32, 1, 33, 1983.
38. Yamada, N., Nonaka, K., Hanafusa, T., Miyazaki, A., Toyoshima, H., and Tarui, S., Preventive and therapeutic effects of large-dose nicotinamide injections on diabetes associated with insulitis, *Diabetes*, 31, 749, 1982.
39. Boitard, C., Timsit, J., Sempe, P., and Bach, J. F., Experimental immunoprevention of type I Diabetes Mellitus, *Diabetes/ Metabolism Rev.*, 7, 1, 15, 1991.
40. Gotfredsen, C. F., Buschard, K., and Frandsen, E. K., Reduction of diabetes incidence of BB Wistar rats by early prophylactic insulin treatment of diabetes-prone animals, *Diabetologia*, 28, 933, 1985.
41. Buschard, K., Brogren, C. H., Röpke, C., and Rygaard, J.: Antigen expression of the pancreatic beta-cells is dependent on their functional state, as shown by a specific, BB rat monoclonal autoantibody IC2, *APMIS*, 96, 342, 1988.
42. Like, A. A., Insulin injections prevent diabetes (DB) in BioBreeding/Worcester (BB/Wor) rats, *Diabetes*, 35, 1, 74A, 1986.
43. Gottlieb, P. A., Handler, E. S., Appel, M. C., Greiner, D. L., Mordes, J. P., and Rossini, A. A., Insulin treatment prevents diabetes mellitus but not thyroiditis in RT6-depleted diabetes resistant BB/Wor rats, *Diabetologia*, 34, 296, 1991.
44. Hunt, U., and Eardley, D. D., Suppressive effects of insulin and insulin like growth factors 1 (IGF-1) on immune responses, *J. Immunol.*, 136, 3994, 1986.
45. Makino, S., Kunimoto, K., Muraoka, Y., Mizushima, Y., Katagiri, K. and, Tochino, Y., Breeding of a non-obese, diabetic strain of mice, *Exp. Anim.*, 29, 1, 1980.
46. Makino, S., Hayashi, Y., Muraoka, Y., and Tochino, Y., Establishment of the nonobese-diabetic (NOD) mouse, *Curr. Top. Clin. Exp. Asp. Diab. Mel.*, 25, 1985.
47. Kolb, H., Mouse models of insulin dependent diabetes: Low-dose streptozotocin-induced diabetes and nonobese diabetic (NOD) mice, *Diabetes/ Metabolism Rev.*, 3, 3, 751, 1987.
48. Leiter, E. H., Prochazka, M., and Coleman, D. L., Animal models of human disease: The Non-obese diabetic (NOD) mouse, *Am. J. Path.*, 128, 2, 380, 1987.
49. Makino, S., Kunimoto, K., Muraoka, Y., and Katagiri, K., Effect of castration on the appearance of diabetes in NOD mouse, *Exp. Anim.*, 30, 137, 1981.
50. Lampeter, E. F., Signore, A., Gale, E. A. M., and Pozzilli, P., Lessons from the NOD mouse for the pathogenesis and immunotherapy of human type I (insulin-dependent) diabetes mellitus, *Diabetologia*, 32, 703, 1989.
51. Fujita, T., Yui, R., Kusumoto, Y., Serizawa, Y., Makino, S., and Tochino, Y., Lymphocyte insulitis in a non-obese diabetic (NOD) strain og mice: an immunohistochemical and electron microscope investigation, *Biochem. Res.*, 3, 429, 1982.
52. Tochino, T., The NOD mouse as a model of type I diabetes, *Crit. Rev. Immunol*, 8, 49, 1987.
53. Kataoka, S., Satoh, J., Fujiya, H., Toyota, T., Suzuki, R., Itoh, K. and, Kumagai, K., Immunologic aspects of the nonobese diabetic (NOD) mouse: abnormalities of cellular immunity, *Diabetes*, 32, 247, 1983.
54. Wicker, L. S., Miller, B. J., and Mullen, Y., Transfer of autoimmune diabetes mellitus with splenocytes from nonobese (NOD) mice, *Diabetes*, 35, 855, 1986.
55. Signore, A., Cooke, A., Pozzilli, P., Butcher, G., Simpson, E., and Beverley, P. C. L., Class II and IL2 receptor positive cells in the pancreas of NOD mice, *Diabetologia*, 30, 902, 1987.

56. Miyazaki, A., Hanafusa, T., Yamada, K., Miyagawa, J., Fujino-Kurihara, H., Nakajima, H., Nonaka, K., and Tarui, S., Predominance of T lymphocytes in pancreatic islets and spleen of prediabetic non obese diabetic (NOD) mice: A longitudinal study, *Clin. Exp. Immunol.*, 60, 622, 1985.

57. Signore, A., Gale, E. A. M., Adreani, D., Beverley, P. C. L., and Pozzilli, P., The natural history of lymphocyte subsets infiltrating the pancreas of NOD mice, *Diabetologia*, 32, 282, 1989.

58. Kanazawa, Y., Komeda, K., Sato, S., Mori, S., Akanuma, K., and Takuku, F., Non-obese-diabetic mice: immune mechanisms of pancreatic B-cell destruction, *Diabetologia*, 27, 113, 1984.

59. Wicker, L. S., Miller, B. J., Coker, L. Z., McNally, S. E., Scott, S., Mullen, Y., and Appel, M. C., Genetic control of diabetes and insulitis in the nonobese diabetic (NOD) mouse, *J. Exp. Med.*, 165, 1639, 1987.

60. Prochazka, M., Leiter, E. H., Serreze, D. V., and Coleman, D. L., Three recessive loci required for insulin-dependent diabetes in nonobese diabetic mice, *Science*, 237, 286, 1987.

61. Komeda, K., and Goto, N., Genetic monitoring of the NOD mice. In *Insulitis and Type I Diabetes — Lessons from the NOD Mouse*, Tarui, S., Tochino, Y. and Nonaka, K., Eds., Academic Press, New York, 1986, 11.

62. Reddy, S., Bibby, N. J., and Elliot, R. B., Ontogeny of islet cell antibodies, insulin autoantibodies and insulitis in the non-obese diabetic mouse, *Diabetologia*, 31, 322, 1988.

63. Pontesilli, O., Carotenuto, P., Gazda, L. S., Pratt, P. F., and Prowse, S. J., Circulating lymphocyte populations and autoantibodies in non-obese diabetic (NOD) mice: a longitudinal study, *Clin. Exp. Immunol.*, 70, 84, 1987.

64. Maruyama, T., Takei, I., Asba, Y., Yanagawa, T., Takahashi, T., Katoka, K., and Ishii, T., Insulin autoantibodies in non-obese diabetic mice and low-dose streptozotocin-induced diabetes in mice, *Diabetes Res.*, 7, 93, 1988.

65. Maruyama, T., Takei, I., Asaba, Y., Tatsuo, Y., Takahashi, T., Itoh, H., Suzuki, Y., Kataoka, K., Saruta, T., and Ishii, T., Insulin autoantibodies in mouse models of insulin-dependent diabetes, *Diabetes Res.*, 11, 61, 1989.

66. Ogawa, M., Maruyama, T., Hasegawa, T., Kanaya, T., Kobayashi, F., Tochino, Y., and Uda, H., The inhibitory effect of neonatal thymectomy on the incidence of insulitis in non-obese diabetic (NOD) mice, *Biomed. Res.*, 6, 103, 1985.

67. Leiter, E. H., Serreze, D. V., Le, P. H., Coleman, D. L., and Shultz, L. D., Autoimmunity in non-obese diabetic (NOD) mice, *J. Cell Biochem.*, 108, S10A, 1986.

68. Harada, M., and Makino, S., Immunological manipulation of diabetes production in NOD mice. In *Insulitis and Type I Diabetes — Lessons from the NOD Mouse*, Tarui, S., Tochino, Y. and Nonaka, K., Eds., Academic Press, New York, 1986, 143.

69. Charlton, B., Bacelj, A., and Mandel, T. E., Administration of silica particles or anti-Lyt2 antibody prevents beta-cell destruction in NOD mice given cyclophosphamide, *Diabetes*, 37, 930, 1988.

70. Kataoka, S., Satoh, J., Fujiya, H., Toyota, T., Suzuki, R., Itoh, K. and, Kumagai, K., Immunologic aspects of the nonobese diabetic (NOD) mouse: abnormalities of cellular immunity, *Diabetes*, 32, 247, 1983.

71. Maruyama, T., Takei, I., Taniyama, M., Katoaka, K., and Matsuki, S., Immunologic aspect of nonobese diabetic mice: immune islet killing mechanism and cell-mediated immunity, *Diabetologia*, 27, 121, 1984.

72. Serreze, D. V., and Leiter, E. H., Lymphokine deficiencies may underlie immunoregulatory defect in NOD mice, *Diabetes*, 36, 68A, 1987.

73. Mori, Y., Suko, M., Okudaira, H., Matsuba, I., Tsuruoka, A., Sasaki, A., Yokoyama, H., Tanase, T., Shida, T., Nishimura, M., Terada, E., and Ikeda, Y., Preventive effects of cyclosporin on diabetes in NOD mice, *Diabetologia*, 29, 244, 1986.

74. Formby, B., Miller, N., Garret, R., and Peterson, C. M., Effects of low-dose cyclosporin prophylaxis in nonobese diabetic mice, *J. Pharm. Exp. Ther.*, 241, 1106, 1987.

75. Harada, M., and Makino, S., Promotion of spontaneous diabetes in non-obese diabetic prone mice by cyclophosphamide, *Diabetologia*, 27, 604, 1984.

76. Nakajima, H., Yamada, K., Hanafusa, T., Fujino-Kurihara, H., Miyagawa, J., Miyazaki, A., Siatoh, R., Minami, Y., Kono, N., Nonaka, K., Tochino, Y., and Tarui. S., Elevated antibody-dependent T cell-mediated cytotoxicity and its inhibition by nicotinamide in diabetic NOD mice, *Immunol. Lett.*, 12, 83, 1987.

77. Vague, P., Vialettes, B., Lassman-Vague, V., and Vallo, J., Nicotinamide may extend remission phase in insulin-dependent diabetes, *Lancet*, 1, 91, 1987.

78. Pozzilli, P., Visalli, N., Ghirlanda, G., Manna, R., and Andreani, D., Nicotinamide increases C peptide secretion in patients with newly-diagnosed type I (insulin-dependent) diabetes, *Diabetic Med.*, 6, 568, 1989.

79. Kato, K., Hamada, N., Mizukoshi, N., Yamamoto, K., Kimura, T., Ishihara, C., Fujioka, Y., Kato, T., Fujieda, K., and Matsuura, N., Depression of delayed-type hypersensitivity in mice with hypothalamic lesion induced by monosodium glutamate: involvement of neuroendocrine system in immunomodulation, *Immunology*, 58, 389, 1986.

80. Nakajima, H., Tochino, Y., Fujino-Kurihara, H., Yamada, K., Gomi, M., Tajima, K., Kanaya, T., Miyazaki, A., Miyagawi, J.-I., Hanafusa, T., Mashita, K., Kono, N., Moriwaki, K., Nonaka, K., and Tarui, S., Decreased incidence of diabetes mellitus by monosodium glutamate in nonobese diabetic (NOD) mouse, *Res. Commun. Chem. Path. Pharm.*, 50, 251, 1985.

81. Atkinson, M. A., MacLaren, N. K., and Luchetta, R., Insulitis and diabetes in NOD mice reduced by prophylactic insulin therapy, *Diabetes*, 39, 933, 1990.

82. Thivolet, C. H., Goillot, E., Bedossa, P., Durand, A., Bonnard, M. and, Orgiazzi, J., Insulin prevents adoptive transfer of diabetes in autoimmune non-obese diabetic mouse, *Diabetologia*, 34, 314, 1991.

83. Toyota, T., Kataoka, S., Oya, K., Shintani, S., Sato, J., Okano, K., Suzuki, S., and Goto, Y., Characterization of abnormalities of immune response in NOD mice as type I diabetes animal model, *Diabetes Res. Clin. Pract.*, suppl 1, S564, 1985.

84. Toyota, T., Satoh, J., Oya, K., Shintani, S., and Okano, T., Streptococcal preparation (OK-432) inhibits development of type I diabetes in NOD mice, *Diabetes*, 35, 496, 1986.

85. Herr, R. R., Eble, T. E., Bergy, M. E., and Jahnke, H. K., Isolation and characterization of streptozotocin, *Antibiotics Annual*, 236, 1959.

86. Rakieten, N., Rakieten, M. L., and Nadkarni, M. V., Studies on the diabetogenic action of streptozotocin, *Cancer Chemother, Rep.*, 29, 91, 1963.

87. Like, A. A., and Rossini, A. A., Streptozotocin-induced pancreatic insulitis: New model of diabetes mellitus, *Science*, 193, 415, 1976.

88. Rossini, A. A., Williams, R. M., Appel, M. C., and Like, A. A., Sex differences in the multi-dose streptozotocin model of diabetes, *Endocrinology*, 103, 1518, 1978.

89. Rossini, A. A., Like, A. A., Dulin, W. E., and Cahill, G. F., Pancreatic beta cell toxicity by streptozotocin anomers, *Diabetes*, 26, 1120, 1977.

90. Yamamoto, H., Uchigata, Y., and Okamoto, H., Streptozotocin and alloxan induce DNA strand breaks and poly (ADP-ribose) synthetase in pancreatic islets, *Nature*, 294, 284, 1981.

91. Wilson, G. L., and Leiter, E. H., Streptozotocin interactions with pancreatic beta cells and the induction of insulin-dependent diabetes, *Curr. Top. Microbiol. Immunol.*, 156, 29, 1990.

92. Kim, Y. T., and Steinberg, C., Immunologic studies on the induction of diabetes in experimental animals: cellular basis for the induction of diabetes by streptozotocin, *Diabetes*, 33, 771, 1984.

93. Paik, S., Fleischer, N., and Shin, S., Insulin-dependent diabetes mellitus induced by subdiabetogenic doses of streptozocin: Obligatory role of cell-mediated autoimmune processes, *Proc. Natl. Acad. Sci*, 77, 6129, 1980.

94. Nakamura, M., Nagafuchi, S., Yamaguchi, K., and Takaki, R., The role of thymic immunity and insulitis in the development of streptozotocin-induced diabetes in mice, *Diabetes*, 33, 894, 1984.

95. Buschard, K., and Rygaard, J., Is the diabetogenic effect of streptozotocin in part thymus dependent?, *Acta Pathol. Microbiol. Scand.*, 86, 23, 1978.

96. Rossini, A. A., Like, A. A., Chick ,W. L., Appel, M. C., and Cahill, G. F., Studies of streptozotocin-induced insulitis and diabetes, *Proc. Natl. Acad. Sci.,* 74, 2485, 1977.

97. Paik, S., Blue, M. L., Fleischer, N., and Shin, S., Diabetes susceptibility of BALB/c BOM mice treated with streptozotocin: inhibition by lethal irradiation and restoration by splenic lymphocytes, *Diabetes*, 31, 808, 1982.

98. Nedergaard, M., Egeberg, J., and Kromann, H., Irradiation protects against pancreatic islet degeneration and hyperglycemia following streptozotocin treatment of mice, *Diabetologia*, 24, 382, 1983.

99. Rossini, A. A., Williams, R. M., Appel, M. C., and Like, A. A., Complete protection from low-dose streptozotocin-induced diabetes in mice, *Diabetologia*, 24, 382, 1983.

100. Hahn, H. J., Barnstorff, K., Nadrowitz, R., and Schmidt, W., The effect of irradiation on the development of low-dose streptozotocin diabetes in mice, *Diabetes Metab.*, 9, 42, 1983.

101. Oschilewski, M., Schwab, E., Kiesel, U., Opitz, U., Stünkel, K., Kolb-Bachofen, V., and Kolb, H., Administration of silica or monoclonal antibody to Thy-1 prevents low-dose streptozotocin induced diabetes in mice, *Immunol. Lett.*, 12, 289, 1986.

102. Kolb, H., Oschilewski, M., Oschilewski, U., Schwab, E., Moume, C. M., Greulich, B., Burkart, V., Zielasek, J., and Kiesel, U., Analysis of 22 immunomodulatory substances for efficacy in low-dose streptozotocin-induced diabetes, *Diabetes Res.*, 6, 21, 1987.

103. Andersson, A., Borg, H., Hallberg, A., Hellerström, C., Sandler, S. and, Schnell, A., Long-term effects of cyclosporin A on cultured mouse pancreatic islets, *Diabetologia*, 27, 66, 1984.

104. Beattie, G., Lonnom, R., Lipsick, J., Kaplan, N. O., and Osler, A. G., Streptozotocin-induced diabetes in athymic and conventional BALB/c mice, *Diabetes*, 29, 146, 1980.

105. Leiter, E. H., Multiple low-dose streptozotocin-induced hyperglycemia and insulitis in C57BL mice: influence of inbred background, sex and thymus, *Proc. Natl. Acad. Sci.*, 79, 630, 1982.

106. Gubbels, E., Poort-Keesom, R., and Hilgers, J., Genetically contaminated BALB/c nude mice, *Curr. Topic. Microbiol. Immunol.*, 122, 86, 1985.

107. Leiter, E. H., Differential susceptibility of BALB/c subline to diabetes induction by multi-dose streptozotocin treatment, *Curr. Topic. Microbiol. Immunol.*, 122, 78, 1895.

108. Paik, S. G., Michelis, M. A., Kim, Y. T., and Shin, S., Induction of insulin dependent diabetes by streptozotocin. Inhibition by estrogens and potentiation by androgens, *Diabetes*, 31, 724, 1982.

109. Pukel, C., Baquerizo, H., and Rabinovitch, A., Destruction of rat islet cell monolayers by cytokines. Synergistic interactions of gamma-interferon, tumor necrosing factor, lymphotoxin and interleukin 1, *Diabetes*, 37, 133, 1988.

110. Nerup, J., Mandrup-Poulsen, T., Molvig, J., Helquist, S., Mogensen, L. and, Egeberg, J., Mechanisms of pancreatic beta cell destruction in type I diabetes, *Diabetes Care*, 11, 16, 1988.

111. Yoon, J. W., Austin, M., Onodera, T., and Notkins, A. L., Virus-induced diabetes mellitus isolation of a virus from the pancreas of a child with diabetic ketoacidosis, *N. Engl. J. Med.*, 300, 1173, 1979.

112. Craighead, J. E., and McLance, M. F., Diabetes mellitus: Induction in mice by encephalomyocarditis virus, *Science*, 162, 913, 1968.

113. Yoon, J. W., McClintock, P. R., Onodera, T., and Notkins, A. L., Virus-induced diabetes mellitus. (XVII). Inhibition by a non-diabetogenic variant of encephalomyocarditis virus, *J. Exp. Med.*, 152, 878, 1980.

114. Yoon, J. W., and Notkins, A. L., Virus-induced diabetes in mice, *Metabolism*, 32, 37, 1982.

115. Bae, Y. S., Eun, H. M., Pon, R. T., Giron, D., and Yoon, J. W., Two amino acids, Phe 16 and Ala 776, on the polyprotein are most likely to be responsible for the diabetogenicity of encephalomyocarditis virus, *J. Gen. Virol.*, 71, 639, 1990.

116. Cohen, S. H., Bolton, V., and Jordan, G. W., Relationship of interferon-inducing particle phenotype to encephalomyocarditis virus-induced diabetes mellitus, *Infect. Immun.*, 42, 605, 1983.

117. Yoon, J. W., Cha, C. Y., and Jordan, G. W., The role of interferon in virus-induced diabetes, *J. Infect. Dis.*, 147, 155, 1983.

118. Kaptur, P. E., Thomas, D. C., and Giron, D. J., Differing attachment of diabetogenic and nondiabetogenic variants of encephalomyocarditis virus to ß-cells, *Diabetes*, 38, 1103, 1989.

119. Craighead, J. E., The role of viruses in the pathogeneis of pancreatic disease and diabetes mellitus, *Prog. Med. Virol.*, 19, 161, 1975.

120. Craighead, J. E., and Steinke, J., Diabetes mellitus-like syndrome in mice infected with encephalomyocarditis virus, *Am. J. Pathol.*, 63, 119, 1971.

121. Notkins, A. L., Yoon, J. W., Onodera, T., and Jenson, A. B., Virus-induced diabetes, *Perspect. Virol.*, XI, 141, 1981.

122. Buschard, K., Hastrup, N., and Rygaard, J., Virus-induced diabetes in mice and thymus-dependent immune system, *Diabetologia*, 24, 42, 1983.

123. Yoon, J. W., The role of viruses and environmental factors in the induction of diabetes, *Curr. Top. Microbiol. Immunol.*, 164, 95, 1990.

124. Buschard, K., Rygaard, J.,and Lund, E., The inability of a diabetogenic virus to induce diabetes mellitus in athymic (nude) mice, *Acta. Path. Microbiol. Scand.* Sect. C, 84, 299, 1976.

125. Jansen, F. K., Thyrneyssen, O.,and Müntefering, H., Virus induced diabetes and the immune system II - Evidence for an immune pathogenesis of the acute phase of diabetes, *Biomedicine*, 31, 1, 1979.

126. Petersen, K. G., Schlüter, K., Kasimir, H., Treiber, A., Müntefering, K., and Kerp, L., Prevention of EMC-virus-induced diabetes by neonatal thymectomized mice, *Excerpta Med. Int. Congr. Ser.*, 481, 184, 1979.

127. Jansen, F. K., Müntefering, H., and Schmidt, W. A. K., Virus induced diabetes and the immune system. I. Suggestion that appearance of diabetes depends on immune reactions, *Diabetologia*, 13, 545, 1977.

128. Dafoe, D. C., Naji, A., Kirby, W., and Barker, C. F., Role in immunity in induction of and recovery from viral immune diabetes, *Surg. Forum,* 31, 51, 1980.

129. Babu, P. G., Huber, S., Sriram, S., and Craighead, J. E., Genetic control of multisystem autoimmune disease in encephalomyocarditis virus infected Balb/cCum and Balb/cBYJ mice, *Curr. Top. Microbiol. Immunol.*, Potter, M., Ed., Springer-Verlag, 154, 1985.

130. Babu, P. G., Huber, S. A., and Craighead, J.E., Contrasting features of T lymphocyte mediated diabetes in encephalomyocarditis virus-infected Balb/cBy and Balb/cCum mice, *Am. J. Pathol.,* 124, 193, 1986.

131. Haynes, M. K., Huber, S. A., and Craighead, J. E., Helper-inducer T-lymphocytes mediate diabetes in EMC-infected BALB/cBYJ mice, *Diabetes*, 36, 877, 1987.

132. Yoon, J. W., McClintock, P. R., Bachurski, C. J., Longstreth, J. D., and Notkins, A. L., Virus-induced diabetes mellitus. No evidence for immune mechanisms in the destruction of ß-cells by the D-variant of encephalomyocarditis virus, *Diabetes*, 34, 922, 1985.

133. Baek, H. S., and Yoon, J. W., Role of macrophages in the pathogenesis of encephalomyocarditis virus-induced diabetes in mice, *J. Virol.*, 64, 5708, 1990.

134. Buschard, K., Rygaard, J., Lund, E., and Röpke, C., Prodromal immune manifestation in EMC-M virus induced diabetes: Islet bound and circulating antibodies and change in lymphocyte subsets, *Diabetes Res.,* 5, 67, 1987.

135. Kanatsuna, T., Lernmark, Å., Rubinstein, A. H., and Steiner, D. F., Block in insulin release from column-perifused pancreatic B-cells induced by islet cell surface antibodies and complement, *Diabetes*, 30, 231, 1981.

Chapter 11

Animal Models in Neuroscience

Jesper Mogensen

CONTENTS

INTRODUCTION

Within all scientific disciplines, studies involving animal models are plagued by problems of theoretical, practical, and ethical nature. Some of these problems, e.g., the ethical question whether human use of subhuman species in the fight against human disease is "speciesism",[1] and whether such speciesism is acceptable or not,[2] are common to all branches of animal model research and will not be dealt with in this chapter. Other issues are more specific to the neuroscientific area and its clinical subdisciplines neurology and psychiatry. A number of these problems are linked to the assumed uniqueness of the human brain, its functions and dysfunctions. While few might challenge that the livers of human and subhuman species are essentially similar, the neuroscientific community is far from reaching consensus about the level of similarity between the brains and "minds" of humans and other species. The question of similarities between structures and functions of the brains of various species is often considered the most basic problem for the use of animal models in studies of diseases of the human brain. However, such endeavours are often impaired by the lack of detailed and objective methods within the areas of clinical and animal experimentation. Finally, some of the confusion and contradiction within experimental neuroscience may spring from uncertainties about the definition of an "optimal", neuroscientific animal model.

SPECIES COMPARISONS

The major task of comparative neuroscience is to go beyond the superficial species differences and identify the basic differences and similarities between species. Many structural differences (e.g., the pattern of cortical sulci and gyri) may be of little or no consequence for the organization of brains. Although anatomical analysis has revealed some basic species differences, there seems to be a growing body of evidence indicating a common "bauplan" for the brains of a broad spectrum of species.

    A number of features have traditionally been believed to mark the major differences between human and subhuman brains. While some such features still appear to be rather unique to the human brain, other aspects of the human brain have been found to be shared with more species than originally believed. Although some aspects of the cortical areas believed to mediate production and perception of speech appear to be present in both humans and certain non-human primates,[3-4] the presence of unilateral, cortical areas specialized in mediation of linguistic functions, including the Broca area, appears likely to be a privilege of the human brain. Animal models of traumatic aphasias are unlikely ever to be developed — even in non-human primates; see, however, the arguments of Noback.[5] Another aspect of the human brain originally believed to be rather specifically "human" is the fact that the prefrontal cortex constitutes approximately one third of the total neocortical surface. The prefrontal cortex has long been believed to be a privilege of mammals and some data seem to indicate that "higher" mammals, e.g., primates, have a relatively larger prefrontal cortex compared to "lower" mammals, e.g., rodents.[6] Partly on the basis of such observations and partly based on the fact that the prefrontal cortex of some species (rodents) differs cytoarchitectonically from the prefrontal area of primates, it has been argued that studies on the functions of the prefrontal cortex should mainly be conducted in primates.[6] More recent studies of the prefrontal cortex have, however, indicated that this structure may be present in a broader variety of species. Both histochemical,[7] biochemical,[8] and functional[9,9a] studies have indicated that the posterodorsolateral neostriatum of the pigeon should be considered equivalent to the prefrontal cortex of mammals. Furthermore, the prefrontal cortex of the echidna (Tachyglossus aculeatus — an egg-laying mammal belonging to the subclass Prototheria) constitutes approximately 50% of the total cortical surface.[10-13] The prefrontal cortex appears to be present in mammals and at least some non-mammals alike. The ratio between prefrontal and non-prefrontal cortical surface is not in itself an "index of evolution".

Comparative studies are of importance to the use of neuroscientific animal models in at least two ways. First, such studies may indicate the areas within which animal models are likely to be useful and the species likely to be acceptable for such studies. As indicated above, animal models of traumatic aphasias are hardly feasible. On the other hand, the prefrontal system seems to subserve functions of rather general survival value and consequently a broad spectrum of species may be available for model experiments in which the focus is on the prefrontal system, its functions and potential prefrontal involvement in pathological conditions. Motivation for developing animal models of aspects of normal and abnormal functions of the human prefrontal cortex may stem from repeated observations of the prefrontal cortex in schizophrenic patients.[14-25]

The second way in which comparative neuroscience may contribute to the development of animal models is by providing the information necessary for making adequate comparisons between structural as well as functional aspects of human and non-human brains. In the case of rat models of processes involving the human prefrontal cortex, the subdivisions of which are functionally heterogeneous,[26-27] it is important that adequate choices are made of the cortical areas to be manipulated in the animal. Detailed analysis of the anatomy (primarily the afferent connections) of the rat prefrontal cortex[28-30] has modified such strategies by redefining the boundaries of subdivisions of the prefrontal cortex.[31] A subcortical example of the ways in which model studies depend upon comparative neuroanatomy, is found in studies of the neostriatum. The neostriata of both rodents and primates are frequently the focus of studies attempting to model aspects of the "extrapyramidal" diseases such as Huntington's chorea, in which the primary cell loss seems to be within the neostriatum, and Parkinson's disease, in which a presumed primary cell loss in the pars compacta of substantia nigra causes a drastic reduction in the striatal concentration of the neurotransmitter dopamine. Although pathological changes may be found in non-striatal brain regions of even early parkinsonian cases, it can hardly be doubted that essential aspects of both conditions can be studied in animal models in which the neostriatum has been affected by mechanical lesion, toxins or local injection of drugs. However, studies on functional aspects of the neostriatum frequently pay insufficient attention to the connectivity and consequent regional specialization within this structure. The neostriatum of all species studied is subdivided into regions each of which receives input from a specific, cortical area with which it is functionally "yoked" in such a way that lesions of a neostriatal region and its associated cortical area are both accompanied by similar patterns of post-lesion symptoms.[32-33] A possible exception to this rule may be found in the "motor" part of the neostriatum.[32] Since the neostriatum is heterogeneous and its regions may indeed be as functionally specialized as the areas of the cortex, knowledge about neostriatal organization is of primary importance when one is to construct or evaluate animal models in which parts of the neostriatum have been manipulated.

FUNCTIONAL ANALYSES

Within psychiatry, and to some extent even neurology, most of the symptoms defining the diseases are aspects of behavior or introspection, and in the case of introspection mainly such that are reflected in verbal behavior. The nature of the symptoms defining such diseases is an obvious problem for the construction of animal models within clinical neuroscience.

Traditionally, the situation in this field has been that the condition of the patient is characterized by subjective and often poorly defined symptoms and the behavior of the subjects of animal modeling is analyzed in a rather crude manner. Such a state of affairs strongly impairs comparisons between the conditions of patient and animal.

SIMILAR TESTS IN PATIENT AND ANIMAL

An important step towards the solution of this problem has been the trend towards applying more detailed behavioral and physiological analyses to not only neurological but even psychiatric patients. Such studies may in themselves provide important information about the structural and functional basis of a certain disease, e.g., the indication by various neuroimaging and functional methods of an association between schizophrenia and dysfunction of the prefrontal system. Additionally, the gathering of objective information about the condition of patients may allow more direct comparisons between patients and animal models. Studies of the "pre-pulse acoustic startle paradigm" in schizophrenics exemplify this type of progress. When exposed to a burst of strong noise, schizophrenic patients as well as normal humans display an objectively measurable startle response. If a pre-stimulus in the form of a weak tone precedes the startle-eliciting noise by 60 to 120 milliseconds, the startle response of normals is significantly reduced, and the degree to which the presentation of the ("warning") pre-pulse is able to inhibit the startle response can be measured as the percentage reduction of startle. Schizophrenics appear to have a significantly less reduced startle response in the presence of the pre-stimulus when compared to normals.[34] Since the acoustic startle paradigm can be applied to non-human species — and the pre-stimulus associated reduction in startle response can be seen in normal subjects from such non-human species — this technique allows essentially identical testing methods to be applied to both schizophrenic patients and animal models. The dominating theory about the neural substrate of schizophrenia is the "dopamine hypothesis"[35] which postulates an association between increased activity of dopamine neurotransmission and the schizophrenic disease (or diseases). The major lines of evidence supporting the dopamine hypothesis are:

- Direct or indirect dopaminergic agonists, e.g., amphetamine, aggravate the symptomatology of schizophrenic patients and can even in normal persons induce a temporary, psychosis-like condition which is indistinguishable from acute paranoid schizophrenia.[35]
- There is a strong positive correlation between the clinical efficacy of antipsychotic drugs and their ability to act as antagonists at the D_2-dopamine receptor.[36]
- Post-mortem studies of schizophrenic patients indicate an increased concentration of

D_2-receptors.[37] The up-regulation of the D_2-receptors may, however, be the consequence of medication rather than a true aspect of a primary disease. Positron emission tomography (PET) studies have indicated that young, non-medicated schizophrenic patients show no measurable change in the concentration of D_2-receptors.[38]

Almost all current animal models of schizophrenia spring from one or another aspect of the "dopamine hypothesis". The rat model focusing on the acoustic startle paradigm[39] accomplishes either regional or global dopamine receptor hypersensitivity by injecting the dopaminergic neurotoxin 6-hydroxy-dopamine into either a limited target area or the cerebral ventricles. The toxin causes destruction of presynaptic dopaminergic neurons and consequently a postsynaptic up-regulation of dopamine receptors. In animals treated this way, systemic injection of the dopamine agonist apomorphine will cause stimulation of all dopamine receptors and consequently dopamine receptor hyperactivity in the region or regions treated with 6-hydroxy-dopamine. In this rat model, it appears that global dopamine receptor hypersensitivity is associated with an impaired effect of the "warning" tone of the acoustic startle paradigm — a pattern similar to that observed for schizophrenic patients. Furthermore, local receptor hypersensitivity in both substantia nigra and the nucleus accumbens (but not in the frontal cortex) seems to be associated with a similar symptom.[39] Such results lend support to theories associating part of the schizophrenic symptomatology and hyperactivity within the dopaminergic system, and the outcome of these studies may even indicate the regional distribution of such dopaminergic abnormalities. On the other hand it should be remembered that the acoustic startle paradigm focuses on only one aspect of the disease and that manipulating other neurochemical or regional systems might have provoked similar symptoms.

INTERPRETATION OF BEHAVIORAL TESTS

While clinicians need to provide more objective information about patients, it is equally important that experimenters working with animal models improve the methods of behavioral analysis. Such analysis must be performed at a level of sophistication that allows the experimenter to establish a detailed and broad-spectred functional profile of the animal. Only such a profile will make it possible to determine the nature of functions that are impaired by a certain neural manipulation (and potentially reinstated by therapy). In determining areas of impairment it is equally important to establish the integrity of functional spheres that are assumed to be spared by the manipulation under investigation. Alternatively, the observed impairments might be secondary to more basic — but unnoticed — dysfunctions. For instance, the observation that prolonged thiamine deficiency in the rat (a potential model for the Wernicke/Korsakoff syndrome) is associated with impaired acquisition and retention of an active, step-through shock-avoidance test[40-42] might not reflect a "cognitive" impairment but rather be secondary to a motoric impairment. This possibility is emphasized by the observation that thiamine deficient rats are impaired in tests of locomotion. The motoric impairment of thiamine deficient rats does not in itself invalidate the model since patients suffering the Wernicke/Korsakoff syndrome may demonstrate ataxia.[43] To establish whether thiamine deficient rats model the learning and memory impairment central to the Wernicke/Korsakoff syndrome, it will be necessary to analyze the performance of such rats in a learning task that is able to reflect acquisition and/or retention in ways that are rather independent of the motoric performance of the animal. Such a task could be a "place learning" task administered in a water-maze (a circular pool of water).[44] In this task, the animal's latency to find a submerged platform may be heavily influenced by the rat's motoric abilities. However, the distance swum and other test parameters (such as the degree to which the animal initially swims directly towards the target position) are rather unaffected by motoric abilities and — if sensory impairment such as blindness can be ruled out — reflect rather truthfully the cognitive aspects of the test.

METHOD-DEPENDENCE OF BEHAVIORAL TESTS

The necessity of multiple, well selected, and detailed behavioral tests was emphasized by Sanberg[45] who compared three animal models: lesions of the neostriatum obtained via the neurotoxins kainic acid, a model of Huntington's disease,[46] and AF64A, which destroys cholinergic neurons selectively[47-48] and is consequently used in animal models of Alzheimer's disease, and cortical as well as neostriatal maldevelopment upon fetal administration of the toxin methylazoxymethanol (MAM).[49-50] The combined analysis of day-time activity and passive avoidance behavior was unable to discriminate between any of the three models, while a subsequent and detailed analysis of aspects of nocturnal locomotion in the same three models allowed discrimination between, on one hand the MAM model and on the other the two other models. Furthermore, the nocturnal locomotion analysis was able to discriminate between the MAM model and a model including subpial aspiration lesions of the cortex.

The importance of an awareness of the characteristics of the behavioral tests employed is underlined by results demonstrating that various measures of what is commonly described as locomotion/exploration or "general activity" reflect the activity of only partly overlapping neural systems,[51] that the nature of the apparatus in which the "delayed alternation" behavior of the rat is tested determines whether this behavior, which is often considered the "Babinsky sign" of the prefrontal system, is able to reflect massive destruction of prefrontal structures,[52] and that while lesions of the parietal association cortex of the rat impair the place learning behavior in a big water-maze[53] similar animals in a smaller water-maze do not differ significantly from sham operated controls.[54]

SPECIES SELECTION

While comparative neuroanatomy is probably the best indicator of which species are available for the creation of a certain animal model, ethical, practical, and financial considerations[55] are likely to determine the species that is actually selected. In the case of the MPTP model of Parkinson's disease, destruction of the dopaminergic cells of substantia nigra by the neurotoxin 1-methyl-4-phenyl-1,2,3,6-tetrahydropyridine (MPTP),[56] the choice between primates and rodents may be determined by several factors. Originally, MPTP-induced destruction of nigral neurons was only believed to be possible in primates,[57-58] but this model has been found to be feasible even in rodents.[59-60] The MPTP concentration necessary for achieving nigral damage in rodents is, however, substantially higher than that required in primates. Although neither this species difference nor the relative lack of Parkinson-like symptoms in MPTP treated rodents necessarily invalidate the rodent MPTP model of Parkinson's disease (or at least of the disease variant which in humans can be induced by MPTP), a number of practical problems remain. The toxicity of MPTP necessitates substantial precautions to be taken whenever the substance itself, injected animals or the cages of such animals are handled.[61] The higher MPTP dosage required if a rodent model is chosen calls for even stricter laboratory procedures than those required for the primate model.

GENERAL STRATEGIES

Once decisions about species selection have been made, all available knowledge about the comparative anatomy of the neural systems under consideration will have to be consulted. As much as possible of the available knowledge about the pathological condition being modeled should be taken into account — especially important are data about objectively measurable conditions. While the majority of studies dealing with animal models in neuroscience have dealt adequately with these issues, more frequent short-comings are found in the area of animal behavioral analysis. It is essential to the future of neuroscientific animal models that more precise and detailed methods of analyzing behavior are developed. Progress in the area of animal models of "global amnesia", including the development of monkeys with combined bilateral lesions of hippocampus and amygdala as a model of this condition, and the subsequent development of theories about the division of the "memory systems" into those subserving "memories" and those subserving "habits",[62-64] has been emphasized as an example of the importance of selecting non-human primates for certain modeling purposes. However, the selection of adequate behavioral tests may have been an even more crucial factor for this successful interaction between clinical observations, animal modeling, and basic neuroscientific studies. Even for non-primates, e.g., rats, available tests can reflect "habits" and "memories" respectively; the latter being impaired by lesions within some of the same neural systems as those necessary for mediation of such tasks in primates.[65,66]

THE ROLE OF ANIMAL MODELS IN NEUROSCIENCE

What should be required of an animal model within neurology or psychiatry? Is the "optimal" neuroscientific animal model — presently — realistically obtainable? And what kind of models should be strived for? The answer to some of these questions may reside with one additional question: What do we want to get out of such models?

HOMOLOGOUS, ISOMORPHIC, AND PARTIAL MODELS

An animal model may, if certain conditions are met, be either "homologous" or "isomorphic".[67] To be considered homologous, the symptoms displayed by the animal and the cause of the condition in the animal should be identical to the human symptoms and the cause of the human disease. Given our relative lack of knowledge of the etiology of most psychiatric and many neurological diseases, such models are within neuroscience only possible in the case of well-defined lesion-syndromes.[68] Even for isomorphic models, it is demanded that the symptoms displayed by patient and animal must be similar, but the animal condition need not be provoked by the same events as those which cause the human condition. If, in a theoretical disease, a specific population of neurons died for unknown reasons, e.g., genetic predisposition, and it would be possible by injection of a neurotoxin into regions of the rat brain to eliminate a neuron population similar to the one lost in humans, the rats lesioned in such a manner might constitute an isomorphic model of the disease. In this case, the final test of whether or not the model could be considered isomorphic would be the degree of similarity between the symptoms displayed by model and disease. As stressed by several authors[2,68] numerous, if not most, neuroscientific animal models are neither homologous nor isomorphic but could be more adequately described as "partial". Such projects make no attempt at modeling the entire disease but focus on more limited aspects of the human condition.

Many systems have been developed to evaluate the quality or "validity" of animal models. While the classification of a model as homologous, isomorphic, or partial constitutes a rather simple and crude system, examples of more elaborate models are those of McKinney[69] and Leonard.[70] McKinney[69] demands of the optimal model: comparable symptomatology, comparable etiology, comparable neurophysiological background, and concordant effects of drugs. Leonard[70] emphasizes the need for comparable symptomatology, normalization of the model condition by drug therapy similar to the pharmacological therapy effective against the human condition, and stresses that the time-course of a drug-induced normalization, e.g., beneficial effects of chronic but not acute medication, should be similar to what is seen in patients. While a number of the issues stressed by McKinney[69] and Leonard[70] are similar to the demands a model would have to fulfil in order to be considered homologous, the most important additional issue taken into account in these systems is the necessity of a model to respond to a given therapy in ways similar to the clinical response to therapy. As emphasized by Willner,[71] the therapies against which neuroscientific models can be tested need not be pharmacological but could include such methods as electroconvulsive stimulation and behavioral therapy. Willner[71] and others have even included separate evaluation of predictive validity, face validity, and construct validity (concepts initially used in the area of psychological testing) in the systems against which neuroscientific animal models are tested.

Given our present level of knowledge, it would be futile to use any of the evaluation systems as a check-list on which every animal model was expected to meet every single demand. The result would in most if not all cases be a rejection of the model. The evaluation systems should rather be seen as guidelines to the directions in which both partial and more complete models should develop. Furthermore, the evaluation systems may highlight the relative strengths and weaknesses of various models of a given condition.

APPLICATION OF ANIMAL MODELS IN NEUROSCIENCE

Neuroscientific animal models mainly serve in two capacities: they are used as a testing ground during early and intermediate phases of the development of new therapies (frequently drugs) and they are used in the process of developing and testing hypotheses about the neurological and psychiatric diseases in general and their neural substrates in particular. For the purpose of testing whether a particular therapy is efficient in preventing, relieving, or eliminating the symptoms of a disease, and whether administration of the therapy is associated with side-effects, one should ideally employ an animal model that mimics as closely as possible all aspects of the disease. A homologous, or at least isomorphic model, is likely to be the optimal choice for evaluation of potential therapies. Given the rareness of such "complete" models, evaluation of drugs and other therapies are frequently performed in models that are only partial. Some such models may, as Willner[71] has argued in the case of some of the models utilized in the testing of antidepressive drugs, be little more than "behavioral receptor assays". Although some of the partial models are far from being a reasonable substitute for the actual disease, valuable pre-clinical evaluation of drugs and other therapies may be achieved through the use of such models — especially if the same therapeutic method is evaluated against a number of different partial models each of which focuses on a different aspect of the disease.

While a homologous or isomorphic model may be optimal for the purpose of therapy evaluation, the models most helpful to the process of studying the mechanisms of diseases are those that lead the experimenter to suspect and eventually realize previously undiscovered processes and relationships. Important aspects of a disease may be discovered in a "simple" animal model which focuses on only a single aspect of the human condition. In fact, such a simple model may provide a better environment for discovery than a model that tries to mimic simultaneously all aspects of the disease. As previously pointed out[2,68] the models most beneficial to the studies of neuropathological conditions are those of the greatest heuristic value, irrespectively of whether or not such models are partial or of a more "complete" nature. The decision whether to select or develop a partial or more complete model must depend on which purpose the model in question is supposed to serve. Partial models may be of substantial value in the gradual process of building a more complete image of the disease and its mechanism, while more complete models, which usually are only possible in case of better understood diseases, may be ideal for the purpose of testing and evaluating drugs or other therapies.

When developing neuroscientific animal models, the experimenter most frequently chooses as the point of departure the dominating theory about the disease under consideration. While such an approach may seem logical, it involves a risk of unwanted conservatism. Clinical studies into the organic substrate of schizophrenia indicate four major areas of abnormalities: dopaminergic hypertransmission, dysfunction of the prefrontal cortex and system, cerebral ventricular enlargement,[72-73] and structural changes in parts of the temporal lobe.[74-77] Since the prefrontal cortex contains the highest cortical amount of dopamine and has the highest cortical concentration of dopamine receptors,[78-79] both the prefrontal abnormalities and the anormalities in dopaminergic transmission may be covered by the "dopamine hypothesis" of schizophrenia.

Almost all animal models of schizophrenia, chronic administration of amphetamine,[80] administration of apomorphine after 6-hydroxy-dopamine induced lesions of dopaminergic neurons or repeated electrical stimulation ("kindling") of the ventral tegmental area in which dopaminergic neurons project to the prefrontal cortex and nucleus accumbens,[80a] focus one way or another on the association between schizophrenia and various parts of the dopaminergic system. Part of the logics of the dopamine hypothesis is that the most potent of the known anti-schizophrenic drugs appear to have a major action on the dopaminergic system. The use of "dopaminergic" animal models in the search for anti-schizophrenic medication may, in this respect, be a self-fulfilling hypothesis. Such models may favor drugs oriented towards the dopaminergic system and neglect "non-dopaminergic" medication, regardless of its potential effects on the actual disease. Furthermore, the process of developing a more complete understanding of the neural substrate of schizophrenia may be seriously impaired by the rather one-sided focus of the "dopaminergic" animal models. An aspect largely ignored by such models is the repeated observation of temporal lobe pathology in schizophrenic patients. Schmajuk[81] has suggested the hippocampally lesioned rat as an animal model of schizophrenia. Although such a model would in itself be highly partial and ignore important aspects of the disease, it represents a step towards widening the focus of animal models of schizophrenia.

An example of a seemingly successful widening of the focus of an animal model comes from work on Alzheimer's disease. This dementia has traditionally been associated with dysfunction (and assumed cell death) within the neural system utilizing acetylcholine as its neurotransmitter, since cholinergic markers are reduced in the brains of Alzheimer patients and the degree of cholinergic reduction seems to correlate with the extent of the cognitive impairment.[82-84] However, it has even been found that in such patients minor changes are present in a number of other neurotransmitter-defined systems, e.g., the serotonergic system.[85,86] Most animal models of Alzheimer's disease have dealt extensively with the cholinergic system, e.g., using the cholinergic toxin AF64A to destroy cholinergic projections from the medial septum and basic forebrain to hippocampus and cortex.[47, 48, 87, 88] In an attempt to establish whether the serotonergic changes seen in the brains of Alzheimer patients contribute significantly to the development of the strongly disabling dementia of Alzheimer's disease, Nilsson et al.[89] studied rats in which the activity of both the cholinergic and the serotonergic systems had been blocked. These animals exhibited a "dementia" that in comparison to the symptoms of rats subjected to cholinergic blockade alone, appeared to be more similar to the human condition in being both chronic and more severe. It appears that the addition of a serotonergic manipulation brought the cholinergic rat model of Alzheimer's disease closer to the human condition and consequently a partial model evolved in the direction of more completeness and validity.

REFERENCES

1. Ryder, R. D., *Victims of Science*. Davis-Poynter, London, 1975.
2. Bond, N. W., Animal models in psychopathology: an introduction, in *Animal Models In Psychopathology*, Bond, N. W., Ed., Academic Press, Sidney, 1984, 1.
3. LeMay, M., and Geschwind, N., Hemispheric differences in the brains of great apes. *Brain Behav. Evol.*, 11, 48, 1975.
4. Petersen, M. R., Beecher, M. D., Zoloth, S. R., Moody, D. B., and Stebbins, W. C., Neural lateralization of species-specific vocalizations by Japanese macaques (Macaca fuscata). *Science*, 202, 324, 1978.
5. Noback, C. R., Neurobiological aspects in the phylogenetic acquisition of speech, in Armstrong, E., and Falk, D., Eds., *Primate Brain Evolution. Methods and Concepts*. Plenum Press, New York, 1982, 279.

6. Fuster, J. M., *The Prefrontal Cortex. Anatomy, Physiology, and Neuropsychology of the Frontal Lobe*. Raven Press, New York, 1980.

7. Divac, I., and Mogensen, J., The prefrontal "cortex" in the pigeon. Catecholamine histofluorescence. *Neuroscience,* 15, 677, 1985.

8. Divac, I., Mogensen, J., and Björklund, A., The prefrontal "cortex" in the pigeon. Biochemical evidence. *Brain Res.,* 332, 365, 1985.

9. Mogensen, J., and Divac, I., The prefrontal "cortex" in the pigeon. Behavioral evidence. *Brain Behav. Evol.,* 21, 60, 1982.

9a. Mogensen, J. and Divac, I., Behavioural effects of ablation of the pigeon-equivalent of the mammalian prefrontal cortex. *Behav. Brain Res.,* 55, 101, 1993.

10. Divac, I., Holst, M.-C., Nelson, J., and McKenzie, J. S., Afferents of the frontal cortex in the echidna (Tachyglossus aculeatus). Indication of an outstandingly large prefrontal area. *Brain Behav. Evol.,* 30, 303, 1987.

11. Divac, I., Pettigrew, J. D., Holst, M.-C., and McKenzie, J. S., Efferent connections of the prefrontal cortex of echidna (Tachyglossus aculeatus). B*rain Behav. Evol.,* 30, 321, 1987.

12. Regidor, J., and Divac, I., Architectonics of the thalamus in the echidna (Tachyglossus aculeatus): Search for the mediodorsal nucleus. *Brain Behav. Evol.,* 30, 328, 1987.

13. Welker, W., and Lende, R. A., Thalamocortical relationships in echidna (Tachyglossus aculeatus), in Ebbesson, S. O. E., Ed. *Comparative Neurology of the Telencephalon.* Plenum Press, New York, 1980, 449.

14. Buchsbaum, M. S., Positron emission tomography in schizophrenia, in Meltzer, H. Y., Ed. *Psychopharmacology: The Third Generation of Progress,* Raven Press. New York, 1987, 783.

15. Buchsbaum, M. S., and Haier, R. J., Functional and anatomical brain imaging: Impact on schizophrenia research. *Schizoph. Bull.,* 13, 115, 1987.

16. Buchsbaum, M. S., Nuechterlein, K. H., Haier, R. J., Wu, J., Sicotte, N., Hazlett, E., Asarnow, R., Potkin, S., and Guich, S., Glucose metabolic rate in normals and schizophrenics during the continuous performance test assessed by positron emission tomography. *Br. J. Psychiat.,* 156, 216, 1990.

17. Goldberg, T. E., Berman, K. F., Mohr, E., and Weinberger, D. R., Regional cerebral blood flow and cognitive function in Huntington's disease and schizophrenia. A comparison of patients matched for performance on a prefrontal-type task. *Arch. Neurol.,* 47, 418, 1990.

18. Goldberg, T. E., Weinberger, D. R., Berman, K. F., Pliskin, N. H., and Podd, M. H., Further evidence for dementia of the prefrontal type in schizophrenia? A controlled study of teaching the Wisconsin Card Sorting Test. *Arch. Gen. Psychiat.,* 44, 1008, 1987.

19. Ingvar, D. H., and Franzén, G., Abnormalities of cerebral blood flow distribution in patients with chronic schizophrenia. *Acta Psychiat. Scand.,* 50, 425, 1974.

20. Karson, C. N., Coppola, R., Morihisa, J. M., and Weinberger, D. R., Computed electroencephalographic activity mapping in schizophrenia. The resting state reconsidered. *Arch. Gen. Psychiat.,* 44, 514, 1987.

21. Mathew, R. J., and Wilson, W. H., Chronicity and a low anteroposterior gradient of cerebral blood flow in schizophrenia. *Am. J. Psychiat.,* 147, 211, 1990.

22. Meltzer, H. Y., Biological studies in schizophrenia. *Schizoph. Bull.,* 13, 77, 1987.

23. Morice, R., Cognitive inflexibility and pre-frontal dysfunction in schizophrenia and mania. *Br. J. Psychiat.,* 157, 50, 1990.

24. Paulman, R. G., Devous Sr., M. D., Gregory, R. R., Herman, J. H., Jennings, L., Bonte, F. J., Nasrallah, H. A., and Raese, J. D., Hypofrontality and cognitive impairment in schizophrenia: Dynamic single-photon tomography and neuropsychological assessment of schizophrenic brain functions. *Biol. Psychiat.,* 27, 377, 1990.

25. Westphal, K. P., Grözinger, B., Diekmann, V., Scherb, W., Reess, J., Leibing, U., and Kornhuber, H. H., Slower theta activity over the midfrontal cortex in schizophrenic patients. *Acta Psychiat. Scand.,* 81, 132, 1990.

26. McAndrews, M. P., and Milner, B., The frontal cortex and memory for temporal order. *Neuropsychology,* 29, 849, 1991.

27. Milner, B., Petrides, M., and Smith, M. L., Frontal lobes and the temporal organization of memory. *Hum. Neurobiol.*, 4, 137, 1985.
28. Divac, I., Kosmal, A., Björklund, A., and Lindvall, O., Subcortical projections to the prefrontal cortex in the rat as revealed by the horseradish peroxidase technique. *Neuroscience*, 3, 785, 1978.
29. Groenewegen, H. J., Organization of the afferent connections of the mediodorsal thalamic nucleus in the rat, related to the mediodorsal-prefrontal topography. *Neuroscience*, 24, 379, 1988.
30. Krettek, J. E., and Price, J. L., The cortical projections of the mediodorsal nucleus and adjacent thalamic nuclei in the rat. *J. Comp. Neurol.*, 171, 157, 1977.
31. Mogensen, J., and Divac, I., Sequential behavior after modified prefrontal lesions in the rat. *Physiol. Psychol.*, 12, 41, 1984.
32. Divac, I., The neostriatum viewed orthogonally, in Ciba Foundation Symposium 107: *Functions of the Basal Ganglia*. Pitman, London, 1984, 201.
33. Divac I., and Mogensen, J., Modularity of the prosencephalon: The vertical systems, in Will, B., Schmitt, P., and Dalrymple-Alford, J., Eds. B*rain Plasticity, Learning, and Memory*. Plenum Press, New York, 1985, 205.
34. Braff, D., Stone, C., Callaway, E., Geyer, M., Glick, I. and Bali, L., Prestimulus effects on human startle reflex in normals and schizophrenics. *Psychophysiology*, 15, 339, 1978.
35. Randrup, A., and Munkvad, I., Special antagonism of amphetamine-induced abnormal behaviour. Inhibition of stereotyped activity with increase of some normal activities. *Psychopharmacology*, 7, 416, 1965.
36. Creese, I., Burt, D. R., and Snyder, S.H., Dopamine receptor binding predicts clinical and pharmacological potencies of antischizophrenic drugs. *Science,* 192, 481, 1976.
37. Seeman, P., Ulpian, C., Bergeron, C., Riederer, P., Jellinger, K., Gabriel, E., Reynolds, G., and Tourtellotte, W., Bimodal distribution of dopamine receptor densities in brain of schizophrenics. *Science,* 225, 728, 1984.
38. Farde, L., Wiesel., F.-A., Hall, H., Halldin, C., Stone-Elander, S., and Sedvall, G., No D_2 receptor increase in PET study of schizophrenia. *Arch. Gen. Psychiat.*, 44, 671, 1987.
39. Swerdlow, N., Braff, D., Geyer, M., and Koob, G., Central dopamine hyperactivity in rats mimics abnormal acoustic startle response in schizophrenics. *Biol. Psychiat.,* 21, 23, 1986.
40. Hemmingsen, R., Mogensen, J., Laursen, H., Barry, D., and Ulrichsen, J., Behavioral effects of thiamine deficiency and ethanol intoxication in rats without structural brain lesion. *Scand. J. Lab. Anim. Sci.*, 16, Supplement 1, 63, 1989.
41. Ulrichsen, J., Laursen, H., Mogensen, J., Clemmesen, L., and Hemmingsen, R., Impaired active avoidance performance in thiamine deficient rats without detectable neuropathological changes. *Neurosci. Res. Commun.*, 1, 65, 1987.
42. Ulrichsen, J., Mogensen, J., Lauersen, H., Barry, D., and Hemmingsen, R., Behavioral impairment during thiamine deficiency and ethanol intoxication in rats without detectable neuropathological changes. *Neurosci. Res. Comm.*, 9, 99, 1991.
43. Victor, M., Adams, R. D., and Collins, G.H., *The Wernicke-Korsakoff Syndrome*. F. A. David, Philadelphia, 1971.
44. Morris, R., Developments of a water-maze procedure for studying spatial learning in the rat. *J. Neurosci. Meth.*, 11, 47, 1984.
45. Sanberg, P. R., Neurobehavioral aspects of some animal models of age-related neuropsychiatric disorders, in Fisher, A., Hanin, I., and Lachman, C., Eds., *Alzheimer's and Parkinson's Diseases. Strategies for Research and Development*. Plenum Press, New York, 1986, 479.
46. McGeer, P. L., and McGeer, E. G., Kainic acid: the neurotoxic breakthrough. *CRC Crit. Rev. Toxicol.,* 10, 1, 1982.
47. Chrobak, J. J., Hanin, I., and Walsh, T. J., AF64A (ethylcholine aziridinium ion), a cholinergic neurotoxin, selectively impairs working memory in a multiple component T-maze task. *Brain Res.*, 414, 15, 1987.
48. Chrobak. J. J., Hanin, I., Schmechel, D. E., and Walsh, T. J., AF64A-induced working memory impairment: behavioral, neurochemical and histological correlates. *Brain Res.*, 463, 107, 1988.

49. Beaulieu, M., and Coyle, J. T., Effects of fetal methylazoxymethanol acetate lesion on the synaptic neurochemistry of the adult rat striatum. *J. Neurochem.*, 37, 878, 1981.

50. Johnston, M. V., and Coyle, J. T., Ontogeny of neurochemical markers for noradrenergic, GABAergic, and cholinergic neurons in neocortex lesioned with methylazoxymethanol acetate. *J. Neurochem.*, 34, 1429, 1980.

51. Geoffroy, M., and Mogensen, J., Differential recovery in measures of exploration/locomotion after a single dosage of reserpine in the rat. *Acta Neurobiol. Exper.*, 48, 263, 1988.

52. Mogensen, J., Iversen, I. H., and Divac, I., Neostriatal lesions impaired rats' delayed alternation performance in a T-maze but not in a two-key operant chamber. *Acta Neurobiol. Exper.*, 47, 45, 1987.

53. Kolb, B., and Walkey, J., Behavioural and anatomical studies of the posterior parietal cortex in the rat. *Behav. Brain Res.*, 23, 127, 1987.

54. Kolb, B., Sutherland, R. J., and Whishaw, I. Q., A comparison of the contributions of the frontal and parietal association cortex to spatial localisation in rats. *Behav. Neurosci.*, 97, 13, 1983.

55. Kolb, B., Functions of the frontal cortex of the rat: a comparative review. *Brain Res. Rev.*, 8, 65, 1984.

56. Burns, R. S., Phillips, J. M., Chiueh, C. C., and Parisi, J. E., The MPTP-treated monkey model of Parkinson's disease, in Markey, S. P., Castagnoli, N., Trevor, A. J., and Kopin, I. J., Eds., *MPTP: A Neurotoxin Producing a Parkinsonian Syndrome*. Academic Press, Orlando, 1986, 23.

57. Jenner, P., Rupniak, N. M. J., Rose, S., Kelly, E., Kilpatrick, G., Lees, A., and Marsden, D., Methyl-4-phenyl-1,2,3,6-tetrahydropyridine-induced parkinsonism in the common marmoset. *Neurosci. Lett.*, 50, 85, 1984.

58. Langston, J. W., Forno, L. S., Rebert, C. S., and Irwin, I., Selective nigral toxicity after systemic administration of 1-methyl-4-phenyl-1,2,5,6-tetrahydropyridine (MPTP) in the squirrel monkey. *Brain Res.*, 292, 390, 1984.

59. Heikkila, R. E., Cabbat, F. S., Manzino, L., and Duvoisin, R. C., Effects of 1-methyl-4-phenyl-1,2,5,6-tetrahydropyridine on neostriatal dopamine in mice. *Neuropharmacology*, 3, 711, 1984.

60. Jenner, P., Marsden, C. D., Costall, B., and Naylor, R. J., MPTP and MPP+ induced neurotoxicity in rodents and the common marmoset as experimental models for investigating Parkinson's disease, in Markey, S. P., Castagnoli, N., Trevor, A. J., and Kopin, I. J., Eds., *MPTP: A Neurotoxin Producing a Parkinsonian Syndrome*. Academic Press, Orlando, 1986, 45.

61. Pitts, S. M., Markey, S. P., Murphy, D. L., Weisz, A., and Lunn, G., Recommended practices for the safe handling of MPTP, in Markey, S. P., Castagnoli, N., Trevor, A. J., and Kopin, I. J., Eds., *MPTP: A Neurotoxin Producing a Parkinsonian Syndrome*. Academic Press, Orlando, 1986, 703.

62. Mishkin, M., A memory system in the monkey. *Philosoph. Trans. Royal Soc.*, London, B 298, 85, 1982.

63. Mishkin, M., Malamut, B., and Bachevalier, J., Memories and habits: two neural systems, in Lynch, G., McGaugh, J. L., and Weinberger, N. M., Eds., *Neurobiology of Learning and Memory*. The Guilford Press, New York, 1984, 65.

64. Mishkin, M., and Petri, H.L., Memories and habits: some implications for the analysis of learning and retention, in Squire, L. R., and Butters, N., Eds., *Neuropsychology of Memory*. The Guilford Press, New York, 1984, 287.

65. Thomas, G. J., and Gash, D. M., Mammillothalamic tracts and representational memory. *Behav. Neurosci.*, 99, 621, 1985.

66. Thomas, G. J., and Spafford, P. S., Deficits for representational memory induced by septal and cortical lesions (singly and combined) in rats. *Behav. Neurosci.*, 98, 394, 1984.

67. Kornetsky, C., Animal models: promises and problems, in Hanin, I., and Usdin, E., Eds., *Animal Models in Psychiatry and Neurology*. Pergamon Press, Oxford, 1977, 1.

68. Mogensen, J., and Holm, S., Basic research and animal models in neuroscience-the necessity of "co-evolution". *Scand. J. Lab. Anim. Sci.*, 16, Supplement 1, 51, 1989.

69. McKinney, W. T., Biobehavioural models of depression in monkeys, in Hanin, I., and Usdin, E., Eds., *Animal Models in Psychiatry and Neurology.* Pergamon Press, Oxford, 1977, 117.
70. Leonard, B. E., From animals to man: advantages, problems and pitfalls of animal models in psychopharmacology, in Hindmarch, I., and Stonier, P. D., Eds., *Human Psychopharmacology: Measures and Methods,* Vol. 2, John Wiley and Sons Ltd., 1989, 23.
71. Willner, P., *Depression. A Psychobiological Synthesis.* John Wiley and Sons, New York, 1985.
72. Raz, S., Raz, N., Weinberger, D. R., Boronow, J., Pickar, D., Bigler, E. D., and Turkheimer, E., Morphological brain abnormalities in schizophrenia determined by computed tomography: A problem of measurement? *Psychiat. Res.,* 22, 91, 1987.
73. Weinberger, D. R., Computed tomography (CT) findings in schizophrenia: Speculation on the meaning of it all. *J. Psychiat.Res.,* 18, 477, 1984.
74. Altshuler, L. L., Conrad, A., Kovelman, J. A., and Scheibel, A., Hippocampal pyramidal cell orientation in schizophrenia. *Arch. Gen. Psychiat.,* 44, 1094, 1987.
75. Bogerts, B., Zur Neuropathologie der Schizophrenien. *Fortschr. Neurol. Psychiat.,* 52, 428, 1984.
76. Falkai, P., and Bogerts, B., Cell loss in the hippocampus of schizophrenics. *Euro. Arch. Psychiat. Neurol. Sci.,* 236, 154, 1986.
77. Scheibel, A. B., and Kovelman, J. A., A neurohistological correlate of schizophrenia. *Biol. Psychiat.,* 19, 1601, 1984.
78. Divac, I., Björklund, A., Lindvall, O., and Passingham, R.E., Converging projections from the mediodorsal thalamic nucleus and mesencephalic dopaminergic neurons to the neocortex in three species. *J. Comp. Neurol.,* 180, 59, 1978.
79. Divac, I., Braestrup, C., and Nielsen, M., Distribution of dopamine and serotonin receptors in the monkey cerebral cortex. *Neurosci. Lett.,* Supp. 5, S99, 1980.
80. Ellinwood, E. H., and Kilbey, M.M., Chronic stimulant intoxication models of psychosis, in Hanin, I., and Usdin, E., Eds., *Animal Models in Psychiatry and Neurology.* Pergamon Press, Oxford, 1977, 61.
80a. Glenthøj, B., Mogensen, J., Laursen, H., Holm, S. and Hemmingsen, R., Electrical sensitization of the meso-limbic dopaminergic system in rats: a pathogenetic model for schizophrenia. *Brain Res.,* 619, 39, 1993.
81. Schmajuk, N. A., Animal models for schizophrenia: the hippocampally lesioned animal. *Schizoph. Bull.,* 13, 317, 1987.
82. Collerton, D., Cholinergic function and intellectual decline in Alzheimer's disease. *Neuroscience,* 19, 1, 1986.
83. Francis, P. T., Palmer, A. M., Sims, N. R., Bowen, D. M., Davison, A. N., Esiri, M. M., Neary, D., Snowden, J. S., and Wilcock, G. K., Neurochemical studies of early-onset Alzheimer's disease: possible influence on treatment. *New Engl. J. Med.,* 313, 7, 1985.
84. Perry, E. K., Curtis, M., Dick, D. J., Candy, J. M., Atack, J. R., Bloxham, C. A., Blessed, G., Fairbairn, A., Tomlinson, B. E., and Perry, R. H., Cholinergic correlates of cognitive impairment in Parkinson's disease: comparisons with Alzheimer's disease. J. *Neurol. Neurosurg. Psych.,* 48, 413, 1985.
85. Mann, D. M. A., and Yates, P. O., Serotonergic nerve cells in Alzheimer's disease. *J. Neurol. Neurosurg.Psychiat.,* 46, 96, 1983.
86. Yamamoto, T., and Hirano, A., Nucleus raphe dorsalis in Alzheimer's disease: neurofibrillary tangles and loss of large neurons. A*nn. Neurol.,* 17, 573, 1985.
87. Fisher, A., and Hanin, I., Potential animal models for senile dementia of Alzheimer's type, with emphasis on AF64A-induced cholinotoxicity. *Ann. Rev. Pharmacol. Toxicol.,* 26, 161, 1986.
88. Walsh, T. J., and Emerich, D. R., Transplantation of fetal cholinergic neurons promotes recovery of AF64A-induced behavioral and neurochemical deficits. *Soc. Neurosci. Abstr.,* 15, 1094, 1989.
89. Nilsson, O. G., Strecker, R. E., Daszuta, A., and Björklund, A., Combined cholinergic and serotonergic denervation of the forebrain produces severe deficits in a spatial learning task in the rat. *Brain Res.,* 453, 235, 1988.

Chapter 12

Animal Models in Pain Research

Arne Tjølsen, Kjell Hole, and Steinar Hunskaar

CONTENTS

INTRODUCTION

Pain is defined by the International Association for the Study of Pain (IASP) as "an unpleasant sensory and emotional experience associated with actual or potential tissue damage, or described in terms of such damage".[1] A noxious stimulus is one that is damaging to normal tissue, and a receptor that is preferentially sensitive to a noxious stimulus, or to a stimulus that would become noxious if prolonged, is called a nociceptor. Activity in the nociceptor and nociceptive pathways and other neurophysiological processes induced by a noxious stimulus is called nociception. Many "pain tests" in animals are in fact tests of nociception. Pain is a subjective and personal psychological experience that at best can be measured only indirectly in animals. Analgesia is the absence of pain in response to stimulation that would normally be painful, while hypoalgesia is a diminished response. An increased response to a stimulus that is normally painful, is called hyperalgesia, the basic concept of inflammatory pain.

ANIMALS, NOCICEPTIVE TESTING, AND ETHICS

Over the years, many tests of nociception and pain in animals have been developed, and the species most frequently used in pain research are rats and mice. The use of animals in this research is necessary for several reasons. Since pain is a complex perceptual experience that can be quantified only indirectly in animals, behavioral measures or nociceptive reflexes in intact animals must be evaluated. Many different methods for testing of pain or nociception in animals have been developed (Table 1). Here, a few of the most commonly used methods will be described, which may illustrate important aspects of investigations of pain in animals. Special emphasis will be put on methodological problems in the tests.

137

138

Table 1. Some animal tests for nociception

Tail-flick*	Chemically induced writhing*
Tail pinch	Formalin test*
Hot-plate*	Chemically induced hyperalgesia*
Increasing temperature hot-plate*	Adjuvant monoarthritis
Paw pressure	Adjuvant arthritis*
Flinch-jump	Intrathecal injection of neurotransmitters*

*discussed in this text

While the use of anesthetics and analgesics are standard in invasive biomedical research involving intact animals, analgesics cannot be used in models where behavioral responses to nociceptive stimulation are studied. Therefore, special considerations must be given to the approval of models and protocols for pain research in animals. The type and intensity of noxious stimulation, and the duration of the stimulus, should be thoughtfully examined. In addition to this, the ability of the animal to terminate or limit the noxious stimulus may be an important factor in evaluating the suitability of nociceptive models.

The Committee for Research and Ethical Issues of the International Association for the Study of Pain has published guidelines for investigations of experimental pain in conscious animals (Table 2).[2] Several tests of nociception measuring acute pain at or close to the pain threshold do not pose problems with respect to these guidelines, while there may be difficulties in applying the present guidelines to chronic pain models. It is not always possible to try the pain stimulus on the experimenter himself, and pain relieving agents most often are prone to interfere with the purpose of the experiments. Adequate evaluations of the intensity and duration of pain necessary to achieve the experimental objective are also difficult.[3] It has been difficult to reach a final agreement about the justification of animal models of chronic pain, and the topic will still have to be thoroughly discussed.

NOCICEPTIVE TESTS
Tail-Flick Test

This test was first described 50 years ago,[4] and it is still an extensively used test of nociception in rats and mice. Radiant heat is focused on the tail, and the time it takes until the animal flicks the tail away from the beam is measured. This tail-flick latency is a measure of the nociceptive sensitivity of the animals, and is prolonged for instance by opioid analgesics. A spinal transection above the lumbar level does not block the tail-flick response. Thus, in this test, a spinal nociceptive reflex is measured, and pain is not measured directly. Still, this is considered a very useful test, both in basic pain research and in pharmacological investigations of analgesic drugs.

This may be a good and useful test of nociception, but only if it is carefully performed and possible sources of error are taken into account. A particular problem with tests that use thermal stimulation is the possible influence of the skin temperature. The tail-flick occurs when the temperature at the level of the nociceptors in the skin reaches a critical value. Obviously, the time required for heating the skin to this critical temperature will depend on the initial temperature of the skin, a parameter determined by local blood flow within the limits given by deep body and ambient temperatures. As a consequence, the tail-flick latency is negatively correlated to the ambient temperature.[5] This may be a source of variation in the test results, even within the same laboratory. More important is the fact that many experimental treatments affect blood flow and thereby the tail skin temperature. A reduction in tail skin temperature may be interpreted as analgesia, and an increase in temperature as hyperalgesia.[6] Thus, the reduced tail-flick latency observed after transection of the spinal cord, selective

Table 2. Ethical guidelines for investigations of experimental pain in conscious animals.

1. Experiments must be reviewed by scientists and lay-persons, and the potential benefit must be made clear.
2. If possible, the investigator should try the pain stimulus on himself.
3. A careful assessment of the animal's deviation from normal behavior should be given.
4. A minimal pain stimulus necessary for the purposes of the experiment should be used.
5. Pain relieving agents or procedures should be used, as long as this will not interfere with the aim of the investigation.
6. The duration must be as short as possible, and the number of animals kept to a minimum.

Adapted from Zimmermann, M., *Pain,* 16, 109, 1983.

lesions of raphe-spinal serotonergic systems, or administration of serotonin receptor blocking drugs systemically or intrathecally can be completely accounted for by an increase in skin temperature due to functional impairment of these systems.

The conclusion is that the tail skin temperature is of great importance for the results of the tail-flick test. The problem may be solved by recording the tail skin temperature and correcting the tail-flick latency data for changes in the temperature. For this purpose, a regression analysis or an analysis of covariance may be performed.[6]

Hot-Plate Test

The hot-plate test was described in 1944,[7] and it is one of the most commonly used tests of nociception and analgesia in rodents. Orginally the test measured nociceptive responses of mice placed on the hot-plate at temperatures varying from 55 to 70°C. Later the test was modified, and a constant temperature of about 55°C was used. Subsequently most researchers have used this temperature. Although there is an extensive literature of studies in which the hot-plate test has been used, there is a paucity of work on the methodological aspects of the test.

The latency to various behavioral responses, including jumping, kicking, and dancing, shaking of a foot, holding the foot tightly against the body and licking the forepaw, the hind paw or both, has been used as a measure of pain sensitivity in mice and rats. In recent years, most investigators have employed either forepaw or hindpaw lick as the end-point. These responses occur in nearly all animals, licking the forepaw usually preceding the hind paw lick.

At a temperature of 55°C, the analgesic effects of morphine and other opiate analgesics are easily identified and quantified in the hot-plate test. However, at this temperature narcotic antagonists and non-narcotic analgesics have no or only weak antinociceptive effects. Various modifications have been made in order to detect the activities of such drugs. When the temperature is reduced to 50°C or lower, the analgesic effects may be detectable, but the variability may be increased so that statistical analysis may be made difficult.[8]

In addition to sensitivity problems, the variability of the results is a major difficulty with the hot-plate test. The response latencies of control animals vary considerably between different research reports, even from the same laboratory.

Increasing Temperature Hot-Plate Test

The increasing temperature hot-plate test[9,10] has several advantages compared to the conventional hot-plate test. In this test, the temperature of the plate is set below pain threshold, and the temperature is gradually increased until a response is observed. The temperature of the plate when the response occurs is recorded as the nociceptive end-point. The licking of a hind paw may be used as the response recorded. Forepaw lick may be a part of heat dissipating mechanisms, and should not be used as an end-point.

The increasing temperature hot-plate test may be performed using a conventional hot-plate that is turned on at a plate temperature of 42 to 43°C, the temperature increasing gradually until the nociceptive response is observed, or a cut-off temperature (50 to 52°C) is reached.

The hot-plate test also involves a thermal stimulus, and the constant temperature hot-plate test may pose problems similar to the tail-flick test, in that the skin temperature may possibly influence the results. In the increasing temperature hot-plate test this problem is reduced, since the end point is the plate temperature when a hind paw lick occurs, regardless of the time it takes before the response occurs. This test will therefore be less, if at all, influenced by the pretest skin temperature. The test has been shown to be more sensitive than the traditional hot-plate test, for instance when studying the analgesic effect of mild analgesics.[9] The nociceptive threshold in this test is similar to that found using other methods.

Chemically Induced Writhing

In this widely used test, the intraperitoneal injection of an irritant induces a syndrome called "writhing", which consists of contractions of the abdomen, twisting and turning of the trunk, and extension of the hind limbs. Several compounds have been shown to elicit this syndrome, such as phenylquinone,[11] acetic acid,[12] bradykinin and acetylcholine, to mention a few. In recent years acetic acid and phenylquinone have been used most frequently. Administration of relatively small doses of non-narcotic drugs, especially the non-steroid anti-inflammatory drugs, abolishes the writhing syndrome in a dose dependent manner. The test is commonly employed as a screening method because of its simplicity and sensitivity.

The main disadvantage of this method is its lack of specificity, as many drugs without certain analgesic effects in humans can effectively inhibit the writhing response.[13] In addition, there is a large variation in the response between mouse strains; ED_{50} values for acetylsalicylic acid have been found to vary from 50 to 200 mg/kg.[14]

The mechanism of the syndrome is not known, but many mediators have been proposed. No significant differences were detected in histamine, serotonin, or prostaglandin content of peritoneal fluid from writhing (using phenylquinone) and control mice, while other reports indicate involvement of the prostaglandin system in writhing induced by at least some irritants. It has been claimed that different irritants may be considered as models of different pain reactions, e.g., distinguishing between inflammatory and non-inflammatory pain.

The writhing test is most widely applied in mice, but it has also been used in a few studies in rats. The test is simple to perform, is sensitive, and is therefore preferred in many laboratories. However, because of the poor specificity, the results of this test should be interpreted with caution.

Formalin Test

In the formalin test,[15] diluted formalin is injected subcutaneously in a paw, and nociceptive behavior (in mice and rats for instance licking and biting of the injected paw) is measured. Two phases of the response are observed: an early phase starting immediately after injection and lasting for 5 to 10 min, and a late phase 15 to 60 min after injection.[16] While the stimulus for the early phase is a direct chemical stimulation of the nociceptors, the stimulus for the late phase involves inflammation. In addition, the response in the late phase is dependent on changes in processing of the information in the spinal cord, due to the afferent barrage during the early phase.[17] It is an interesting aspect of this test that two principally different stimuli are employed in the same test, with the possibility to study different analgesic effects of a drug in the two phases of the test. It may also be claimed that this test is a better model of clinical pain than the hot-plate and tail-flick tests.

It has recently been shown that in mice, the late phase is very sensitive to changes both in ambient temperature and to drugs and lesions that influence peripheral blood flow and skin temperature.[18] Hence, also in the formalin test changes in blood flow and skin temperature may be interpreted in terms of analgesia or hyperalgesia. Drugs may influence blood flow as a "side effect", and CNS lesions and stress may also affect peripheral blood flow. For studies of the late phase, which is most commonly studied, it may be recommended to use ambient temperatures that are not too low (above 23°C) and formalin concentrations of 1 to 5 % (0.4 to 2 % formaldehyde). The early phase seems not to be sensitive to moderate changes in ambient temperature, and in this phase the use of lower concentrations of formalin (0.02 to 0.1 % formaldehyde) may increase the possibility of observing an increase as well as an attenuation of the response.[19,20] These recommendations are clearly valid for mice, and although the role of skin temperature in the formalin test has not been investigated in rats, it is likely that similar mechanisms may apply in this species.

Rats show a more complex behavioral response than mice in this test. The method of scoring the behavioral response in rats is usually an adaptation of the original method described by Dubuisson and Dennis.[16] A rating scale is used for different behaviors, and a total pain rating is calculated with the ratings weighted according to the time spent in each rating category. The main assumption made is that the animal has a one-dimensional nociceptive experience, and that each behavioral category adds to this experience. However, pain in animals as well as in humans may rather be a multidimensional perceptual experience. Different behaviors displayed by the animal may express different aspects of nociception, and not necessarily only different intensities of one nociceptive modality. The importance of observing the integrated motor performance when evaluating the complex perception of pain in animals has been emphasized.[21] For this type of data, the adequate treatment may be a multivariate statistical analysis.[22] This type of analysis may also make it possible to separate nociceptive and non-nociceptive (for instance motor) behavioral changes, improving both the amount and the relevance of the information obtained from the data in future studies.

Chemically Induced Hyperalgesia

In rats, subcutaneous injections of carrageenan or yeast cause localized inflammation. Pressure is applied to the inflamed area by means of a metal cylinder and the force at which the animals begin to vocalize or struggle is recorded. Several modifications of the test have been described.[23,24] Drugs can be administered before, at the time of, or after the injection of the inducing agent. Edema and hyperalgesia do not seem to be correlated in this model. The contralateral, non-injected paw may be used as a control. Thus, the test has been used to distinguish between drugs acting in the CNS and locally at the site of inflammation. The test is sensitive to the non-narcotic analgesics and is relatively simple to perform.

Carrageenan or uric acid injected intra-articularly in the knee or ankle joint of rats induces a monoarthritis, with dysfunction that lasts 2 to 3 days. The dysfunction, protective ("nocifensive") behavior, and hyperalgesia may be used as models of joint pain.[25,26]

Adjuvant-Induced Arthritis

Intradermal injection of heat-killed Mycobacterium tuberculosis in Freund's complete adjuvant into the tail of rats induces polyarthritis.[27] This disease in rats shows many similarities to various human arthritic conditions, and most anti-inflammatory drugs are effective in adjuvant arthritis. The drugs have the same rank order of potency as in humans,[28] and results from the test are predictive for the effect of such agents in humans.

In this chronic model, the stimuli are tonic rather than phasic in nature. Thus, the model may elucidate possible changes in neurochemistry, metabolism, and drug tolerance in test animals compared to normal animals. However, the animals suffer from an immunological disease that does not necessarily reflect all chronic pain conditions. Drug effects are usually measured as the amount of foot swelling and this may not be indicative of nociception. The vocalization response induced by manipulation of the tarso-tibial joint has been used to indicate the nociceptive threshold. Simultaneous measurement of edema (paw volume) and recording of vocalizations have also been claimed to separate anti-inflammatory from antinociceptive activity of drugs.

Intrathecal Injection of Nociceptive Neurotransmitters

The excitatory amino acids glutamate and aspartate and the neuropeptide substance P are important neurotransmitters in primary sensory nociceptive neurons. If these substances, or capsaicin releasing substance P, are injected intrathecally in the lumbar region in rats or mice, biting and scratching directed towards the caudal part of the body occur.[29] In this way, a centrally induced state of pain may be studied, and it may be possible to investigate central as opposed to peripheral effects of analgesic drugs.

MODELS OF NOCICEPTION IN TISSUE PREPARATION OR IN ANESTHETIZED ANIMALS

Although the concept of pain can only be studied by means of behavioral measures in awake, intact animals, important elements of the nociceptive systems may be studied in preparations where the animals cannot experience pain. The responses of neurons to noxious stimulation of peripheral tissues have been studied in several areas of the CNS: in the spinal cord, the brain stem, the thalamus, and the cerebral cortex. Electrical recordings can be made from neurons in all these areas in intact, anesthetized animals, and their response to noxious stimulation and pharmacological treatment may be investigated. From the spinal cord, tissue slices can be prepared with intact dorsal roots, in such a way that the response of neurons in the dorsal horn to stimulation of the root may be subject to study.

SOME COMPARATIVE ASPECTS OF TESTS OF NOCICEPTION

Fundamental functions of the nervous system of animals are to detect and avoid noxious stimuli. It is, therefore, not surprising that similar regulatory systems for nociception are found over a wide range of animal species. The vast majority of studies of nociception has been performed in rodents, and hence the knowledge of systems involved in nociception and nociceptive signal processing are based on these species. Other species have occasionally been used; the formalin test was originally described in cats as well as in rats, and it has been adapted also for monkeys.

Some focus has been put on the advantages of utilizing non-mammalian species, in that these are lower on the phylogenetic spectrum.[30] It has been assumed that reptiles and amphibia have less capacity to experience pain or distress than mammals. In the crocodile, however, both the hot-plate and the formalin tests have been shown to be useful tests of nociception, and in these tests, crocodiles were also very sensitive to the analgesic effect of morphine.[31] Crocodiles also showed a marked nociceptive response to instillations into the eye of diluted capsaicin, unlike birds and amphibians.

Several amphibian models of nociception have been described, and it has generally been difficult to show antinociceptive effects of reasonable doses of opioids. However, a model using cutaneous application of various concentrations of acetic acid in frogs has been developed,[30] and in this model, opioid analgesia seems to be more conveniently studied. The model involves the application of progressively higher concentrations of acetic acid on the hind limb, and the end-point is defined as the concentration that elicits a characteristic wiping response.

SUMMARY

By definition, pain is a psychological experience.[1] In animals, pain can at best be assessed indirectly, by behavioral measures. Investigation of behavioral responses in animals is an important and necessary part of the study of pain, and this type of research necessitates the use of intact, unanesthetized animals. Animal models of pain pose ethical problems, and ethical guidelines have been recommended by the International Association for the Study of Pain (Table 2). Parts of the nociceptive systems may also be studied in animal preparations, both in anesthetized animals and in *in vitro* preparations.

REFERENCES

1. Merskey, M., Pain terms: a list with definitions and notes on usage. Recommended by the IASP Subcommittee on Taxonomy, *Pain, 6, 249, 1979.*
2. Zimmermann, M., Ethical guidelines for investigations of experimental pain in conscious animals, *Pain, 16, 109, 1983.*
3. Roberts, V.J., Ethical issues in the use of animals for pain research. In Chapman CR, Loeser JD (eds): *Advances in Pain Research and Therapy, Vol. 12.* Raven Press, New York, 1989.
4. D'Amour, F.E., Smith, D.L., A method for determining loss of pain sensation, *J. Pharmacol. Exp. Ther., 72, 74, 1941.*
5. Berge, O-G., Garcia-Cabrera, I., Hole, K., Response latencies in the tail-flick test depend on tail skin temperature. *Neurosci. Lett., 86, 284, 1988.*
6. Tjølsen, A., Lund, A., Berge, O-G., Hole, K., An improved method for tail flick testing with adjustment for tail skin temperature. *J. Neurosci. Meth., 26, 259, 1989.*
7. Woolfe, G., MacDonald, A.D., The evaluation of analgesic action of pethidine hydrochloride (demerol), *J. Pharmacol. Exp. Ther. 80, 300, 1944.*
8. Taber, R.I., Predictive value of analgesic assays in mice and rats. pp. 191–211. In Braude MC, Harris LS, May EL, Smith JP, Villarreal JE (eds): *Narcotic Antagonists. Advances in Biochemical Psychopharmacology, Vol. 8.* Raven Press, New York, 1974.
9. Hunskaar, S., Berge, O-G., Hole, K., A modified hot-plate test sensitive to mild analgesics, *Behav. Brain Res., 21, 101, 1986.*
10. Tjølsen, A., Rosland, J.H., Berge, O-G., Hole, K., The increasing temperature hot plate test: an improved test of nociception in mice and rats. *J. Pharmacol. Meth., 25, 241, 1991.*
11. Siegmund, E., Cadmus, R., Lu, G., A method for evaluating both non-narcotic and narcotic analgesics. *Proc. Soc. Exptl. Biol. Med., 95, 729, 1957.*
12. Koster, R., Anderson, M., deBeer, E.J., Acetic acid for analgesic screening. *Fed. Proc., 18: 412, 1959.*
13. Chernov, H.I., Wilson, D.E., Fowler, F., Plummer, A.J., Non-specificity of the mouse writhing test, *Arch. Int. Pharmacodyn., 167, 171, 1967.*
14. Brown, D.M., Hughes, B.O., Practical aspects of strain variation in relation to pharmacological testing. *Pharmac. Pharmacol., 14, 399, 1962.*
15. Tjølsen, A., Berge, O-G., Hunskaar, S., Rosland, J.H., Hole, K., The formalin test: an evaluation of the method, Review article. *Pain, 51, 5, 1992.*
16. Dubuisson, D., Dennis, S.G., The formalin test: a quantitative study of the analgesic effects of morphine, meperidine, and brain stem stimulation in rats and cats. *Pain, 4, 161, 1977.*
17. Coderre, T.J., Vaccarino, A.L., Melzack, R., Central nervous system plasticity in the tonic pain response to subcutaneous formalin injection. *Brain Res., 535, 158, 1990.*
18. Rosland, J.H., The formalin test in mice: the influence of ambient temperature. *Pain, 45, 211, 1991.*
19. Shibata, M., Ohkubo, T., Takahashi, H., Inoki, R., Modified formalin test: characteristic biphasic pain response. *Pain, 38, 347, 1989.*

20. Rosland, J.H., Tjølsen, A., Mæhle, B., Hole, K., The formalin test in mice – effect of formalin concentration. *Pain, 42, 235, 1990.*
21. Chapman, C. R., Dubner, R., Foley, K.M., Gracely, R.H., Reading, A. E., Pain measurement: an overview. *Pain, 22, 1, 1985.*
22. Tjølsen, A., Berge, O-G., Hole, K., Lesions of bulbo-spinal serotonergic or noradrenergic pathways reduce nociception as measured by the formalin test. *Acta Physiol. Scand., 142, 229, 1991.*
23. Randall, L.O., Selitto, J.J., A method for measurement of analgesic activity on inflamed tissue. *Arch. Int. Pharmacodyn., 111, 409, 1957.*
24. Vinegar, R., Truax, J.F., Selph, J.L., Quantitative comparison of the analgesic and antiinflammatory activities of aspirin, phenacetin and acetaminophen in rodents. *Eur. J. Pharmacol., 37, 23, 1976.*
25. Okuda, K., Nakahama, H., Miyakawa, H., Shima, K., Arthritis induced in cat by sodium urate: a possible animal model for tonic pain. *Pain, 18, 287, 1984.*
26. Coderre, T.J., Wall, P.D., Ankle joint urate arthritis (AJUA) in rats: an alternative animal model of arthritis to that produced by Freund's adjuvant. *Pain, 28, 379, 1987.*
27. Costa, M. de C., Sutter, P., Gybels, J., van Hess, J., Adjuvant-induced arthritis in rats: a possible animal model of chronic pain. *Pain, 10, 175, 1981.*
28. Pircio, A.W., Fedele, C.T., Bierwagen, M.E., A new method for the evaluation of analgesic activity using adjuvant-induced arthritis in the rat. *Eur. J. Pharmacol., 31, 205, 1975.*
29. Aanonsen, L.M., Wilcox, G.L., Nociceptive action of excitatory amino acids in the mouse: Effects of spinally administered opioids, phencyclidine and sigma agonists. *J. Pharmacol. Exp. Ther., 243, 9, 1987.*
30. Stevens, C.W., Alternatives to the use of mammals for pain research. *Life Sci., 50, 901, 1992.*
31. Kanui, T.I., Hole, K., Miaron, J.O., Nociception in crocodiles — capsaicin instillation, formalin and hot plate tests. *Zool. Sci., 7, 534, 1990.*

Chapter 13

Animal Models in Virology

Hans Mogens Kerzel Andersen

CONTENTS

INTRODUCTION

Animals were widely used in virology before viruses could be cultivated in cell cultures. Often viral diseases were diagnosed by transmitting the disease to laboratory animals; for instance, material from herpes simplex virus lesions was inoculated into mice or rabbit's eyes. Similarly, many vaccines were produced by infecting animals and harvesting virus from lesions or organs. This was the case with vaccinia virus produced in the skin of young calves after scarification of the skin and infection with vaccinia virus. Foot-and-mouth-disease vaccine was produced in cows in a similar way by harvesting viruses from infected tongue epithelium and other lesions in experimentally infected animals.

After the introduction of modern techniques for cultivating viruses for diagnostic, serological, and vaccine purposes, animals were only used for cultivation of a very few species of viruses that still cannot be propagated in tissue culture. An example is chicken embryos for isolation and vaccine production of influenza virus. A substantial number of animals are, however, still used for safety testing of vaccines and in model studies of the pathogenesis of viral diseases.

As it is not possible to cover the more than thousand known viruses that can infect humans and animals, this chapter will focus on a few, but very important viruses of current interest, namely cytomegalovirus, human immunodeficiency virus, the cause of AIDS, and the agent of transmissible spongiform encephalopathy, although the exact nature of the filtrable agent responsible for this disease is still not known.

GUINEA PIG AND MOUSE CYTOMEGALOVIRUS INFECTION

Human cytomegalovirus (HCMV) belongs to the ß-herpes virus group, the members of which are characterized by being very host-restricted, slow growing-viruses causing a wide range of diseases. The infected cells frequently become enlarged, containing a Cowdry type A nuclear inclusion — "cytomegalic cells". The latent infection is usually lifelong and can be reactivated during immunosuppression.

Although most human infections with HCMV are asymptomatic, a febrile infection, CMV-Mononucleosis, resembling Infectious Mononucleosis or kissing disease caused by Epstein-Barr virus, can be seen after a primary HCMV infection. This is a self-limiting disease in immunocompetent individuals, but severe and sometimes fatal infections occur in immuno-suppressed patients after organ and bone-marrow transplantation (BMT) and in AIDS. These infections are seen in connection with primary as well as reactivated HCMV infections, but at least in kidney transplant patients they are often a result of superinfection with a new strain of HCMV. The symptoms in these patients include fever, lymphadenopathy, interstitial pneumonia, diarrhea (gastro-intestinal ulcerative disease), and CMV retinitis. The importance of CMV infections in these patients is well-documented: in one study 20% of bone marrow transplant patients died of CMV pneumonitis.[1] CMV retinitis is a severe complication in AIDS patients, often causing impaired vision or even blindness.

Due to a primary infection or reactivated infection of the mother, the fetus can be infected with HCMV. About 0.5 to 2.5% of all babies are born with congenital CMV infection causing mild or severe symptoms in about 10% of the infected infants. The severe symptoms may be hepato-splenomegali, bleedings and encephalitis (microcephaly), and hearing defects.

Infections with HCMV in immunocompetent patients do not call for specific antiviral treatment. Nucleoside analogues like ganciclovir and foscovir are used in the treatment of the most severe diseases such as retinitis and interstitial pneumonitis in immunosuppressed patients. Unfortunately, treatment has to be repeated or continued for the rest of the patient´s life because virus synthesis and cell destruction appear in many patients after discontinuation of the treatment.

The species specificity of HCMV prevents the study of this virus in animals and necessi-tates appropriate animal models. A great variety of animal species become infected with their own specific cytomegaloviruses. Most model studies have been performed in mice and guinea pigs using mouse cytomegalovirus (MCMV) and guinea pig cytomegalovirus (GPCMV), respectively. Both viruses cause tissue lesions with formation of characteristic cytomegalic cells; hence, these models can be studied using light microscopy, electron microscopy as well as isolation of virus in tissue culture.

THE GUINEA PIG MODEL

Cytomegalic cells were recognized in the salivary gland of naturally infected guinea pigs as early as 1920.[2] The cells resembled cells found in humans, but at that time they were thought to be of a parasitic nature. Cole and Kuttner performed transmission experiments between guinea pigs using gland homogenates and suggested in 1926 that these cells had a viral etiology as the lesion resembled herpes simplex lesions in humans and the agent could pass bacteria-tight filters.[3] In 1957, Hartley et al. succeeded in isolating a virus from infected guinea pig salivary glands.[4] Since then, most experiments have been performed with this strain of GPCMV, being propagated by transmission in animals and harvested from salivary glands (GPCMV-SG) or being passaged in tissue culture (GPCMV-TC). The method for virus production is very important for the outcome of the experiments. GPCMV-SG and GPCMV harvested from lungs of animals with pneumonia are more virulent and produce more specific lesions than GPCMV produced in tissue culture. After a number of passages in tissue culture, GPCMV become more or less attenuated and hence less pathogenic. This type of virus has been used in vaccine studies.

A comparison of GPCMV and HCMV DNAs reveals similarities and differences. DNA from the two viruses are similar in size and G+C content and, indeed, there is some DNA homology between the two DNAs. GPCMV DNA, however, is considerably less complex than that of HCMV.[5] Middelkamp et al. studied the morphogenesis of GPCMV in salivary gland cells and in embryonic guinea pig tissue culture cells and found that nucleocapsids are produced in the cell nucleus and the viral envelope is achieved by passing the nucleolemma.[6] Interestingly, they also noted membrane-bound electron-dense bodies containing amorphous material within the cell cytoplasm. These "dense bodies", also seen in human embryonic cells infected with HCMV, are free of infectious virus, but contain viral antigens.[7] They are interesting candidates for vaccine production. GPCMV can cause lytic as well as non-lytic cell infection depending on the cell type infected. During lytic infection, the whole virus genome is expressed, resulting in production of all viral antigens and infective viral particles. In non-lytic infection, the virus genome is only partly expressed, and infective particles are not produced. Thus, the infection can only be traced by testing for GPCMV genome or GPCMV antigens.

The immune system reacts in a classical manner to CMV infection with production of humorally and cellularly mediated immunity. Based on experiments, Andrews was able to show in 1930 that serum from immune animals contained virus neutralizing antibodies that could neutralize the infectious agent before inoculation into animals.[8] Passive immunization by injecting serum containing neutralizing antibodies, however, could not protect animals from infection by challenge. The outcome of the infection is dependent on the cellular immune system, but the humoral immune system may be important and it also participates in the eradication of virus and virus infected cells.

Animals may be infected by different routes, intratracheally, subcutaneously, intravenously, and intraperitoneally. During the second week after subcutaneous inoculation, animals become viremic, with the virus initially located in the serum, later associated to leukocytes. During the viremia, virus is spread to cells in different organs such as brain, kidney, liver, lung, pancreas, spleen, thymus, and salivary gland. The severity of infectious lesions is dependent not only on the type of virus used for infection (GPCMV-SG vs. GPCMV-TC), the size of the inoculum, and the strain of guinea pigs, but also on the route of inoculation. For details, see Bia et al.[9] The virus may be cleared from blood and the various organs after some weeks, but may persist for months or even years, especially in salivary glands as is the case with human CMV infection. The infection may be transmitted by blood with a low level of virus not detectable by co-cultivation. This is also well-known in human CMV infection, but the transmission is prevented by transfusion of leukocyte-depleted blood.

A disease resembling CMV-Mononucleosis in humans can be experimentally induced in guinea pigs. During acute infection, the hematopoietic and lymphoid systems of the animals are involved, resulting in anemia, leukopenia and relative lymphocytosis. Also, atypical lymphocytes are often visualized in the peripheral blood of these animals.[10] An important finding during these experiments, and of major diagnostic importance for the human CMV infection, was the recovering of GPCMV from citrated as opposed to heparinized blood. Like in humans, virus can persist in some subsets of blood cells for months and is often recoverable from the spleen, lymph nodes, bone marrow, and thymus. The reaction to the infection can be visualized histopathologically in lymph nodes in which germinal centers with B-cells are developed. Likewise, an increase in T cell-dependent periarteriolar sheets can be observed. During infections, granulocyte functions are restrained. Thus, this model might offer some clues to the understanding of alterations in host defence mechanisms that predispose to bacterial, parasitic, and fungal superinfection being so important for the CMV infection in immunosuppressed patients.

Studies of GPCMV infection in pregnant guinea pigs have shown that the placenta is infected during the viremic phase and its role in determining the outcome of fetal CMV infection was assessed by Griffith and Hsiung.[11] As great similarities between the human and guinea pig placental structures are seen, it is not surprising that placental infection results in transmission to the fetus, from which GPCMV can be isolated. This model can also be used to study the pathogenesis of CMV infection in the auditory system, since it has been shown that a significant number of congenitally infected guinea pigs develop significant auditory defects.[12] Within the inner ear, GPCMV infection can be localized in auditory nerve spiral ganglion cells, endothelial cells, and cochlear cells. Infection of female guinea pigs also results in increased cervical excretion of GPCMV during pregnancy as seen in pregnant women with CMV infection.

THE MURINE MODEL

A comprehensive review of this model has been given by Hudson.[13] In many respects, good agreement is seen between findings in the mouse and guinea pig models, but at least in one field differences have been found relating to variations in the cellular structure of the placentas of the two species. The barrier between the circulatory systems of the mother and the mouse fetus is thicker than in guinea pigs. Congenital infection in mice is therefore difficult to produce, unless pregnant animals are infected *in utero*.[14] Using this non-physiological route of infection, it is of course possible to infect embryos and obtain pathological lesions, but abortion and stillbirth can also be seen after infection of pregnant mice by other routes. However, as mouse cytomegalovirus (MCMV) can only very rarely be isolated from or demonstrated in the outcome of the pregnancy, it may be assumed that the findings are more likely caused by nutritional deprivation than by transmission of MCMV to the fetuses.

The mouse model has given valuable information on the influence of genetically determined factors of MCMV infection. Mice of the $H-2^b$ and $H-2^d$ haplotypes appear to have the highest rate of lesions, correlating with high virus titres and high mortality. However, genes outside the H-2 complex also contribute to the detailed histopathology. More resistant strains like $H-2^k$ only show scattered foci of infection, which are resolved sooner after infection.[13]

It was first determined in the mouse model that CMV-infected animals had reduced responsiveness to foreign antigens or interferon-inducing agents, explaining perhaps the higher susceptibility of CMV-infected patients to infection with fungi, protozoa, and bacteria.[15] The murine model also offers possibilities to study the effect of various reactivation stimuli on latently infected animal. In mice as well as in humans, cortisone can reactivate latent infections and suppress inflammatory cell responses resulting in expanding areas of inflammation and higher mortality.[1,16]

Studies of the two models of HCMV infection performed *in vivo* as well as *in vitro* have offered much information on the pathogenesis of CMV infections. Much of this information has also been of practical importance for management of human infections and for diagnostic procedures.[17]

INFECTION WITH AIDS VIRUS IN MICE, MONKEYS, AND CHIMPANZEES

The recent epidemic of AIDS caused by the human immunodeficiency viruses HIV-1 and HIV-2 is well-known. Although the spread of the infection initially occurred only among homosexual men and drug addicts due to sexual practice or blood injections, the infection is now a threat to heterosexual men and women as well as to children, since millions of people have been infected during the decade this disease has been on the scene. Therefore, we can expect to see the number of cases continuing to grow, not only in western countries where the epidemic was first recognized, but also in developing countries in Africa and Asia, where protection is uncommon or difficult to practise. Thus, already in 1990 in sub-Saharan Africa, 1 out of every 50 men and women was thought to be infected, and in some African countries as many as 30% of pregnant women are HIV-1 seropositive.[18] As the two human viruses cannot provoke disease in animals, although chimpanzees can be subclinically infected, much interest has been concentrated on studies of simian immunodeficiency virus (SIV), which is believed to be the ancestor of HIV.

HIV and related viruses like SIV are retroviruses related to lentiviruses, which cause maedi/visna in sheep, caprine arthritis in goats, and infectious equine anemia in horses. The functions required by the virus are encoded in an RNA genome, situated in the core of the virus particle together with the core proteins, including the group antigens and an enzyme — reverse transcriptase — able to produce DNA copies of RNA. The core is surrounded by a lipid membrane to which the envelope glycoproteins (gp) gp 160, gp 120, and gp 41 are attached.

The virus genome encodes other proteins including the regulatory proteins *tat, nef,* and *rev*. There are great antigenic variations between strains. HIV can infect cells expressing the CD4 molecule on their surface, mainly CD4 positive lymphocytes and macrophages.

SIV has been isolated from various species of monkeys, but the African green monkey is apparently the natural host of SIV as more than 30 to 70% of wild green African monkeys are seropositive.[19] As they do not show any signs of disease, it looks as if SIV in this species of monkey is well-adapted. Transmission of SIV to other monkeys, macaques and rhesus, by injection or accidently by bites, can provoke a lethal disease like AIDS in humans, called simian AIDS (SAIDS).

SIV is approximately 50% related to HIV at the nucleotid sequence level. The organization of structural and regulatory genes is virtually identical in SIV and HIV. The two diseases are both characterized by depletions of CD4-lymphocytes with ensuing immunosuppression and opportunistic infections. Serological cross-reaction occurs between the two viruses, as infected monkeys and AIDS patients develop cross-reacting antibodies against the highly conserved proteins of the inner core of the two viruses (p55 and p24). Humans also produce antibodies against HIV envelope glycoproteins (gp 160 and 120) and monkeys against the homologous SIV glycoproteins, but without cross-reactivity. As the retroviruses are known for their ability by mutations to change the amino acids of the envelope-proteins, this is not a drawback for the simian model. The ability to mutate is a trick that many parasites (viruses, worms) use to overcome the host's specific immunoreactive T-lymphocytes. Fortunately, antigen instability has not been typical of infections like polio and other infectious diseases that can be controlled by vaccination. This mode of escaping the immune reaction occurring in the host is very important for the pathogenesis of HIV infection and stresses the difficulties in producing an effective vaccine.

By studying mutant strains of SIV in which the regulatory gene *nef* is not transcribed, it was found that these mutant strains could infect monkeys without causing SAIDS, whereas those infected with the parent strain containing *nef* with full expression died from SAIDS. Thus, in this model af AIDS, *nef* seems to be necessary for full pathogenesis. Transfer of human cytotoxic T-lymphocytes specific for *nef* peptides confers partial protection against HIV-1. These interesting observations are in conflict with earlier *in vitro* studies showing that *nef* could down-regulate HIV gene expression. The findings emphasize the importance of animal model studies.[20]

Another genetic determinant of replicative efficiency is the viral long terminal repeat (LTR). This part of the HIV genome has been studied *in vitro*, but it is necessary as with *nef* to use a simian model to determine which LTR sequences govern transcription *in vivo*, and particularly to study the interaction with other viruses like cytomegalovirus in the host.

Another animal gaining in popularity is the SCID mouse with reconstituted immunity based on injection of human fetal lever, bone marrow, or peripheral blood mononuclear cells (PBMC). The mouse reconstituted with PBMC can be infected with a low inoculum of HIV and provides a convenient model for studying prototype vaccines. Thus, partial protection against challenge with HIV was seen in SCID mice reconstituted with PBMCs from healthy human volunteers vaccinated with a vaccinia-virus coding for HIV gp160. Unfortunately, however, the protection did not correlate to the level of neutralizing antibody detected in volunteers.[20]

News concerning gp160 is not all gloomy, though. Thus, chimpanzees vaccinated with recombinant gp120, but not with gp160, were protected against challenge.[21]

The unique property of HIV of escaping immune surveillance by changing amino acids in the envelope proteins has initiated studies of the antigenic importance of peptides as vaccine constituents. The third hypervariable domain (V3) of the HIV-1 envelope gp120 has interesting immunogenic properties. The domain is constructed as a loop consisting of 30 amino acids, which bind and elicit anti-HIV-1 type specific virus-neutralizing antibodies. Protection of chimpanzees against HIV-1 persistent infection seems to correlate with the presence of anti-V3 domain antibody. Protection of chimpanzees against challenge with HIV using a V3 domain specific monoclonal antibody supports efforts to develop vaccine immunogens designed to induce broad reactive anti-V3 loop antibodies.[22] Time will show whether such immunogens may be active not only in preventing infection in high risk groups but also in serving as post infection immuno-prophylactic agents. The problem today and in the future is not only to prevent the spread of AIDS by vaccination, but also to find better and cheaper methods than the present chemotherapy to treat HIV-infected patients before they develop AIDS. Post-exposure vaccination can prevent development of a disease like rabies, where post-exposure vaccination is the specific treatment to avoid clinical symptoms and death.

It will probably still take some years before an effective HIV vaccine will appear on the market. A major problem in designing an effective vaccine is that T-cell depletion in AIDS is not understood. As only a very small proportion of CD4 cells (1:10,000) is actually infected during HIV infection, it is not conceivable that the T-cell depletion is merely due to direct viral cell lysis. Several theories have been brought up to explain the tremendous loss of T-cells. Recently, it has been proposed that a superantigen encoded by HIV may cause the progressive immune cell depletion that leads to collapse of the patients´ immune system.[23] This opens up further studies in animals.

TRANSMISSIBLE SPONGIFORM ENCEPHALOPATHIES IN ANIMALS AND HUMANS

In 1986, a bovine spongiform encephalopathy (BSE) in dairy cattle, "mad cow disease", was identified in England and since then an epidemic of this disease has developed. More than 50,000 cases in more than 12,000 herds have been diagnosed. Although a reduction in the number of cases is expected, this epidemic has renewed the interest in transmissible spongiform encephalopathies. Several comprehensive reviews of this disease and related diseases like Scrapie in sheep, transmissible mink encephalopathy, and the human counterparts, Kuru, Creutzfeldt-Jacob Disease (CJD) and Gerstmann-Sträussler Syndrome (GSS) have been published recently.[24]

In spite of a long history of intense investigation, the transmissible spongiform encephalopathies remain a poorly understood family of neuro-degenerative diseases. Transmission between humans was originally recognized in the unique epidemiology of Kuru in New Guinea tribesmen, where the disease was related to ingestion of organs and brains from diseased family members.[25] Cessation of the practice of ritual cannibalism as a rite of mourning and respect for dead kinsmen stopped the transmission to new members of the tribe, although new cases continue to appear because the incubation period of transmissible spongiform encephalopathies is in the order of 1 to >30 years. Since the beginning of Kuru investigations in 1956, over 2,500 cases have been recorded. Kuru mortality has declined continuously and the disease no longer appears in younger people. Now only 5 to 10 patients all over 35 years of age still die of the disease every year.

The precise nature of the agents of these diseases remains unknown, although it is clear they resemble each other, if they are not identical. The agents are filtrable, but morphologically not like classical viruses. Thus far, infectivity can only be assayed by serial transmission to new individuals of the same species or other species ranging from mice to monkeys and chimpanzees. The list of animals in Table 1 to which the various spongiform encephalopathies can be transmitted is not complete. Due to problems with interspecies transmission, only a few animal models have been tested. Firstly, the incubation period for the first transmission from one species to another is usually very long compared with later passages, and often survivors are seen. Secondly, interspecies barriers exist. Thus, it has not been possible to transmit Scrapie to mice from infected mink brains although minks are infected by ingestion of food

Table 1. Animal models in transmissible spongiform encephalogpathies

Disease	Natural host	Transmission	Epidemiological pattern	Transmissible to:
Scrapie	Sheep Goats	Vertical and via ingestion of fetal membranes	Endemic in most countries	Goats, mice, Syrian Hamsters
Transmissible mink encepha-lopathy	Mink	Via ingestion of food containing sheep carcases	Sporadic	Monkeys, sheep, goats, ferrets (not to mice)
Bovine spongiform encephalopathy	Cattle and some zoo ruminants	Via improper sterilized meat and bone meal produced on sheep carcases	Sporadic	Mice, cats, pigs
Kuru	Humans	Via ritual cannibalistic consumption of dead relatives	Endemic in New Guinea	Chimpanzees, monkeys, goats, minks, and ferrets
Creutzfeldt-Jakob disease	Humans	Iatrogenic, familial	Sporadic (incidence: $1:10^6$ population per year)	Chimpanzees, Monkeys, cats, goats, guinea pigs, Syrian hamsters, mice
Gerstmann-Sträusslers syndrome	Humans	Familial	Sporadic, genetic disorder	Chimpanzees, mice

containing carcases from Scrapie-infected sheep. Some tissue cultures, however, allow production of agents, but in low titres, whereas infectivity titres of brains from infected animals can be in the order of 10^8/gram of tissue. Accidental transmission from human to human has occurred in a recipient of a corneal graft that was taken from a donor who was diagnosed retrospectively as having pathologically confirmed CJD. Eight patients have also developed CJD after being treated with pituitary-derived human growth hormone, and cases have appeared after brain surgery where cadaveric grafts were inserted. The agent is extremely resistant to inactivation by heat, chemicals, and irradiation. This property creates significant biohazards during exposure to infected tissue and is the reason why accidental human-to-human transmission has been seen even after use of 70% alcohol and formaldehyd vapor disinfected instruments for brain surgery.[26]

The transmissible encephalopathies have pathomorphological generalities in common with many other neurodegenerative diseases. They present progressive, symmetrically distributed, selective degenerations of neuronal systems. The pathology of Scrapie, CJD, GSS, and BSE includes vacuolar degenerations (spongiosis) of neurons, astrocyte reaction, and amyloidogenic accumulations of an altered neuronal membrane glycoprotein. There may be agent and interspecies variations in the degree of spongiosis. Pathological homologies between the diseases include characteristic Scrapie associated fibrils consisting of the major fibril protein, the proteinase resistant protein (PrP). This protein may be part of a virus that may also contain a small piece of nucleic acid (virino hypothesis). The infectious agent may, however, also be an abnormally modified membrane fragment that can initiate production of proteins in the host responsible for the neurological lesions. In CJD and GSS families, several mutations resulting in several different amino acid substitutions have been found in the human homology of the Scrapie PrP.[27] No immunological reactions such as formation of specific antibodies are detectable in infected hosts, rendering epidemiological studies difficult.

CJD is a rare, usually sporadic, presenile dementia; it has a familial pattern of inheritance in about 10%. The typical clinical picture includes rapid progressive dementia, myoclonus, and marked motor dysfunction. The disease is usually fatal in less than 1 year. GSS is probably a variant of CJD as patients have a progressive cerebellar ataxia and regularly — like CJD patients — show deposits of unusual amyloid plaques in their brains. GSS has a longer duration from onset to death. In this respect, GSS-cases are more like Kuru cases.[26] Scrapie and BSE are characterized by slowly developing neurological abnormalities of 1 to 6 months duration. The symptoms are apprehensive behavior, hyperesthesia, and ataxia. Severe pruritus is a typical sign of Scrapie that causes the sheep to rub against any upright post — hence the name Scrapie.

As infected animals do not develop an immunological response, and tissue culture systems for diagnostic purposes are not available, the only diagnostic method is to await clinical signs of disease after transmission to laboratory animals.

ANIMAL MODEL STUDIES OF SPONGIFORM ENCEPHALOPATHIES

In the initial studies, it was shown that Kuru was an infectious disease by transmitting the disease to monkeys. CDJ is regularly transmissible to chimpanzees and monkeys and some but not all strains, together with the Scrapie agent, are transmissible to laboratory mice, Syrian hamsters, and domestic cats. Human brain material injected into goats produces a disease that is also histologically indistinguishable from Scrapie, but there have been problems provoking the disease in sheep, indicating strain differences. The long incubation period — in monkeys infected with Kuru about 2 to 4 years — raises some serious experimental problems.[26] A mouse and Syrian hamster model is now available for the human diseases as it has been for Scrapie. With mouse-adapted strains, the incubation period is reduced to about 4 months, and it has therefore been possible to study the pathogenesis of these diseases. The agents of the human diseases replicate in lymph nodes and spread with the blood. Control of infectivity is difficult and demands a lot of mice as infectivity is tested in mice by titration. Histological and ultrastructural studies of amyloidogenesis in infected mice have revealed that the mice regularly develop plaques with the same pattern of amyloid fibril formation as in Scrapie-infected mice. After passage in mice, it is possible to provoke infection in monkeys.[26] The mouse and hamster models also offer an opportunity to test resistance of CDJ agent to physical and chemical agents, which is very important to minimize iatrogenic transmission.[28]

Other presenile dementias, like Alzheimer's disease, have also been tested for transmissibility by transferring material to chimpanzees, monkeys, and laboratory animals with hitherto negative results. It is, however, possible that some of these diseases also have an infectious background, as a substantial number of cases histologically show amyloid plaques like the plaques seen in transmissible encephalopathies. Co-cultivation of brain explants with tissue culture of nerve cells have also given disappointing results.[26]

Concerning BSE, there is epidemiological and experimental evidence available that the epidemic is of dietary origin: the sudden occurrence of this disease coincides with the introduction of specific changes in the manufacturing of meat and bone meal about 10 years ago. Due to the long incubation periods, this correlates to the appearance of the first cases in 1986. The two major changes that may have been important in altering the exposure are (1) a move away from batch rendering of material to continuous processes, and (2) the reduction in the use of hydrocarbon solvent extraction of fat from meat and bone meal.[29] This change in processing had a reduced sterilizing effect on Scrapie agent from sheep carcasses whereby foodstuff containing meat and bone meal became infectious.

The future will show whether cattle-to-cattle transmission will occur due to adaption of Scrapie strains to cattle or the epidemic will die out because the food-borne route has been curtailed by legislation. Molecular characterization of the BSA-agent and use of mice as models for direct transmission of the disease[30] may help solve this problem.

REFERENCES

1. Skinhøj, P., Andersen, H. K., Møller, J., and Jacobsen, N., Cytomegalovirus infection after bone marrow transplantation: Relation of pneumonia to postgrafting immunosuppressive treatment, *J. Med. Virol.*, 14, 91, 1984.
2. Jackson, L., An intracellular protozoan parasite of the ducts of the salivary glands of the guinea-pig, *J. Infect. Dis.*, 26, 347, 1920.
3. Cole, R., and Kuttner, A. G., A filterable virus present in the submaxillary glands of guinea pigs. *J. Exp. Med.*, 44, 855, 1926.
4. Hartley, J. W., Rowe, W. P., and Huebner, R. J., Serial propagation of the guinea pig salivary gland virus in tissue culture, *P.S.E.B.M.*, 96, 281, 1957.
5. Isom, H. C., and Yin, C. Y., Guinea pig cytomegalovirus gene expression, in *Cytomegaloviruses*, McDougall, J. K. Ed., Current Topics in Microbiology and Immunology, Springer-Verlag, Berlin, 1990, 154, 101, 1990.
6. Middlekamp, J. N., Patrizi, G., Reed, C. A., Light and electron microscopic studies of the guinea pig cytomegalovirus, *J. Ultrastruc. Res.*, 18, 85, 1967.
7. Sarov, I., and Abady, I., The morphogenesis of human cytomegalovirus, isolation and polypeptide characterization of cytomegalovirus and dense bodies, *Virology*, 66, 464, 1975.
8. Andrewes, C. H., Immunity to the salivary virus of guinea pigs studied in the living animal, and in tissue culture, *Br. J. Exp. Pathol.*, 11, 23, 1990.
9. Bia, F. J., Griffith, B. P., Fong, C. K. Y., and Hsiung, G. D., Cytomegaloviral infections in the guinea pig: Experimental models for human disease, *Rev. Inf. Dis.*, 5, 177, 1983.
10. Griffith, Brigitte P., Lucia, H. L., Bia, F. J., and Hsiung, G. D., Cytomegalovirus induced mononucleosis in guinea pigs, *Infect. Immun.*, 32, 857, 1981.
11. Griffith, Brigitte P., and Hsiung, G. D., Cytomegalovirus infection in guinea pigs. IV. Maternal infection of different stages of gestation, *J. Infect. Dis.*, 141, 787, 1980.
12. Woolf, N. K., Koehrn, F. J., Harris, J. P., and Richman, D. D., Congenital cytomegalovirus labyrinthitis and sensorineural hearing loss in guinea pigs, *J. Infect. Dis.*, 160, 929, 1989.
13. Hudson, J. B., The murine cytomegalovirus as a model for the study of viral pathogenesis and persistent infections, *Arch. Virology*, 62, 1, 1979.
14. Baskar, J. F., Stanat, S. C, Sulik, K. K., and Huang, E. S., Murine cytomegalovirus-induced congenital defects and fetal maldevelopment, *J. Infect. Dis.*, 148, 836, 1983.
15. Osborn, June E., Blazkovec, A. A., and Walker, D. L., Immunosuppression during acute murine cytomegalovirus infection. *J. Immunol.*, 100, 835, 1968.
16. Henson, D., Smith, R. D., Gehrke, J., and Neapolitan, Carole, Effect of cortisone on nonfatal mouse cytomegalovirus infection., *Amer. J. Pathol.*, 51, 1001, 1967.
17. Osborn, June E., and Walker, D. L., Enhancement of infectivity of murine cytomegalovirus *in vitro* by centrifugal inoculation, *J. Virol.*, 2, 853, 1968.
18. Anderson, R. M., May, R. M., Boily, M. C., Garnett, G. P., and Rowley, J. T., The spread of HIV-1 in Africa: sexual contact patterns and the predicted demographic impact of AIDS, *Nature*, 352, 581, 1991.
19. Essex, M., and Kanki, Phyllis J., The origins of the AIDS virus, *Scient. Amer.*, 259, 44, 1988.
20. Groopman, J. E., Of mice, monkeys and men, *Nature*, 349, 568, 1991.

21. Berman, P. W., Gregory, T. J., Riddle, L., Nakamura, G. R., Champe, M. A., Porter, J. P., Wurm, F. M., Hershberg, R. D., Cobb, E. K., and Eichberg, J. W., Protection of chimpanzees from infection by HIV-1 after vaccination with recombinant glycoprotein gp 120 but not gp160, *Nature,* 345, 622, 1990.

22. Emini, E. A., Schleif, W. A., Nunberg, J. H., Conley, A. J., Eda, Y., Tokiyoshi, S., Putney, S. D., Matsushita, S., Cobb, K. E., Jett, C. M., Eichberg, J. W., and Murthy, K. K., Prevention of HIV-1 infection in chimpanzees by gp120 V3 domain-specific monoclonal antibody, *Nature,* 355, 728, 1992.

23. Imberti, Luisa, Sottini, Allessandra, Bettinardi, Allessandra, Puoti, M., Primi, Daniele, Selective depletion in HIV infection of T cells that bear specific T cell receptor V_β sequences, *Science,* 254, 860, 1991.

24. Transmissible spongiform encephalopathies, in *Current Topics in Microbiology and Immunology,* Chesebro, B. W., Ed., Springer-Verlag, Berlin, 1991, 172.

25. Gajdusek, D. C., and Gibbs, C. J. Jr., Subacute and chronic diseases caused by atypical infections with unconventional viruses in aberrant hosts, *Perspect. Virol.,* 8, 279, 1973.

26. Gajdusek, D. C., Subacute spongiform encephalopathies: transmissible cerebral amyloidoses caused by unconventional viruses, in *Virology,* Fields, B. N, and Knipe, D. M., Eds., Sec. Ed., Raven Press, New York, 1990, chap. 80.

27. Hsiao, Karen, Baker, H. F., Crow, T. J., Poulter, M., Owen, F., Terwilliger, J. D., Westaway, D., Ott, J., and Pruisner, S. B., Linkage of a prion protein missense variant to Gerstmann-Sträussler syndrome, *Nature,* 338, 342, 1989.

28. Taguchi, F., Tamai, Y., Uchida, K., Kitajima, R., Kojima, H., Kawaguchi, T., Ohtani, Y., and Miura, S., Proposal for a procedure for complete inactivation of the Creutzfeldt-Jakob disease agent, *Arch. Virol.,* 119, 297, 1991.

29. Wilesmith, J. W., and Wells, G. A. H., Bovine spongiform encephalopathy in *Transmissible Spongiform Encephalopathies,* Current Topics in Microbiology and Immunology, Chesebro, B. W., Ed., Springer-Verlag, Berlin, 172, 21, 1991.

30. Barlow, R. M., Middleton, D. J., Dietary transmission of bovine spongiform encephalopathy to mice, *Vet. Rec.,* 126, 111, 1990.

Chapter 14

Animal Models in Bacteriology

Andrew N. Rycroft

CONTENTS

INTRODUCTION

Animals have been used in the study of bacteria that cause disease since the germ theory of disease was proposed in the latter part of the 19th century. Currently, animal models of bacterial infection are used in three primary areas of bacteriological research: the evaluation of the efficacy of prophylactic vaccines and antimicrobial agents *in vivo,* the diagnosis of specific infectious diseases, and basic research towards understanding the processes of bacterial infection and mechanisms of bacterial pathogenicity.

There have been a vast number of different animal models developed for experimental bacteriological purposes. Different animal species respond in different ways to a given organism and the quest to find models that more closely mimic the features and consequenses of natural bacterial infections is a continuing one. It would not be possible or indeed helpful to include examples of all of these animal models, and therefore only representative examples that are currently used or that are considered to have particular purposes or value, will be included. Models of bacterial infections will be grouped according to the site of the experimental infection: gastrointestinal infections, respiratory disease, systemic or non-localized disease, etc. In addition, animals are used occasionally for the cultivation of bacteria and for the analysis of bacterial toxins *in vivo.*

ANIMAL MODELS OF BACTERIAL INFECTION

ANIMAL MODELS OF GASTROINTESTINAL INFECTIONS

The primary gastrointestinal infections of humans that have a bacterial aetiology include cholera, salmonellosis, shigellosis (dysentery), *Campylobacter* infection, and infection by enterotoxigenic or enteropathogenic strains of *Escherichia coli.*

Cholera and Enterotoxigenic *Escherichia coli* Diarrhea

There has been considerable research over the past few decades to understand the mechanisms of disease production and to attempt to improve prophylaxis and treatment of these diseases. Research on cholera has made extensive use of animal models for the study of colonization of the gut and the mechanisms of pathogenicity of *Vibrio cholerae.* Human volunteers have been used in some experiments, but important animal models have been developed in the rabbit and suckling mouse.

The Adult Rabbit Ligated Ileal Loop Model

This model, first described in 1953 by De and Chattergee,[1] involves fasting the animal, general anaesthesia, and laparotomy. The small intestine is tied off in alternating 2 and 10 cm lengths proximal to the mesoappendix. Inocula of bacteria or bacterial product are introduced into the lumen of the 10 cm segments of the gut with a fine gauge needle. The abdomen is then closed for a number of hours until the rabbit is killed at a predetermined time to observe the pathological effects of the inoculum. The 2 cm segments should be free of fluid if the ties have held correctly preventing the passage of contents from one segment to another. Inoculated segments may be each treated in different ways to include treatment or antibody, etc. It is usual to do each experiment using triplicate segments to verify the reproducibility of results.

The RITARD Model

Another model, known by the acronym RITARD (removable intestinal tie adult rabbit diarrhea model), was described by Spira et al. in 1981.[2] This model did not replace the rabbit ileal loop model, but it superseded the use of the dog and the chinchilla as models of bacterial intestinal disease because dogs are expensive and chinchillas do not suffer from true diarrhea. In this procedure, laparotomy under general anaesthesia is again performed. The large, blind caecum is ligated to prevent it from taking up fluid secreted by the small intestine. Also, a temporary, reversible obstruction (slip knot) is introduced into the ileum at the mesoappendix. Bacterial challenge is introduced into the small intestine and the wound is closed. The slip knot is retained long enough to allow the challenge bacteria to colonize the gut. This is usually taken as two hours after introduction of the bacteria into the lumen, at which time the slip knot is removed. *Vibrio cholerae* produces a fatal dehydrating diarrhea in this model. It is also suitable for the study of enterotoxigenic *Escherichia coli* which produces a less explosive watery diarrhea and for reproduction of *Campylobacter jejuni* enteritis.

The Suckling Mouse Model

The suckling mouse model was developed as a less expensive, and more convenient alternative to the rabbit ileal loop model.[3] Since the latter is a closed system, it was not considered ideal for the study of an infective process that occurs naturally in an open gastrointestinal tract. Early versions of the model were improved and the fluid secretion into the gut was expressed as a fluid accumulation (FA) ratio: the weight of gut against the remaining body weight.[4] The infant mouse was also used extensively in the discovery and description of the heat-labile and heat-stable toxins of enterotoxigenic *Escherichia coli*.[5]

Some putative enteric pathogens are unable to colonize and cause disease in normal experimental animals. In order to study, or to improve the chances of such colonization in mice, the animals can be pre-treated with the antimicrobial streptomycin. This reduces the competing flora and has been used with experimental infections such as enterohemorrhagic *E. coli* enteritis in which a streptomycin-resistant mutant of the test bacterial strain was used.[6]

Salmonellosis

Salmonella typhimurium is a natural pathogen of the mouse infection, causing a severe typhoid-like illness.[7] Immunosupression is known to increase the susceptibility of mice to wild-type salmonellae. Immunosupression is achieved by sublethal irradiation with X-rays or by the use of mice with a homozygous *xid* mutation. Irradiated mice are unable to supress the growth of salmonellae in the reticuloendothelial system in the early stages of the infection. The X-linked defect *xid* causes a B-lymphocyte defect, which is expressed in F1 male mice from crosses of homozygous CBA/N females with male mice from other inbred strains.[8]

Campylobacter Enteritis

Campylobacter jejuni causes diarrhea, colitis, and abortion in humans. It is among the most common agents of human enteritis and has overtaken *Salmonella* infection as a public health problem in some parts of the world. It also affects domestic animal species, particularly when they are raised in relatively hygienic environmental conditions: early exposure to infection generates immunity, which prevents further disease.

A wide variety of animal models has been used in attempts to reproduce *Campylobacter* enteritis. Most animals fail to develop serious infection under natural conditions. It has been found necessary to flush the intestine or to use germ-free animals. The RITARD procedure in the rabbit has been successfully used with *Campylobacter jejuni*[9] and oral immunization experiments by gastric feeding have also utilized the rabbit in immunization experiments.[10] The ferret has been proposed as the model of choice because natural infection of these animals reproducibly generates diarrhea and abortion.[11] The infant mouse,[12] hamsters,[13] and primates[14] have also been used in *Campylobacter* research. In primates, the clinical course of diarrhea and the presence of colitis is reported to be similar to the diarrheal disease in humans. In addition, the 3- to 4-week duration of excretion of *C. jejuni* is similar to that observed in humans after foodborne infection. Hamsters were reported by Humphrey et al. to develop diarrhea upon infection with *C. jejuni*.[13] However, other workers have been unable to reproduce this result, achieving an asymptomatic infection of the gut in this species.[15]

Shigella Infection (Dysentery)

Shigellosis and the closely similar syndrome caused by enteroinvasive *Escherichia coli* are diseases of humans and some non-human primates. The bacteria invade the epithelial cells of the colonic mucosa causing damage to the intestinal tissue with a resulting bloody mucous diarrhea. Protracted efforts to understand the pathogenicity of *Shigella* strains and to develop an effective vaccine against the disease have been made.

Initial testing of vaccines requires immunization and subsequent challenge of human volunteers or primates (eg. rhesus monkey, *Macaca mulatta*), usually by the oral route.[16] Such studies are difficult to perform, costly, and ethically tenuous. The ability of the Shigella bacteria to invade the corneal epithelium of the guinea pig and other rodents causing a keratoconjunctivitis (Sereny test), has provided a model system that mimics the invasive process occurring in the mucosal epithelium.[17,18] This has been used extensively in testing the virulence of *Shigella* strains and has been used infrequently to test the efficacy of potential vaccines used for immunization.[19]

Swine Dysentery

Serpulina (Treponema) hyodysenteriae is an anaerobic spirochaete causing Swine Dysentery, an endemic, large intestinal disease of pigs. Although the pig itself provides the prime model of infection, small animal models of infection have included guinea pigs, mice, and young chickens.[20-22]

Helicobacter pylori

An organism that has risen to prominence in recent years is the Gram-negative *Campylobacter*-like curved rod *Helicobacter pylori*. This organism has been implicated in inflammatory and ulcerative conditions of the gastric mucosa, the site of colonization in humans. A tentative association between infection with this organism and human gastric carcinoma has been shown to exist. Rats, mice, and guinea pigs cannot be colonized by *H. pylori* unless they are gnotobiotic or the immune system of those animals is manipulated.[23] Gnotobiotic dogs have also been infected with the organism.[24] However, such unnaturally raised animals are less than satisfactory in the study of colonization. The ferret, which has a similar anatomical and physiological gastrointestinal tract to humans, is naturally colonized by *H. mustelae* shortly after birth. This related but immunologically distinct organism has been used in a ferret model of the infection.[25] More recently, the barrier-born pig has been used as the animal model of choice.[26] This displays many of the features of *H. pylori* gastritis, including a systemic antibody response, seen in human cases and may be used to observe animals with the infection over a period of several months.

RESPIRATORY INFECTIONS
Pertussis

Bordetella pertussis is the cause of Pertussis (whooping cough) in humans. Vaccination against this disease has been successfully practised in the developed world for many years but controversy over the safety of the killed, whole cell vaccine in the 1970s led to renewed interest in the pathogenicity factors of the organism as components of an acellular vaccine. There is no ideal model for the reproduction of human pertussis. The conventional method of testing overall virulence has been lethality for newborn mice following intranasal challenge.[27] An aerosol challenge model in the mouse, described by Sato et al.,[28] has benefits over the basic challenge model because it includes some of the features of pertussis seen in humans such as specific attachment of the organism to the ciliated epithelium of the respiratory tract, increased severity of the disease in neonates, pneumonia, and leukocytosis.[29]

Streptococcal Pneumonia

The mouse has long been the animal used for demonstrating infection with *Streptococcus pneumoniae*, the agent of bacterial lobar pneumonia.[30] The LD50 for the mouse is 1000-fold greater by intranasal inoculation of live bacteria than by intraperitoneal inoculation. Mouse infection by the intraperitoneal route was once the method used to improve the isolation of *S. pneumoniae* when other, contaminant organisms were present in the material for culture. It has also been widely used for the study of pneumococcal pathogenicity and immunity and the development of antimicrobial therapies and vaccines.[31]

Mouse Pneumonitis Agent

This organism, murine *Chlamydia trachomatis*, has been used to produce a model of murine pneumonia.[32] The organism is introduced by the intranasal route in athymic (*nu/nu*) BALB/c mice. This model has been developed in efforts to understand the role of cellular and cytokine factors in the host defense against infectious agents in the respiratory tract.

Murine Respiratory Mycoplasmosis

Natural or experimental infection of the rat with *Mycoplasma pulmonis* provides a useful model for the study of immunological and inflammatory mechanisms operating in the respiratory tract. The infection, known as murine respiratory mycoplasmosis (MRM) results in the development of otitis, rhinitis, tracheitis, and bronchopneumonia.[33] The infection begins in the upper respiratory tract and progresses downward into the lungs with a mononuclear cell accumulation in all the mucosal regions of the respiratory tract. The differential response of rats to vaccination by different routes suggests that this model offers a means of studying interactions between the systemic and mucosal immune systems, including the upper and lower respiratory tracts in a naturally occurring infection.[34]

URINARY TRACT INFECTION

The development of a reliable, accurate model of human urinary tract infection (UTI) holds certain difficulties in that UTI in humans is influenced by body posture, age, mobility, and other factors. Bladder infection in rodents is relatively simple to reproduce by inoculation of the bacterial culture into the bladder by catheterization. The natural ascent of organisms to the renal pelvis is more difficult to achieve reliably. Murine models of pyelonephritis such as the rat model[35] and the BALB/c mouse model have been used with a variety of urinary pathogens including *Proteus mirabilis* and *Escherichia coli*.[36,37]

GENITAL TRACT INFECTION
Syphilis

Syphilis is a venereal disease that initially causes lesions of the genital tract before disseminating throughout the body. It is caused by the spirochaete *Treponema pallidum*. The standard model of syphilis infection is by intratesticular infection of rabbits with approximately 10^8 *Treponema pallidum* bacteria. These animals must be free of *Treponema paraluiscuniculi* infection, which would cause immunological interference with the experimental disease. As an alternative to this, a more observable method is intradermal challenge in rabbits. Injection of *Treponema pallidum* into the skin of a susceptible rabbit leads to the development of erythematous, indurated lesions which progress to ulceration.[38]

Vertical transmission of *T. pallidum* in utero is important as a route of infection in humans. Infection of the fetus before birth results in stillbirth or fatal disease, or latency, or apparent absence of the disease. Clear diagnosis of congenital syphylis is difficult and there is a lack of understanding of the immunological response of the fetus to infection. Maternal transmission of *T. pallidum* has been studied in the rabbit over a long period,[39] but the rabbit model fails to mimic human congenital transmission because a natural resistance to the disease is apparent in the rabbit fetus. Recently, infection of the guinea pig during pregnancy has been shown to resemble more closely the congenital infection of human infants.[40] This offers a better means of examining the factors involved in asymptomatic infection, seen in human neonatal syphilis, for the development of a means of diagnosing asymptomatic, infected infants.

Chlamydia

Chlamydia trachomatis is an important genital tract pathogen of pelvic inflammatory disease, infertility, and ectopic pregnancy.[41] An improved model is the mouse chlamydial salpingitis and subsequent infertility model in which the chlamydia bacteria are inoculated directly into the ovarian bursa.[42] This causes acute inflammation of the genital tract. Mice are then monitored for a number of weeks to demonstrate their infertility compared with controls and the immune response and pathology can be examined.

As an alternative, a guinea pig model has been used.[43] Instead of *Chlamydia trachomatis*, these studies have used *Chlamydia psittaci*, the agent of guinea pig inclusion conjunctivitis, which has been shown to produce infections of the eye and genital tract that resemble human chlamydial genital infections in their pathogenesis, immunology, and pathology.[44]

MAMMARY GLAND INFECTION

Bovine mastitis, and mastitis in the sheep and the pig, are economically important bacterial diseases. Experimental mastitis in the natural host is expensive and problematical. A laboratory animal model of mastitis in the lactating mouse was developed by Chandler in which *Staphylococcus aureus* and other mastitis pathogens were inoculated directly into the mammary gland.[45] The appearance and histological effects of infection with different bacterial species resembled the characteristic mastitis produced in the bovine mammary gland by those same bacterial species. The model has been used in a number of studies of the fundamental pathogenesis of mastitis,[46] and the virulence factors of the causative bacteria.[47]

ORAL INFECTION
Periodontitis

Human periodontal disease, inflammation of the gingival crevice, has become an important area of microbiological research. The aetiology of these infections is clearly bacterial, but a vast number of different bacterial species occupy this niche and the roles of the different species in periodontal disease is unclear. Animal models in a number of species have been developed in rodents[48,49] and in non-human primates.[50,51] In rodent models, there is the constant difficulty of relating periodontal disease progression in the rodent to that in humans. Rodents have a dentition and microflora very different from that of humans. Primates such as the squirrel monkey (*Saimira sciureus*) have a human-like dentition. In order to initiate periodontal disease, silk ligatures are placed around the teeth.[52] This species has become the model of choice for the study of the bacterial aetiology of periodontal disease.

Because many of the bacteria implicated in periodontal disease are of relatively low pathogenicity in the whole body, models have been attempted that demonstrate their low levels of virulence. For example, *Wolinella recta*, a member of the pathogenic subgingival microbiota has been examined in a murine abcess model in BALB/c mice. Using dexamethasone to supress neutrophil function[53] or simultaneous treatment with galactosamine,[54] the bacteria were injected subcutaneously into the posterior dorsolateral surface with the development of gangrenous, necrotic skin lesions.[55]

Dental Caries

Dental caries are the result of bacteriologically induced decalcification of the dental enamel. Models of dental caries in the young gnotobiotic rat have been described. The diet of these animals is manipulated so that a proportion of the diet (between about 5 and 50%) is sucrose and they are infected with a test strain of bacteria — usually *Streptococcus mutans*. After a number of days or weeks, the animals are sacrificed and the mandibles are removed for caries analysis.[56,57]

ANIMAL MODELS OF SYSTEMIC DISEASE AND OTHER INFECTIONS
Lyme Disease

A useful model of Lyme disease has been developed in the mouse. This is a spirochaetal infection (*Borrelia bergdorferi*) of humans and some animal species, particularly the dog, which results in a combination of musculoskeletal, cardiac, and neurological diseases. Initial work on the disease used infection models in rats, guinea pigs, and mice but infection of C3H/He mice has been found to result in the arthritis and carditis which effectively mimicks the human disease.[58] Another model described as resembling the human arthritis of Lyme disease is the irradiated hamster model. Inbred, immunocompetent LSH hamsters develop histologically demonstrable arthritis after inoculation of the hind paw with *Borrelia bergdorferi*. However, when the same animals are first irradiated with 600 rads of gamma radiation and infected with the Lyme disease spirochaete, the damage to the bone marrow tissues diminishes the immune response to the infection which results in severe, prolonged inflammation of the hind paws with destructive and errosive bone changes resembling Lyme arthritis in humans.[59]

Listeriosis

Listeria infection is a cause of bacterial meningitis, abortion, and stillbirth in humans. It also causes a very severe septic illness: granulomatosis infantisepticum. *Listeria* strain virulence can be measured in the mouse.[60] Neonatal mice are highly susceptible to the organism while adult animals are much less sensitive.

Listeria infection in the mouse is also widely used as a model for the development of protective immunity to infections by facultative intracellular pathogens.[61]

Haemophilus influenzae Type B

This organism has become one of the most important causes of meningitis in infants and young children in the developed world. Experimental models of the disease have been very important in understanding the pathogenesis of this disease that has led to the development of a safe and apparently very effective vaccine. Models of *Haemophilus influenzae* type B disease include intranasal[62] and intraperitoneal[63] inoculation of the rat, and also the rabbit[64] in which the role of subcellular components of the organism in disease have been studied.

Anthrax

Anthrax is a severe, frequently fatal, infection of humans and a variety of domestic animals caused by the Gram-positive spore-forming *Bacillus anthracis*. Animals (sheep and cattle) were used in the classical experiments of Pasteur in 1881. In the 1950s work on this organism led to the discovery of a three-component toxin and the finding that the toxin was only produced during growth *in vivo*.

Considerable work is proceeding to improve vaccination against anthrax since it remains a problem in the developing world. Animals differ in their susceptibility to anthrax and among the laboratory animals, mice and guinea pigs are susceptible while rats are relatively resistant. Guinea pigs are therefore frequently used to reproduce the disease.[65] They are challenged with

162

an appropriate intramuscular dose of spores. Mice are also used in the study of both specific and non-specific resistance, and mechanisms of pathogenesis.[66] They are challenged subcutaneously; some strains of mouse (A/J mice) are extremely sensitive showing a 50% lethal dose of less than 1 spore while others are less susceptible with between 10 and 100 spores as the LD50 depending on the strain of mouse and the strain of *B. anthracis*.

Staphylococcal Toxic Shock Syndrome

Toxic shock syndrome (TSS) was recognized in the late 1970s. It is an acute illness characterized by fever, hypotension, rash, and other features attributed to Staphylococcus aureus strains expressing TSS toxin 1. To mimic the disease, pre-prepared TSS toxin is continuously pumped from a miniosmotic pump implanted subcutaneously in the flank of a rabbit and the animals are monitored for a number of days.[67]

Francisella tularensis

The mouse has been shown to be a useful model of host immune response during tularaemia. A relatively avirulent Francisella strain, the live vaccine strain in the U.S., causes a lethal infection in mice that is indistinguishable from human disease.[68] This has provided another murine model for the study of cell-mediated immunity.[69]

Bacterial Arthritis

There have been many models of bacterial arthritis reported and suggested.[70] Most of these models have used the rabbit, and the bacteria have been administered directly into the joint. However, human bacterial arthritis is spread via the bloodstream. Spontaneous bacterial arthritis is sometimes seen in mice and *Staphylococcus aureus* strains are often isolated from the infected joints. Using intravenous injection via the tail vein, but not the ip. or sc. routes tested, it was possible to reproducibly induce arthritis in mice with a naturally occuring arthritis strain of *S. aureus*.[71]

Non-living bacterial products can also induce experimental arthritis. A single systemic injection of rats with an aqueous suspension of purified peptidoglycan-polysaccharide polymers from cell walls of group A streptococci can induce inflammation of peripheral joints characterized by repeated episodes of waxing and waning and progression over a period of several months to joint destruction. Includes spontaneous recurrence of inflammation; a feature of human rhumatoid arthritis. A more predictably timed arthritis can be achieved by reactivation of a previously sensitized joint with a small systemic dose of cell wall polysaccharide or lipopolysaccharide.[72]

ANIMALS USED FOR THE CULTIVATION OF BACTERIA

A very few bacterial species have not been cultivated on laboratory media. While some of these organisms have been reported to be cultivable *in vitro*, the unreliability and technical difficulties of this mean that animals are still used to grow these organisms for research purposes, vaccines, and for the harvesting of antigens.

MYCOBACTERIUM LEPRAE

Mycobacterium leprae is not cultivable in artificial medium, nor in most laboratory animals. It is necessary to culture it in the armadillo, e.g., the nine banded armadillo (*Dasypus novemcinctus* Linn.). The organism is harvested from the liver and spleen after a number of months incubation.[73] As a means of reproducing infection, the mouse footpad can be used. Alternatively the organism can be grown in and harvested from the footpad of athymic (*nu/nu*) mice over a period of approximately 12 months.[74]

TREPONEMA PALLIDUM

It is not possible to cultivate this organism *in vitro* and the method commonly used to prepare the treponemal antigen for use in serodiagnostic tests and bacteriological research is by growth in the rabbit testicle. This involves the intratesticular injection of 5×10^7 virulent T. pallidum (e.g., Nichols strain). Rabbits develop orchitis after 7 to 12 days and the organisms are then harvested from the infected tissues.

DETECTION AND MEASUREMENT OF BACTERIAL TOXINS IN ANIMALS

ENDOTOXIN (LIPOPOLYSACCHARIDE)

Lipopolysaccharide (LPS) is a component of the outer membrane of all Gram-negative bacteria. Its effects on the body are many and varied and it is considered to be an important mediator of host damage *in vivo* during infection with Gram-negative organisms. Although biological assays of endotoxin activity are available (e.g., *Limulus* amoebocyte lysate assay) mice are still used in measuring the protective effects of compounds or antibody against the lethal effects of endotoxin. It was found by Galanos et al.[54] that when injected simultaneously with LPS, galactosamine abrogates reticuloendothelial system function of the liver which is critical for LPS detoxification. It increases the sensitivity to endotoxin (and the apparent virulence of endotoxin-producing bacteria). In contrast, hydrazine sulphate, a specific inhibitor of gluconeogenesis, protects mice against lethal endotoxaemia.[75]

Endotoxin non-responder mice have been useful in attempts to understand the mechanism of endotoxin (lipopolysaccharide) action. The first LPS-resistant mouse strain (C3H/HeJ) was used in genetic studies, which showed the existance of a gene for LPS responsiveness.[76] The Lps locus, located on mouse chromosome 4, occurs in two allelic forms: Lpsn for normal responsiveness and Lpsd for defective responsiveness. Lpsn mice exhibit normal sensitivity to the biological effects of LPS while Lpsd mice are highly resistant due to a spontaneous mutation of the Lps locus. Three Lpsd strains of mouse are recognized: C3H/HeJ, C57BL/10ScCr, and C57BL/10ScN. These strains, in contrast to responsive mice, survive when injected with large amounts of lipopolysaccharide.

BOTULINUM TOXIN

Botulism is a rare disease of humans but it occurs, usually in sporadic outbreaks, in some animal species. It is diagnosed by demonstration of the neurotoxin in foodstuff, serum, or filtered fecal material from the affected animal. Demonstration of the toxin activity is by intraperitoneal injection of mice, and protection of some of the mice with specific antitoxin antibody to identify which of the six types of toxin is involved.

DERMONECROTIC TOXIN OF *BORDETELLA PERTUSSIS*

This toxin, also known as Heat Labile Toxin, causes necrotic lesions after intradermal injection. It is detected and assayed in preparations from *Bordetella pertussis* by infant mouse nuchal injection model of Cowell et al.[77] The toxin material is applied subcutaneously into the nuchal areas of 4 day old mice. After 20 hours at 30°C this area is observed for darkening.

REFERENCES

1. De, S.H. and Chatterjee, D.N., An experimental study of the mechanisms of action of *Vibrio cholerae* on the intestinal mucous membrane. *J. Pathol. Bacteriol.*, 46, 559. 1953.
2. Spira, W.M., Sack, R.B. and Froehlich, J.L., Simple adult rabbit model for *Vibrio cholerae* and enterotoxigenic *Escherichia coli* diarrhea. *Infect. Immun.*, 32, 739, 1981.

164

3. Dean, A.G., Ching, Y-C., Williams, R.G. and Harden, L.B. Test for *Escherichia coli* enterotoxin using infant mice: application in a study of diarrhea in children in Honolulu. *J.Infect. Dis.*, 125, 407. 1972.

4. Baselski, V., Briggs, R., and Parker, C. Intestinal fluid accumulation induced by oral challenge with *Vibrio cholerae* or cholera toxin in infant mice. *Infect. Immun.*, 15, 704. 1977.

5. Jacks, T.M. and Wu, B.J. Biochemical properties of *Escherichia coli* low-molecular-weight, heat-stable enterotoxin. *Infect. Immun.*, 9, 342. 1974.

6. Wadolkowski, E.A. Burris, J.A. and O'Brien A.D. Mouse model for colonisation and disease caused by enterohemorrhagic *Escherichia coli* O157:H7. *Infect. Immun.*, 58, 2438. 1990.

7. Heffernan, E.J., Fierer, J., Chickami, G. and Guiney, D.G., Natural history of oral *Salmonella dublin* infection in BALB/c mice: effect of an 80 kilobase-pair plasmid on virulence. *J.Infect. Dis.*, 155, 1254. 1987.

8. Scher, I., Steinberg, A.D. and Paul, W.E. X-linked B lymphocyte immune defect in CBA/N mice. II. Studies of the mechanisms underlying the immune defect. *J. Exp. Med.*, 142, 637. 1975.

9. Caldwell, M.B., Walker, R.I., Stewart, S.D. and Rogers, J.E. Simple adult rabbit model for *Campylobacter jejuni* enteritis. *Infect. Immun.*, 42, 1176. 1983.

10. Burr, D.H., Caldwell, M.B., Bourgeois, A.L., Morgan, H.P., Wistar, R. and Walker, R.I. Mucosal and systemic immunity to *Campylobacter jejuni* in rabbits after gastric inoculation. *Infect. Immun.*, 56, 99. 1988.

11. Fox, J.G., Ackerman, J.I., Taylor, N., Claps, M. and Murphy, J.C. *Campylobacter jejuni* infection in the ferret: an animal model of human campylobacteriosis. *Am. J. Vet. Res.*, 48, 85. 1987.

12. Abimiku, A.C. and Dolby, J.M. The mechanisms of protection of infant mice from intestinal colonisation by *Campylobacter jejuni*. *J. Med. Microbiol.*, 23, 339, 1987.

13. Humphrey, C.D., Montag, D.M. and Pittman, F.E. Experimental infection of hamsters with *Campylobacter jejuni*. *J. Infect. Dis.*, 151, 485. 1985.

14. Russell, R.G., Blaser, M.J., Sarmiento, J.I. and Fox, J. Experimental *Campylobacter jejuni* infection in *Macaca nemestrina*. *Infect. Immun.*, 57, 1848. 1989.

15. Aguero-Rosenfeld, M.E., Yang, X.-H. and Nachamkin, I. Infection of adult syrian hamsters with flagellar variants of *Campylobacter jejuni*. *Infect. Immun.*, 58, 2214. 1990.

16. Formal, S.B., Hale, T.L., Kapfer, C., Cogan, J.P., Snoy, P.J., Chung, R., Wingfield, M.E., Elisberg, B.L. and Baron, L.S. Oral vaccinaton of monkeys with an invasive *Escherichia coli* K-12 hybrid expressing *Shigella flexneri* 2a somatic antigen. *Infect. Immun.*, 46, 465. 1984.

17. Sereny, B. Acquired natural immunity following recovery from keratoconjunctivitis shigellosa. *J. Hygi., Epidemiol., Microbiol. Immunol.*, 3, 292. 1959.

18. Mackel, D.C., Langley, L.F. and Venice, L.A. The use of the guinea pig conjunctivae as an experimental model for the study of virulence of *Shigella* organisms. *Am. J. Hyg.*, 73, 219. 1961.

19. Verma, N.K. and Lindberg, A.A. Construction of aromatic dependent *Shigella flexner* 2a live candidate strains: deletion mutations in the *aroA* and *aroD* genes. *Vaccine*, 9, 6. 1991.

20. Joens, L.A., Songer, J.G., Harris D.L., and Glock, R.D. Experimental infection with *Treponema hyodysenteriae* in guinea pigs. *Infect. Immun.*, 22, 132. 1978.

21. Joens, L.A. and Glock, R.D. Experimental infection in mice with *Treponema hyodysenteriae*. *Infect. Immun.*, 25, 757. 1979.

22. Sueyoshi, M. Adachi, Y. and Shoya, S. Enteropathogenicity of *Treponema hyodysenteriae* in young chicks. *Zentralbl. Bakteriol. Mikrobiol. Hyg. Reihe A.* 266, 469. 1987.

23. Engstrand, L. & Gustavvsson, S. 1991. Gastric CLO, ulcer disease and gastritis in animals and animal models of *Helicobacter pylori* gastritis, p. 55-65. In B.J. Marshall, R.W. McCallum and R.L. Guerant (Ed.), Helicobacter Pylori in *Peptic Ulceration and Gastritis*. Blackwell scientific publications, Cambridge, Mass.

24. Radin, M.J., Eaton, K.A., Krakowka, S., Morgan, D.R., Lee, A., Otto, G. and Fox, J. *Helicobacter pylori* gastric infection in gnotobiotic beagle dogs. *Infect. Immun.,* 58, 2606. 1990.
25. Fox, J.G., Pelayo, C., Taylor, N.S., Lee, A., Otto, G., Murphy, C. and Rose, R. *Helicobacter mustelae*-associated gastritis in ferrets: an animal model of *H. pylori* gastritis in humans. *Gastroenterology,* 99, 352. 1990.
26. Engstrand, L., Gustavsson, S., Jörgensen, A. Schwan, A. and Scheynius, A. Inoculation of barrier born pigs with *Helicobacter pylori*: a useful animal model for gastritis type B. *Infect. Immun.,* 58, 1763. 1990.
27. Weiss, A.A. and Falkow, S. Genetic analysis of phase change in *Bordetella pertussis*. *Infect. Immun.,* 43, 263. 1984.
28. Sato, Y., Izumiya, H., Sato, H., Cowell, J.L. and Manclark, C.R. Aerosol infection of mice with *Bordetella pertussis*. *Infect. Immun.,* 29, 261. 1980.
29. Sato, Y. and Sato, H. Animal models of pertussis. p.309-325. In A.C. Wardlaw and R. Parton (Ed.), *Pathogenesis and Immunity in Pertussis*. John Wiley and Sons Ltd, Chichester, UK.
30. Avery, O.T., Cole, R., Doche, A.R. and Chickering, H.T. *Acute Lobar Pneumonia. Prevention and Serum Treatment*. Rockerfeller Institute for Medical Research, New York. 1917.
31. Austrian, R. Pneumococcal vaccine: development and prospects. *Am. J. Med.,* 67, 547. 1979.
32. Williams, D.M., Schachter, J., Drutz, D.J. and Sumaya, C.V. Pneumonia due to *Chlamydia trachomatis* in the immunocompromised (nude) mouse. *J. Infect. Dis.,* 143, 238. 1981.
33. Lindsay, J.R., Baker, H.J., Overcash, R.G., Cassell, G.H. and Hunt, C.E. Murine chronic respiratory disease. Significance as a research complication and experimental production with *Mycoplasma pulmonis*. *Am. J. Pathol.,* 64, 675. 1971.
34. Cassell, G.H. and Davies, J.K. Protective effect of vaccination against *Mycoplasma pulmonis* respiratory disease in rats. *Infect. Immun.,* 21, 69. 1978.
35. Silverblatt, A.B. Host parasite interactions in the rat renal pelvis: a possible role of pili in the pathogenesis of pyelonephritis. *J. Exper. Med.,* 140, 1696. 1974.
36. Moayeri, N., Collins, C.M. and O'Hanley, P. Efficacy of a *Proteus mirabilis* outer membrane protein vaccine in preventing experimental Proteus pyelonephritis in a BALB/c mouse model. *Infect. Immun.,* 59, 3778. 1991.
37. O'Hanley, P., Lark, D., Falkow, S. and Schoolnik, G.K. Molecular basis of *Escherichia coli* colonisation of the upper urinary tract in BALB/c mice. *J. Clin. Invest.,* 75, 347. 1985.
38. Champion, C.I., Miller, J.N., Borenstein, L.A., Lovett, M.A. and Blanco, D.R. Immunization with *Treponema pallidum* endoflagella alters the course of experimental rabbit syphilis. *Infect. Immun.,* 58, 3158. 1990.
39. Kemp, J.E. and Fitzgerald, E.M. Studies in experimental syphilis and the transfer of immunity from immune syphilitic female rabbits to their offspring. *J. Invest. Derm.,* 1, 353. 1938.
40. Wicher, V., Wicher, K., Rudofsky, V., Zabek, J., Jakubowski, A. and Nakeeb, S. Experimental neonatal syphilis in a susceptible (CD4) and a resistant (Albany) strain of guinea pig. *Clin. Immunol. Immunopathol.,* 55, 23. 1990.
41. Moore, D.E., Spadoni, L.R., Foy, H.M. et al. Increased frequency of serum antibodies to *Chlamydia trachomatis* in infertility due to disal tube disease. *Lancet* ii, 574. 1982.
42. Landers, D.V., Erlich, K., Sung, M. and Schachter, J. Role of L3T4-bearing T-cell populations in experimental murine chlamydial salpingitis. *Infect. Immun.,* 59, 3774. 1991.
43. Howard, L.V., O'Leary, M.P. and Nichols, R.L. Animal model studies of genital chlamydial infections. Immunity to re-infection with guinea-pig inclusion conjunctivitis agent in the urethra and eye of male guinea-pigs. *Br. J. Vener. Dis.,* 52, 261. 1976.
44. Rank, R.G. Role of the immune response, p. 217-234. In A.L. Barron (Ed.), *Microbiology of* Chlamydia. CRC Press, Boca Raton, FL.
45. Chandler, R.L. Experimental bacterial mastitis in the mouse. *J. Med. Microbiol.,* 3, 273. 1970.

46. Anderson, J.C. Pathogenesis of experimental mastitis in the mouse caused by a strain of *Staphylococcus aureus* of low virulence and its modification by endotoxin. *J. Compar. Pathol.*, 85, 531. 1975.

47. Haraldsson, I. and Jonsson, P. Histopathology and pathogenesis of mouse mastitis induced with *Staphylococcus aureus* mutants. *J. Compar. Pathol.*, 94, 183. 1984.

48. Taubman, M.A., Yoshie, H., Ebersole, J.L., Smith, D.J. and Olson, C.L. Host response in experimental periodontal disease. *J. Dent. Res.*, 63, 455. 1984.

49. Sanavi, F., Listgarten, M.A., Boyd, F., Sallay, K. and Nowotney, A. The colonisation and establishment of invading bacteria in periodontium of ligature-treated immunosuppressed rats. *J. Periodontol.*, 56, 273. 1985.

50. Brecx, M.C., Nalbandian, J., Kornman, K.S. and Robertson, P.B. Morphological studies on periodontal disease in the cynomolgus monkey. III. Electron microscopic observations. *J. Periodontal Res.*, 21, 137. 1986.

51. Holt, S.C., Ebersole, J., Felton, J., Brunsvold, M. and Kornman, K.S. Implantation of *Bacteroides gingivalis* in non-human primates initiates progression of periodontitis. *Science*, 239, 55. 1988.

52. Heijl, L. Rifkin, B.R. and Zander, H.A. Conversion of chronic gingivitis to periodontitis in squirrel monkeys. *J. Periodontol.*, 47, 710. 1976.

53. Hajime, S., Takashi, W. and Horikawa, Y. Effects of *Lactobacillus casei* on *Pseudomonas aeruginosa* infection in normal and dexamethasone-treated mice. *Microbiol. Immunol.* 30, 249. 1986.

54. Galanos, C., Freudenburg, M.A. and Feutter, W. Galactosamine induced sensitisation to the lethal effects of endotoxin. *Proc. Nat. Acad. Sci. U.S.A.* 76, 5939. 1979.

55. Kesavalu, L., Holt, S.C. Crawley, R.R., Borinski, R. and Ebersole, J.L. Virulence of *Wolinella recta* in a murine abscess model. *Infect. Immun.*, 59, 2806. 1991.

56. Barletta, R.G., Michaelek, S.M. and Curtiss, R. Analysis of the virulence of *Streptococcus mutans* serotype *c gftA* mutants in the rat model system. *Infect. Immun.*, 56, 322. 1988.

57. Ooshima, T., Izumitani, A., Sobue, S., Okahashi, N. and Hamada, S. Noncariogenicity of the disaccharide palatinose in experimental dental caries of rats. *Infect. Immun.*, 39, 43. 1983.

58. Barthold, S.W. Infectivity of *Borrelia bergdorferi* relative to the route of inoculation and genotype of laboratory mice. *J. Infect. Dis.*, 163, 419. 1991.

59. Schmitz, J.L., Schell, R.F., Hejka, A., England, D.M., Konick, L. Induction of Lyme arthritis in LSH hamsters. *Infect. Immun.*, 56, 2336. 1988.

60. Gaillard, J.L., Berche, P. and Sansonetti, P. Transposon mutagenesis as a tool to study the role of haemolysin in the virulence of *Listeria monocytogenes. Infect. Immun.*, 52, 50. 1986.

61. Hahn, H. and Kauffmann. The role of cell-mediated immunity in bacterial infections. *Rev. Infect. Dis.*, 3, 1221. 1981.

62. Moxon, E.R., Smith, A.L., Averill, D.R. and Smith, D.H. *Haemophilus influenzae* meningitis in infant rats after intranasal inoculation. *J. Infect.Dis.*, 129, 154. 1974.

63. Smith, A.L., Smith, D.H., Averill, D.R., Marino, J. and Moxon, E.R. Production of *Haemophilus influenzae* b meningitis in infant rats by intraperitoneal inoculation. *Infect. Immun.*, 8, 278. 1973.

64. Syrogiannopoulos, G.A., Hansen, E.J., Erwin, A.L. Munford, R.S., Rutledge, J., Reisch, J.S. and McCracken, G.H. *Haemophilus influenzae* type b lipooligosaccharide induces meningeal inflammation. *J. Infect. Dis.*, 157, 237. 1988.

65. Turnbull, P.C.B., Broster, M.G., Carman, J.A., Manchee, R.J. and Melling, J. Development of antibodies to protective antigen and lethal factor components of anthrax toxin in humans and guinea pigs and their relevance to protective immunity. *Infect. Immun.*, 52, 356. 1986.

66. Welkos, S.L., Trotter, R.W., Becker, D.M. and Nelson, G.O. Resistance to the Sterne strain of *B. anthracis*: phagocytic cell responses of resistant and susceptible mice. *Microb. Pathog.* 7, 15. 1989.

67. Parsonnet, J., Gillis, Z.A., Richter, A.G. and Pier, G.B. A rabbit model of toxic shock syndrome that uses a constant, subcutaneous infusion of toxic shock syndrome toxin 1. *Infect. Immun.,* 55, 1070. 1987.

68. Anthony, L.S.D. and Kongshavn, P.A.L. Experimental murine tularemia caused by *Francisella tularensis*, live vaccine strain: a model of acquired cellular resistance. *Microb. Pathog.,* 2, 3. 1987.

69. Eigelsbach, H.T., Hunter, D.H. Janssen, W.A. Dangerfield, H.G. and Rabinowitz, S.G. Murine model for study of cell-mediated immunity: protection against death from fully virulent *Francisella tularensis* infection. *Infect. Immun.,* 12, 999. 1975.

70. Goldenberg, D.L., Chisholm, P.L. and Rice, P.A. Experimental models of bacterial arthritis. *J. Rheumatol.,* 10, 5. 1983.

71. Bremell, T., Lange, S., Yacoub, A., Ryden, C. and Tarkowski, A. Experimental *Staphylococcus aureus* arthritis in mice. *Infect. Immun.,* 59, 2615. 1991.

72. Schwab, J.H., Anderle, S.K., Brown, R.R., Daldorf, F.G. and Thompson, R.C. Pro and anti-inflammatory roles of interleukin-1 in recurrence of bacterial cell wall-induced arthritis in rats. *Infect. Immun.,* 59, 4436.

73. Wheeler, P.R. Oxidation of carbon sources through the tricarboxylic acid cycle in *Mycobacterium leprae* grown in armadillo liver. *J. Gen. Microbiol.,* 130, 381. 1984.

74. Franzblau, S.G. and Hastings, R.C. Rapid in vitro metabolic screen for antileprosy compounds. *Antimicrob. Agents Chemother.,* 31, 780. 1987.

75. Silverstein, R., Christoffersen, C.A. and Morrison, D.C. Modulation of endotoxin lethality in mice by hydrazine sulphate. *Infect. Immun.,* 57, 2072. 1989.

76. Rosenstreich, D.L. Genetic control of endotoxin response: C3H/HeJ mice, p 82-122 In R.A. Proctor and L.J. Berry (Eds.) *Handbook of Endotoxin*, vol. 4. Elsevier, Amsterdam.

77. Cowell, J.L., Hewlett, E.L. and Manclark, C.R. Intracellular localisation of dermonecrotic toxin of *Bordetella pertussis*. *Infect. Immun.,* 37, 1278. 1979.

Chapter 15

Animal Models in Mycology

Henrik Elvang Jensen

CONTENTS

INTRODUCTION

The development and application of experimental animal models in mycology are indispensable and used extensively in the study of a wide range of aspects such as pathogenesis, pathology, virulence, transformative properties, defense mechanisms (immunity), therapy, and prophylaxis. For diagnostic purposes, animal models are important for the isolation and identification of some fungi from both clinical and environmental materials and in the standardization of immunodiagnostic assays. Although some fungi are almost host-specific, i.e., the anthropophilic dermatophytes which only very rarely infect animals and *Histoplasma capsulatum* var. *farciminosum*, which naturally is restricted to equines, fungi are generally not host-specific in contrast to many other invasive microorganisms. Therefore, a variety of different animal species are suitable for infection with most of the fungi which are of importance in both medical and veterinary medicine.

For the establishment of experimental mycotic infections in animals, a number of different routes for challenge is used. The route of choice is strictly dependant on the goal of the study which also must reflect the animal, fungus, and disease-model applied. In general, disseminated infections are produced after intravascular administration, usually intravenous (i.v.), or by intraperitoneal (i.p.) and per oral (p.o.) challenge. For a number of fungi, the latter two routes will only produce localized mycosis, which, however, are more regularly established subsequently to intracerebral (i.cer.), intranasal (i.n.), intratracheal (i.t.), intratesticular (i.test.), intracorneal (i.cor.), intramuscular (i.m), intracutaneous (i.c.), subcutaneous (s.c.), and intravaginal (i.vag.) inoculation.

In addition to causing infection, a number of fungi are deleterious to human and animal health because of their formation of mycotoxins, some of which are among the most toxic (e.g., ochratoxin) and carcinogenic (e.g., aflatoxin) substances known. Moreover, fungi are potent sources of antigens and some of these (allergens) are the cause of immediate hypersensitivity response (Type I allergy). Fungal allergy is usually characterized by respiratory diseases and a high serum level of IgE to the allergens. The most important source of fungal allergens seems to be spores of especially *Cladosporium* and *Alternaria,* but allergy may also result from exposure to hyphae as seen in, e.g., allergic bronchopulmonary aspergillosis.

In the present chapter, only the infective aspects of animal models in mycology are covered.

ANIMAL MODELS OF MYCOSES

ANIMAL MODELS OF DERMATOPHYTOSIS

In dermatophytosis, the fungi are usually superficially located in keratinized layers of skin, hair, and nails. In severe cases, however, the infection may lead to granuloma formation in the subcutis or become disseminated to internal organs.[1,2] Animal models of dermatophytoses are especially used in the evaluation of new therapeutic agents, but are also applied in the study of pathogenicity, immune responses, and pathology.

Experimental animal infections in a variety of animal species have particularly been performed with zoophilic dermatophytes, especially *Trichophyton mentagrophytes* var. *mentagrophytes* and var. *granulare, Trichophyton verrucosum,* and *Microsporum canis.*[3,4] Infections with the geophilic and anthropophilic dermatophytes, e.g., *Microsporum gypseum* and *Trichophyton rubrum*, are generally difficult to establish in laboratory animals. *T. rubrum,* the fungus most often isolated from human ringworm, unfortunately has a rather low ability to induce experimental ringworm in laboratory animals.[1,3] However, certain strains with a high virulence, selected by, e.g., passage in animals, produce exothrix as well as endothrix infection in guinea pigs.[4,5] Infection of rabbits with *T. rubrum* has also been reported, but the lesions produced were not homogeneous and prior to inoculation, the animals were exposed to irradiation or were castrated.[6] Models using the natural ringworm dermatophyte of mice *T. mentagrophytes* var. *quinckeanum* are also used in the study of infection and immunity, because of the close resemblance to human dermatophytosis.[7,8]

Generally, in the study of experimental dermatophytosis, the guinea pig is the animal of choice in favor of the mouse, rat, hamster, rabbit, and dog because these animals make their toilet by licking or scratching and bite itching or irritated lesions intensively.[9] In the study of skin lesions due to dermatophytosis, hairless strains of guinea pigs are preferred as the lesions produced in these are like those seen in humans.[10] Moreover, hairless animals are more suitable for the application of topical antifungal agents. Studies of infections in dogs are few but dermal inoculations by zoophilic and geophilic dermatophytes produce uniform and long lasting infections (3 to 4 months), presumably mongrels being more sensitive to infection than beagles.[9]

Epidermal inoculation of dermatophytes is the classical way of inoculation and may be done in a number of ways, e.g., by abrasion with sandpaper, a scalpel, or a lancet after which the inoculum is applied. Repeating putting on and pulling off tape on a hair cut area in guinea pigs has also been used for getting the skin more suitable for the inoculation.[4] Depilation with sodium sulfide (36%) for 30 min is also useful.[9] Prick inoculation is performed with a needle smeared with inoculum. An advantage of this method is that the enlargement of the process can be expressed numerically, which is important when testing the effect of therapeutic agents.[4] A disadvantage, however, is that the rate of positive infections is less in comparison with the results of the abrasive methods. A non-traumatizing method used on guinea pigs is by the occlusive dressing method, where the area is kept moist after plucking off the hair and the inoculum is applied under a polyethylene film and an elastic bandage.[11,12] In this model, the severity of lesion increases proportionally with the time of occlusion.

A general disadvantage of the experimental dermatophytosis models is that they are not long-lasting. However, a prolonged infection in guinea pigs can be maintained by using highly virulent strains of *T. mentagrophytes,* or by transplantation of their skin, which subsequently is infected, into athymic nude mice.[4,13] However, administration of steroids and other immunosuppressants, and the use of germ free animals are not effective for prolonging an infection.[14]

The i.v. route for the establishment of dermatophytosis is also widely used especially as a model in the testing of new therapeutic agents.[9,15-17] As in skin inoculations, especially the zoophilic dermatophytes exhibit a trophism for infecting the skin after i.v. inoculation (Figure 1). A disadvantage of the i.v. route for dermatophytes is that also internal organs, especially the lungs, are regularly invaded, too. Moreover, in these models, relapse of ringworm in animals that were cured is often seen and is thought to originate from lesions in internal organs.[9] Concerning reproductivity of skin lesions after i.v. inoculation with *T. mentagrophytes* as an example, the guinea pig is also the animal of choice with the rabbit and dog being of intermediate value, whereas the chicken, mouse, and rat are considered useless due to a very low susceptibility.[4,9] Intravenous inoculation of non-dermatophytes, e.g., *Candida albicans, Cryptococcus neoformans, Rhizopus spp.,* and *Absidia corymbifera* may also result in mycotic folliculitis and skin eruptions.[9,18-20]

Routes of infection other than the cutaneous and intravenous are usually not successful or only sporadically so. However, intraperitoneal inoculation of mice with *T. rubrum* may result in the development of granulomatous lesions.[21]

Apart from laboratory animals, domestic animals, e.g., goats, pigs, cattle, and horses, are also used for experimental inoculations.[4] However, the course of infection in these animals is often too short to be compared with the chronic spontaneous infections found in humans and animals. Particular attention has been paid to the development of a vaccine against trichophytosis in cattle based on a killed or an attenuated strain of *T. verrucosum*.[22,23] However, in humans, the result of vaccination against different types of superficial mycoses including dermatophytosis has been rather disappointing.[24] Experimental dermatophytosis has also been produced in volunteers, and when their course of infection is compared to the spontaneous infections, they always resolve quickly like experimental infections in most animals.[25] When dealing with laboratory animals with ringworm, whether received experimentally or naturally, one must always pay attention to the risk of being infected as many of the zoophilic dermatophyte species also easily cause ringworm in humans.

ANIMAL MODELS OF SUBCUTANEOUS MYCOSES

In this group of mycoses, a number of heterogeneous fungi are responsible for infection. Generally, the infections are the result of traumatic implantation of the fungus into the skin, and the infection is only slowly spreading into surrounding tissues.[26] In some infections, extension by lymph vessels is frequent (sporotrichosis), in other diseases also hematogenous spread may be seen (chromoblastomycosis).

172

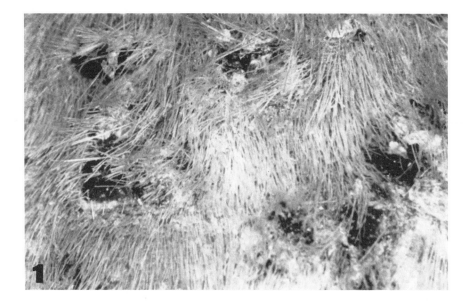

Figure 1. Experimental trichophytosis in the guinea pig by i.v. challenge with *Trichophyton mentagrophytes*. (1) Ringworm lesions on the back 3 weeks after infection. (From Van Cutsem, J. *Current Topics in Medical Mycology*, Vol. 3, Springer-Verlag, New York, 1, 1989. With permission.)

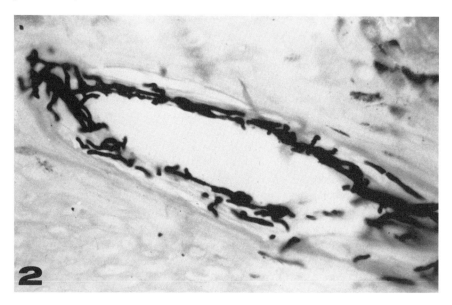

Figure 1. (2) Fungi in the hair root sheath. (From Van Cutsem, J. *Current Topics in Medical Mycology*, Vol. 3, Springer-Verlag, New York, 1, 1989. With permission.)

Chromomycosis

Chromoblastomycosis encompasses a specific clinical entity (verrucous dermatitis) and is caused by a limited series of soil-inhabiting dematiaceous fungi, showing sclerotic cells as the parasitic form, of which *Fonsecaea spp.* are most important.[4,26,27] Other clinical types of infection with dematiaceous fungi are termed phaeohyphomycosis (hyphal forms in infected tissue) and may be manifested in a variety of clinical types. In humans, the infection may be

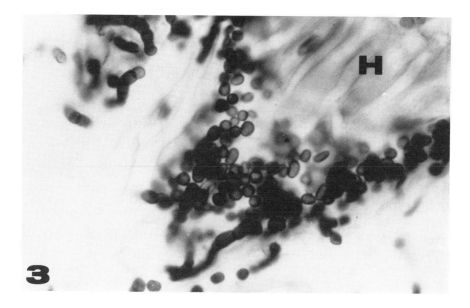

Figure 1. (3) Fungal elements in the hair shaft (H).

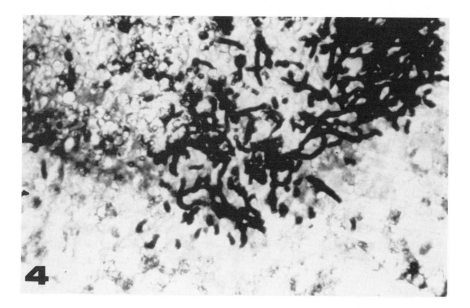

Figure 1. (4) Granulomatous mycotic pneumonia.

caused by a variety of fungi belonging to several genera, e.g., *Wangiella spp.* and *Cladosporium spp.*[4,26] Chromoblastomycosis and pheohyphomycosis is collectively referred to as chromomycosis. Mice, rats, rabbits, hamsters, guinea pigs, and monkeys are susceptible to experimental chromomycosis, with mice and rats having the highest susceptibility.[28] Both localized dermal and systemic infections with reactions that resemble those observed in humans have been produced in a number of animal models by inoculation by different routes, e.g., s.c., i.v., and i.p.[4,26,29] Moreover, animal inoculations are used to distinguish *Cladosporium carrionii* from *Cladosporium bantianum,* the latter being highly neurotropic.[26]

Lobomycosis

Lobomycosis is caused by a yeast-like organism referred to as *Loboa loboi,* which has not been cultured *in vitro.*[26] Clinically, lobomycosis is a chronic localized subepidermal infection. Experimental infections have been established successfully in hamsters by inoculation of clinical material resulting in a clinical picture similar to that seen in humans.[30] In turtles, tortoises, and armadillos the lesions develop more rapidly and are accompanied by liquifactive necrosis.[26] In mice, i.p., i.c., and i.test inoculations have been unsuccessful, whereas transfer of the infection through generations of mice is feasible by using the hind footpad as inoculum site.[26,30]

Mycetoma

Mycetoma s. maduromycosis is a clinical syndrome of localized indolent, deforming, swollen lesions, and sinuses, involving cutaneous and subcutaneous tissues, facia, and bone.[31] The infection is established by a variety of bacteria (actinomycetoma) and true fungi (eumycetoma). Experimental actinomycotic granules due to *Norcardia spp.* and *Actinomadura spp.* have been produced in a variety of animals, e.g., mice, hamsters, rabbits, goats, and guinea pigs.[4] Subcutaneous lesions are generally produced after s.c. inoculations, whereas granules in internal organs and on the abdominal wall are produced after i.v. and i.p. inoculation, respectively. With eumycotic agents establishment of animal models has had limited success, and reports of experimental animal inoculations are few.[4,31] Inoculation of eumycotic fungi i.p. into mice only produces granules in a small number of the animals challenged.[32,33] However, s.c. nodules with granules similar to those in humans are formed in rabbits inoculated s.c. with *Exophiala jeanselmei.*[34] Only rarely are fungi such as *Aspergillus fumigatus* and *T. rubrum* the causative agents in mycetomas. However, i.p. inoculation of mice with these fungi may result in the formation of granules, too.[35,36]

Rhinosporidiosis

Rhinosporidiosis is a chronic granulomatous disease of the mucocutaneous tissue and is caused by *Rhinosporidium seeberi.* Although many attempts to transfer the disease to laboratory animals have been done, a model for prolonged and chronic disease has not yet been developed.[26] In a few instances, granulomata have been produced, but sustained and progressive disease as seen in humans have not occurred.[26]

Sporotrichosis

Sporotrichosis is caused by the dimorphic fungus *Sporothrix schenckii.* Clinical types of sporotrichosis are cutaneous, lymphocutaneous, extracutaneous, and disseminated.[26,37] In laboratory animals, infection with *S. schenckii* may be established in mice, rats, gerbils, hamsters, rabbits, guinea pigs, dogs, cats, and monkeys.[4,26] The disease is seen after challenge by the i.p., i.v., i. test., s.c., and i.m. routes. Mice and rats are particulaly susceptible and a systemic infection is established after, e.g., i.p. inoculation, a course of infection only rarely seen in humans.[37] In rabbits and guinea pigs, the course of disease is more variable than in mice and rats.[4] A lymphatic infection that in many aspects resembles the course of human infection is produced in cats, hamsters, and monkeys after s.c. footpad inoculation.[38-41] Histopathologically, characteristic asteroid bodies surrounding the fungal cells are sometimes seen in testicular tissue of mice, rats, hamsters, and guinea pigs.[26] Furthermore, differences in thermophilia for colony formation (35°C and 37°C) of *S. schenckii* isolate the fungus and, depending on the temperature under which the animals are kept, will grow in different organs of mice and rats.[42] Therefore, when working with experimental infections due to *S. schenckii,* it is mandatory that the temperature under which the animals are kept is fully controlled. Some investigators recommend that the animals are kept at 20°C as the rate of infection is higher at this temperature.[43,44]

ANIMAL MODELS OF MYCOSES DUE TO TRUE PATHOGENIC FUNGI

Mycoses in this group are caused by species that have the ability to elicit disease in normal hosts when the inoculum has a sufficient size.[45] Therefore, cultures of these fungi should be handled in the most rigorous of containment facilities by experienced personal only. The mycoses are usually systemic and occur in restricted geographic areas primarily in North and South America and Africa.[45] The true pathogenic fungi are dimorphic and exhibit a morphological transition from a mycelial (saprophytic) form to a budding/yeast-like (parasitic) form seen in infected tissue where chronic granulomatous processes are formed.[45,46]

Blastomycosis

Blastomycosis is caused by *Blastomyces dermatitidis,* and is characterized by having a primary pulmonary stage that may be followed by dissemination to other body sites especially the skin and bones.[45] Mice are highly susceptible to yeasts of *B. dermatitidis,* but the maturity of mice (body weight and age) is a critical factor in resistance, as is the strain of mice used, because they influence both the course of infection and lethality in mice when challenged with *B. dermatitidis.*[47,48] Mice are preferably infected by the aerogene route as it is the natural portal of entry in humans. Following i.n. challenge, an acute to chronic pulmonary infection is established and dissemination to other organs may be seen.[48,49] In this model, the course of infection and the pathological reactions seen are comparable to human blastomycosis.[50] By experiments in hamsters, which are more susceptible to infection than mice, a female:male lethal ratio of 1:7 is observed, which corresponds to the 1:9 ratio in humans.[46,51,52] Moreover, treatment of ovariectomized hamsters with testosterone will render them as susceptible as male hamsters, and castrated males are more resistant than normal ones.[51] These results with experimental blastomycosis strongly point to the importance of always giving full information on the models used. More rarely, guinea pigs and dogs are also used as models of blastomycoses.[46]

Coccidioidomycosis

Coccidioidomycosis is usually a mild respiratory infection due to *Coccidioides immitis.* Rarely, the infection is an acute or chronic disseminating and fatal mycosis.[45,46]

Experimental disease may be produced in most laboratory animals. Mice are usually used, and according to inoculum, port of entry, and strain, the course of disease may vary from acute fatal to chronic.[46] In the i.p. and i.n. model of coccidioidomycosis, like in blastomycosis, a marked difference in susceptibility has been found in a variety of genetically different but defined mice.[53,54] Also, the course of coccidioidomycosis in mice is highly age-dependent but not sex-dependent.[54] The pulmonary model in mice mimics the infection of humans with a characteristic formation of granulomas.[46] As immunized mice restrict extrapulmonary dissemination,[55,56] which seldom is seen in human cases, this model should be considered in, e.g., pathogenicity studies. Apart from mice, also guinea pigs, dogs, and monkeys are applicable in the study of different aspects of coccidioidomycosis.[46]

Histoplasmosis

Histoplasmosis capsulati, a granulomatous disease, is caused by *Histoplasma capsulatum* var. *capsulatum* and has a worldwide distribution. Clinically, the disease may vary from subclinical/completely benign to a chronic progressive lung disease, a chronic cutaneous or systemic disease, or an acute fulminant and fatal systemic infection.[57]

While there may be no good animal model of the more chronic forms of infection by *H. capsulatum* var. *capsulatum,* reproductive animal models of acute pulmonary, disseminated, and ocular forms have been developed and are applied extensively in studies concerning therapy.[45,46] Experimental histoplasmosis is easily produced by challenge i.v. and i.n. in mice and dogs, whereas guinea pigs, hamsters, rabbits, and rats vary considerably in their susceptibility to infection.[45] The self-resolving infection of the murine lung after i.t. inoculation of yeast cells is an essential model for the most frequent human form of subclinical infection.[58] Because as little as 1 to 10 yeast cells or even a single macroconidium will infect a mouse, it is a useful means of isolation of the fungus from patient material and soil samples, for which a standardized procedure is devised.[45] Also, monkeys and poikilothermic animals have been used as experimental models of histoplasmosis.[45] In the latter group, it was found that the lesions of animals incubated at 25°C contain mycelium and those at 37°C contained yeast cells regardless of the infectious material.

Histoplasmosis farciminosi is caused by a variant called *Histoplasma capsulatum* var. *farciminosum* and is the cause of epizootic lymphangitis in horses, donkeys, and mules. Experimental disease by i.d. and i.p. inoculation of mice and rabbits has been produced.[59,60] However, in these animals, the disease had not caused what is seen in the equines, i.e., formation of lymphangitis.

Histoplasmosis duboisii (African histoplasmosis) is caused by *Histoplasma capsulatum* var. *duboisii* and the disease evoked by this fungus is characterized by granulomatous and suppurative lesions, primarily of the cutaneous, subcutaneous, and osseous tissues.[45] Because the time between infection and clinical symptoms in natural infection with *H. capsulatum* var. *duboisii* is long, the disease has sometimes been imported through primates to countries outside the African continent.[61,62] Experimental infections in animals have been studied in a number of species, e.g., mice, hamsters, guinea pigs, rabbits, and pigeons and in comparison to *H. capsulatum* var. *capsulatum* the *duboisii* variant is of relatively low virulence.[45,63] In laboratory animals, the course of infection is comparable to human cases.[45,63] Histologically, the reaction is initially histiocytic, which is later replaced by giant cells that are also dominant in the human granulomatous lesions of African histoplasmosis.

Paracoccidioidomycosis

Paracoccidioidomycosis is caused by *Paracoccidioides brasiliensis* and is a chronic granulomatous disease that, after nidation in the lung, disseminates to form ulcerative granulomas of especially the head and gastrointestinal mucosa.[45] Also lymph nodes are often involved. As for *H. capsulatum* var. *capsulatum* and *B. dermatitidis,* the fungus may be isolated from clinical material by inoculation into laboratory animals where, e.g., i. test. inoculation of rats, of which especially the mountain rat (*Proechimys guayanensis*) is particulary susceptible to infection should be used.[45] Next to mice, hamsters, which are more susceptible than guinea pigs, have been used most extensively in the study of paracoccidioidomycosis.[46,64,65] In mice and other laboratory animals, acute systemic infections are seen after i.v. and i.p. challenge with the yeast form of the fungus. However, as for blastomycosis and coccidioidomycosis, the maturity of the mice is essential when used for experimental infection.[66] Rabbits are relatively resistant to infection.[67]

A chronic progressive model in hamsters inoculated i. test. with yeast cells is somewhat analogous to the human disease.[68,69] However, the pulmonary route of infection with dissemination to other organs, which is the natural route of infection in humans, is established in immunosuppresed mice by inoculation of elements of the saprophytic form of *P. brasiliensis*.[70] Therefore, this model is the most suitable model for the study of paracoccidioidomycosis with respect to, e.g., pathogenesis.

ANIMAL MODELS OF MYCOSES DUE TO OPPORTUNISTIC PATHOGENIC FUNGI

Infection due to fungi in this group is normally only established when predisposing factors are present.[71] The number of factors promoting the development of opportunistic mycotic infections is quite large and comprises aspects regarding the fungus (e.g., dose of exposure and virulence of strain) but much more important are predisposing, favoring, or stimulating factors in the host.[72] Among predisposing conditions in humans the most important ones are diseases like diabetes mellitus, acute lymphoblastic leukemia, and other hematological neoplasms, and the acquired immunodeficiency syndrome (AIDS).[72,73] Also, the use of therapeutics that compromise the immunological status of humans and animals or comprise the normal bacterial flora of the outer surfaces and the gastrointestinal tract, e.g., corticosteroids, broad-spectrum antibiotics, and chemotherapeutics are conductive to opportunistic fungal infections.[73] Some agents directly stimulate the growth of fungal agents, e.g., deferoxamine (or administration of iron) in aspergillosis, candidosis, and zygomycosis.[72,74,75] In women, pregnancy or the use of high-estrogen-containing oral contraceptives are predisposing factors for developing vaginal candidosis.[76,77]

A number of immunodepressed animal models has been developed in order to obtain models related to the conditions described in humans and animals. Induced immunosuppression by treatment with, e.g., X-irradiation, corticosteroids, cyclophosphamide, mechlorethamine, and splenectomy is frequently used.[72,73,78,79] Spontaneous immunosuppressive animal models like congenitally athymic nude mice or New Zealand Black (NZB) mice (defective in T-lymphocytes) and AKR/J leukemic mice are used in order to mimic the infections in humans under immunocompromised conditions, but also in the study of the defense mechanisms involved during different mycoses.[27,73,80] Endocrinological disturbance models such as diabetic models are routinely produced in various animals by administration of alloxan or streptozotocin.[72,73] It should also be noted that sex-hormones are of significant influence on the establishment of some systemic mycoses, e.g., blastomycosis. Likewise, in the model of vaginal candidosis, it is essential to use oophorectomized animals, usually rats and mice, which are treated with estrogen to bring them in a permanent state of pseudoestrus.[8,18,72,77]

Aspergillosis

Aspergillosis refers to a number of diseases in which *Aspergillus spp.* are involved. Generally the disease results from toxicity due to contaminated food; allergy mainly due to spore allergens; pulmonary colonization without extension, and invasion with or without subsequent dissemination.[71] *Aspergillus fumigatus* is the most important pathogen with *Aspergillus flavus, Aspergillus niger,* and *Aspergillus terreus* being less frequent in a decreasing manner.[73] In humans, the lung is the most common site affected, and preexisting or concurrent lung diseases are a major factor predisposing a host to infection.[71] However, most of the predisposing factors mentioned in the introduction to the present section dealing with the opportunistic pathogenic fungi are also responsible for the development of aspergillosis.[71,73] Especially in severely debilitated persons, the course of infection may be dissemination with localization in a variety of internal organs. In veterinary medicine, avian aspergillosis and bovine proventriculitis and placentitis with subsequent abortion due to especially *A. fumigatus* are of great importance.[81-83] Invasive lung aspergillosis may be established in mice, chicks, ducks, rabbits, rats, and other laboratory animals when used as inhalation models (challenged i.n or i.t.) where the conidia are given in aerosols either in a dry or wet form.[73,84,85] In these models, the mouse is preferred and treatment with cortisone is essential for the development of a high incidence of fatal pulmonal aspergillosis as murine alveolar macrophages are capable of preventing germination and can kill spores.[86-88] However, in the cortisone treated animals, the lysosomal membranes within macrophages are stabilized making the animals more susceptible to infection.[89,90] An experimental pulmonary aspergilloma model in rabbits is established by artificial bronchostenosis, ligature of pulmonary artery, and injection of *Aspergillus* spores into the distal bronchus. In this model, bronchiectasis, cavity and cyst, and a massive laminated growth of hyphae are found within the bronchial lumen which is similar to the human aspergilloma.[91] The aerogene route of entry to the body is, compared to i.v. and i.p. inoculations, compatible to the natural entry in humans where the lungs are the most frequent portal of entry. By the i.v. route, disseminated forms of aspergillosis are formed regularly

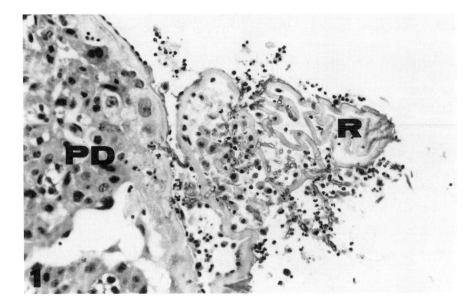

Figure 2. Experimental aspergillosis in a pregnant mouse (day 16 of pregnancy) inoculated i.v. with *Aspergillus fumigatus* on day 10 of pregnancy. (1) The growth of hyphae in the periphery of the placental disc (PD) and Reichert's membrane (R) is accompanied by necrosis and polymorphonuclear cell infiltration. (From H. E. Jensen and J. Hau, *In vivo,* 4, 247, 1990. With permission.)

whereas dissemination after i.p. challenge often requires treatment by cortisone or cyclophosphamide.[73] The i.v. model of disseminated aspergillosis, however, has the advantage that a precise dose-related course of infection can be established, which is important in the evaluation of virulence parameters (ID_{50} and LD_{50}) of different fungal strains and the estimation of therapeutic parameters such as TD_{50}, ED_{50} and PD_{50}; see pg. 188. In the systemic aspergillosis model, the kidneys are the target organs. However, when pregnant animals (cows, sheep, and mice) are inoculated i.v. by spores from *A. fumigatus,* the placenta is also a target organ (Figure 2).[92-95]

Next to the mouse, the rabbit is the dominant animal species used in the study of experimental aspergillosis.[73] By i.v. challenge, the course of disseminated infection may vary from acute to chronic depending on the size of inoculum. As in mice, administration of immunosuppressive agents will turn the infection into extensive aspergillosis. The rabbit lung has a high susceptibility to aspergillosis. Primary pulmonary aspergillosis in rabbits is established by i.t. inoculation of spores and, as in mice, the use of immunosuppressive drugs is essential for the establishment of fatal infections. In this model, a primary and predominant involvement of the lung tissue is seen with subsequent spread to especially the liver, spleen, and kidneys.[73] Moreover, among laboratory animals, natural occurrence of aspergillosis seems to have been reported only in rabbits.[96]

Localized aspergillosis models of endophthalmitis and endocarditis have also been described. In the latter model, the fungal spores are introduced i.v. into animals that have received an intracardial catheter.[97] From the occlusive vegetations formed on the heart valves, infected emboli are carried to other organs in which subsequent aspergillosis develop.

Rats have also been extensively used as models for aspergillosis and show no significant differences in the course of infection compared to the other animal species.[73]

A primate model in rhesus monkeys of allergic bronchopulmonary aspergillosis (ABPA) was established by Golbert and Patterson.[98]

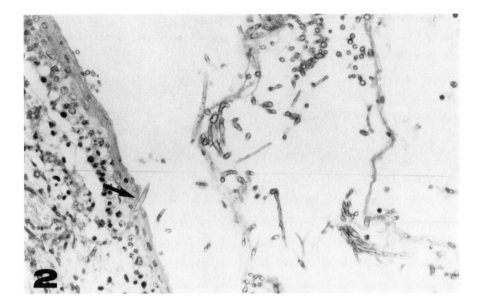

Figure 2. (2) Hyphae are seen around amnion and within the fetal skin (arrow). (From H. E. Jensen and J. Hau, *In vivo,* 4, 247, 1990. With permission.)

Candidosis

Candidosis is an opportunistic infection caused by yeasts of the genus *Candida* and predominantly of the species *Candida albicans*.[71,73] The manifestations of candidosis are ranging from acute, subacute to chronic and may involve the skin, mucous membranes, or more rarely become systemic. Here, only experimental infections with *C. albicans* will be considered as it is the dominant cause of human candidosis and infections by other pathogenic *Candida* spp. show comparable events in laboratory animals. Disseminated infections have been produced in a number of different species (e.g. rats, rabbits, and guinea pigs) by challenge i.v. and i.p.[73] The mouse is the most often used model for systemic candidosis. It should be noted, however, that guinea pigs are particularly resistant to i.p. challenge with blastospores of *Candida,* and that rabbits are more susceptible to infection than mice.[73] Among strains of mice, there are prominent differences in the susceptibility to *C. albicans* infections after i.v. challenge with C57BL/6, C57BL/6J, and Sec/1Rej being most resistant and the C57C57BL/Hej, BALB/c, and CBA/J mice moderately susceptible, while the highest susceptibility is found in AKR/J, CBA/CaJ, DBA/1J, DBA/2J, A/J, and RF/J mice.[73,99] These differences in susceptibility probably reflect different properties in the release of lymphokines, the degrees of natural killer cell activity, and function of the complement system.[99,100]

Systemic candidosis is also seen after i.a. and i. cra. challenge of rabbits and rats with blastospores.[101-103] In systemic infection models, the kidneys are the target organs which seem to reflect an initial protection from inflammatory cells by intraluminal localization in the tubuli (Figure 3).[104] However, recently it was shown that the placenta of pregnant mice showed an even higher susceptibility to infection, which may be a general feature, after i.v. challenge of pregnant animals with opportunistic pathogenic fungi (see also aspergillosis) (Figure 4).[105] In Figure 5, the pathogenesis of murine mycotic placentitis is shown. Localized organ manifestations may also be seen after i.v. and i.p. challenge of animals, e.g., endophthalmitis in rabbits and dermatitis in guinea pigs.[18,73] Localized exogenous candidosis models of endophthalmitis, dermatitis, arthritis, cystitis, and endocarditis (see aspergillosis) have all been established in rabbits and other animals.[18,72,73,106] Cutaneous candidosis can be produced in a wide range of animals, but the guinea pig is especially susceptible, and when diabetic animals (alloxan

180

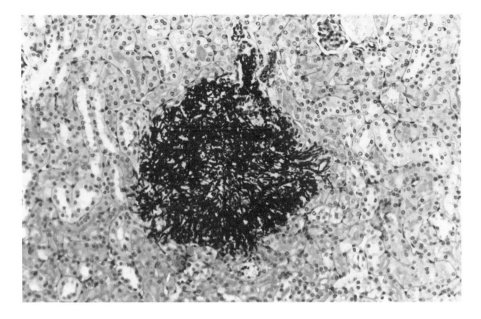

Figure 3. Experimental renal candidosis in a mouse after i.v. challenge with *Candida albicans* blastospores.

treated) are used, the lesions formed are compatible to the human form, and therefore the model is commonly used in the screening of new antifungal agents.[9,18,72,73] The model of chronic vaginitis usually established in rats is also widely used in the evaluation of new antifungal agents. The infection is established by i. vag. inoculation of blastospores into animals that are oophorectomized and kept in a permanent state of pseudoestrus by weekly injections of estrogen.[9,73,77] Localized oral candidosis in rats ("thrush") and in the crop of several avian species are produced after p.o. challenge with blastospores. The disease is favored by a carbohydrate rich diet, antibiotic treatment, or/and use of germ-free or SPF-animals.[73,106,107] Also, localized candidosis in air-filled subcutaneous cysts imitating "thrush" is used in the testing of antifungal agents.[108] Intragastric challenge of infant mice results in systemic spread of candidosis, whereas the same course of infection in adult animals requires some compromising treatment with, e.g., antibiotic and cytotoxic agents.[73,109,110]

In murine models of candidosis, an enhancement of infection is seen after treatment with an overload of iron.[74] Iron also enhances the course of aspergillosis and zygomycosis, and seems to be a result of saturation of fungal siderophores, iron-transport cofactors, which bind iron and form a chelate that is essential for the growth of the fungi.[72,73,75] Generally, also X-irradiated, corticosteroid treated, and diabetic animals have a lowered tolerance to challenge with *Candida* blastospores.[18,72,73]

Finally, it should be mentioned that i.m. injection of *C. albicans* blastospores (viable, heat-killed, or lyophilized) is a well-recognized experimental model of murine amyloidosis, which may be used in studying pathogenesis and treatment of amyloidosis.[111]

Cryptococcosis

Cryptococcosis is a subacute or chronic, rarely acute, pulmonary, systemic, or meningeal infection caused by the yeast *Cryptococcus neoformans*.[71,73]

Mice are highly susceptible to cryptococcosis and are frequently used as a model in the study of the disease as it shows a number of similarities to the disease in humans. Dissemination to internal organs is seen after i.v., i.cer., and i.p. challenge of mice with an appropriate

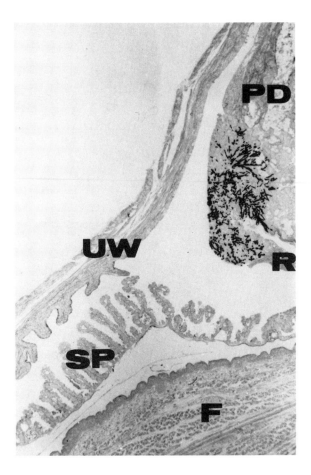

Figure 4. Experimental candidosis in a pregnant mouse. The fungi are characteristically restricted to the perifery of the placental disc (PD) and the degenerated Reichert's membrane (R). UW: Uterine wall. SP: Splanchnopleura. F: Foetus. (From H. E. Jensen et al., *APMIS*, 99, 829, 1991. With permission.)

amount of *C. neoformans* cells.[73] As for *C. albicans,* variations in susceptibility to infection are seen in mice of different strains. In the disseminated disease models, the histopathological findings are characterized as either granulomatous or cystic, reflecting the presence of macrophages in the different organs.[27,112,113] *C. neoformans* has a propensity for infecting the brain, lungs, and kidneys.[73] Cryptococcal meningitis is so accurately developed in mice after i.v. inoculation of appropriate numbers of cells that this model is used in the differentiation of *C. neoformans* from other *Cryptococcus* species and in the evaluation of antifungal agents.[71] However, when the respiratory system is the portal of entry, dissemination to other organs is delayed (especially to the brain) and allows a more preferable exploration of the course of infection in humans. Mice and rats are the preferred animals, and rabbits and guinea pigs are almost resistant to cryptococcal infections, although chronic cryptococcal meningitis has been developed in cortisone treated rabbits after i. cer. inoculation.[114-117] In addition to its similarity to the human disease, this rabbit model has the advantage in comparison with the murine model that the larger size of the animal allows repeated aspiration of larger volumes of cerebrospinal fluid for analysis.[73]

Localized cryptococcal infection models are produced in other organs after local application, e.g., cutaneous and ocular cryptococcosis.[9,73] After administration of *C. neoformans* cells to mice p.o. some will have the gastrointestinal tract colonized and dissemination to other

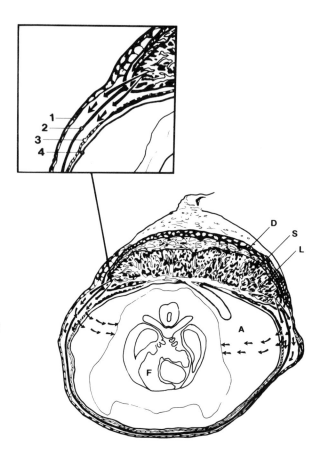

Figure 5. The pathogenesis of murine placental candidosis. Arrows indicate the origin and extent of murine candidosis. A: Amniotic cavity. D: Decidua. F: Foetus. L: Labyrinth. S: Spongiotrophoblasts. 1: Uterine wall. 2: Reichert's membrane. 3: Splanchnopleure. 4: Amnion. (From H. E. Jensen et al., *APMIS*, 99, 829, 1991. With permission.)

organs may occur, however infrequently, and the course is not influenced by treatment compromising the immunological status of the animal.[73,118] Colonization of the nasal mucosa of mice may also be seen after i.n. inoculation of cells of some strains of *C. neoformans*.[119]

Scedosporiosis

Scedosporiosis is caused by *Scedosporium apiospermum (Pseudallescheria boydii)* and *Scedosporium inflatum,* and the infection may vary from local infection of especially the lung, skin, and cornea to disseminated mycosis.[120] Comparable animal models of local scedosporiosis include granulomas, keratitis, and arthritis in rabbits.[71] Mice are often used in the production of disseminated infections developing subsequent to i.v. inoculation of conidia.[121]

Zygomycosis

Zygomycosis refers to infections caused by fungi of the class *Zygomycetes* of which the family *Mucoraceae* of the order *Mucorales* is most important in medical and veterinary mycology.[122,123] The course of infection may be acute to long-term chronic. The localization of the infection may be in the cutis or subcutis, the lung, the nose with subsequent spread to the brain (rhinocerebral zygomycosis) or more rarely the disease may turn out in a disseminated form.[71,122] *Absidia corymbifera, Rhizopus spp.* and *Mucor spp.* are most often found as

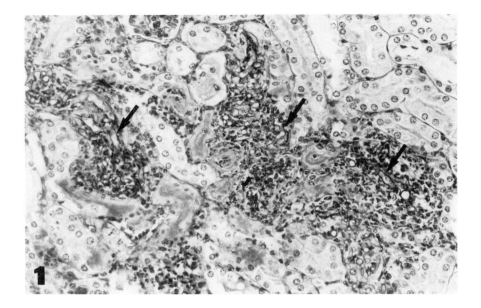

Figure 6. Murine zygomycosis due to *Absidia corymbifera*. (1) Acute renal zygomycosis after i.v. challenge. Arrows: hyphae.

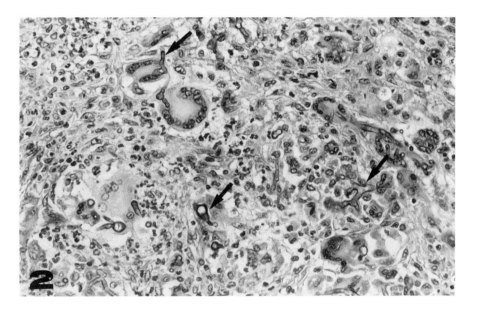

Figure 6. (2) Chronic subcutaneous granulomatous zygomycosis after s.c. challenge. Arrows: hyphae.

a causative organism of human and animal zygomycosis.[122,123] Disseminated acute systemic infections by these fungi are easily established in most animals after i.v. challenge (Figure 6). Mice, rats, rabbits, and guinea pigs are often used, with guinea pigs being the most appropriate.[19,73] However, these infections are not likely to be used as models as this course of infection is seen only rarely in humans. The i.v. route of challenge is, however, used extensively in studies of etiology, immunology, histopathology, and assessment of new antifungal agents.[19,72,73]

184

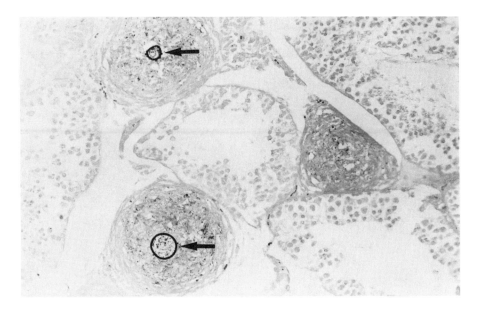

Figure 7. Adiaspiromycotic granulomatous orchitis in a hamster after i.test. inoculation of culture material. Arrows: Adiaspores.

Inoculation of spores i.n. and i.t. into cortisone-treated or streptozotocin-diabetic animals results in pulmonary and cerebral zygomycosis with a course of infection and pathology close to that of human cases of pulmonary zygomycosis.[73,124,125] Also, treatment of mice with deferoxamine and iron (Fe^{+++}) will render them more susceptible to infection, and p.o. challenge of guinea pigs pretreated with aspirin will cause gastric invasion.[72,126,127] Localized chronic pyogranulomatous infections in most animals may also be produced after cutaneous, subcutaneous, or orbital inoculations (Figure 6).[73]

ANIMAL MODELS OF MISCELLANEOUS MYCOSES AND ALGOSES
Miscellaneous fungi
Geotrichum spp. may be the cause of mucocutaneous infections. In laboratory animals, it is very difficult to establish infection by the fungi; however, inoculation of mice i.v. and i.p. with clinical isolates of *Geotrichum candidum* may result in systemic infection.[71,128,129]

Penicillium spp. are very common in the environment but are only rarely the cause of infection.[71] However, one exception is *Penicillium marneffei,* which have been recovered from a number of human and animal (especially the bamboo rat *Rhizomys pruinosus)* infections particulary in Asian countries.[130,131] In humans, infections are often progressive, and disseminated forms similar to those seen in histoplasmosis are formed. A comparable course of disease occurs in mice, rats, and hamsters challenged i.v. or i.p. with the fungus.[130]

Pityrosporum ovale (Malassezia furfur) a lipophilic fungus, is an etiological agent in the development of pityriasis versicolor, folliculitis, and seborrheic dermatitis in humans.[9] Faergemann has successfully infected volunteers by cutaneous infection under occlusive dressing and additional application of olive oil. The positive effect of olive oil was also demonstrated by using the inside of ears of rabbits.[132,133] A number of more low-pathogenic fungi, e.g., *Rhodotorula rubra, Candida glabrata* and other *Candida spp.* different from *C. albicans* produce a moderate skin infection when inoculated onto the back of diabetic (alloxan pretreated) guinea pigs.[9]

Adiaspiromycosis, which is seen especially in the lungs of wild living rodents, is caused by the inhalation of conidia of the fungal genus *Chrysosporium (Emmonsia).*[71] In humans,

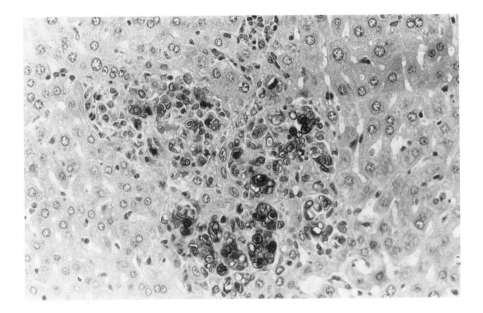

Figure 8. Murine hepatic granulomatous protothecosis after i.v. challenge by cells of *Prototheca zopfii*. In the process uni- and multicellular organisms are seen.

adiaspiromycosis is rare but the knowledge of the infection is especially important as a differential diagnosis to other fungi in tissues of rodents. Injection of conidia into mice, rabbits, rats, and dogs may result in the development of systemic infection.[71] Localized granulomatous orchitis is produced after i. test. inoculation of the fungi in hamsters (Figure 7).

Mycotic keratitis in humans is often caused by members of the genera *Candida* and *Aspergillus*, but in rare situations infection by more low-pathogenic fungi, e.g., *Fusarium spp.* may occur as well. A variety of rabbit and rat models of mycotic keratitis due to these fungi is used preferably in the testing of new antifungal agents.[73]

Algae

Human and animal infections due to algae are rare. However, infection by *Prototheca spp.*, especially *Prototheca zopfii* (an achloric alga), may be the cause of superficial or deep cutaneous infections and bursitis in humans and more frequently mastitis in cattle.[134,135] Reports also have been given on disseminated infections in cows and dogs.[136,137] Some cases of bovine lymphadenitis due to infection with green algae of the order *Chlorococcales* are reported, too.[138] Mice inoculated i.v. with *Prototheca zopfii* develop systemic granulomatous infections (Figure 8) and skin infections appear in guinea pigs after i.d. inoculation.[139] In rats, i.p. challenge by green algae results in the formation of slowly progressive infection of the serosal peritoneal surface.[138]

APPLICATION OF MODIFIED ANIMAL MODELS IN MYCOLOGY

To obtain more homogeneous infections with pathogenic fungi, and to establish an infection with opportunistic pathogenic or poorly invasive fungi a variety of methods are used to enhance the susceptibility of animals to infection. Furthermore, some modified models are also used in order to mimic the conditions under which humans are infected especially with the opportunistic pathogenic fungi. In the section dealing with these infections, factors were listed that were predisposing, favoring, and stimulating for the growth of fungi. Here some other modified models applied in the study of transformative fungal changes and defense mechanisms involved in mycoses are given.

Some fungi adapt themselves by transformation into a parasitic form when growing in tissues, a phenomenon called dimorphism, a unique factor in the pathogenicity of these fungi. In order to study this phenomenon, a number of *in vitro* methods have been used. *In vivo* fungal transformation can be followed by consecutive histopathology following challenge, e.g., i.v., s.c., and i.p. In these models, heavy cell and humoral defense mechanisms will often mask the details of transformation. In the "agar implantation" model, blocks of agar containing the saprophytic stages of fungi are implanted into the abdominal cavity of mice.[27] From series of mice, the agar blocks are removed after adequant intervals and subjected to histo- and electronmicroscopy. In this model, the development and transformation of fungi are only influenced by humoral defense factors of the host.[27] Based on results from the agar implantation model, the study of fungal infections after, e.g., i.v, s.c., and i.p. challenge and naturally fungal infections in humans and animals, the pathogenic fungi have been classified into two categories according to their parasitic forms:[27] (1) Fungi that are mycelial in their saprophytic stage and spherical in their parasitic stage. The transformation of these fungi is either via the stage of arthroconidiae (e.g., *T. rubrum, C. immitis,* and *P. marneffei),* the stage of chlamydospores (e.g., *B. dermatitidis, P. brasiliensis,* and *Fonsecaea pedrosoi,* a common cause of chromomycosis), or by direct budding from hyphae (*S. schenckii, H. capsulatum* var. *capsulatum,* var. *duboisii,* and var. *farciminosum.* (2) Fungi whose parasitic forms are similar to the saprophytic form either in the form of mycelia (e.g., *Aspergillus, Absidia, Mucor, Rhizopus, Fusarium,* and *Scedosporium species),* the form of mycelial and yeast forms (e.g., *Candida* spp.) or yeast (e.g., *Cryptococcus neoformans).*

In the study of specific aspects of pathogenicity and defense mechanisms involved in mycotic infections, a number of modified animal models has been used. By these models, important differences of the cell-mediated reactions and the influence of complement in the defense against fungal infections have been elucidated.

Inbred strains of mice that are genetically deficient in the 5th factor of the complement system (C5), e.g., DBA/ZN and B.10.D2/oSn mice and C4D guinea pigs (congenitally deficient in component C4) have been used to study the possible role of the alternative complement pathway in cryptococcosis and candidosis.[27,73]

In the study of the defensive role of T-lymphocytes, congenital athymic mice (nu/nu BALB/c mice), New Zealand Black (NZB) mice which often become defective in their T-lymphocytes, and thymectomized mice are used. The number and function of polymorphonuclear (PMN) cells are decreased and suppressed, respectively, by X-irradiation and administration of nitrogen mustard.[27] In these models, the sessile macrophages of the RES-system usually remain intact, and the importance of the PMN cells can be analyzed. The defensive role of mononuclear cells in mycoses can be analyzed by challenge of mice treated i.v. with dextran sulfate or silica, which saturate the phagocytic function of monocytes and sessile macrophages.[27] Histopathological examination of tissues from these modified mycotic animal models has contributed greatly to the understanding of which defense mechanisms are involved against different fungi. Table 1 is a review of differences in the susceptibility (lethal dose, severity of lesions, and efficacy in killing the fungus) of congenitally athymic nude mice (nu/nu) vs. their heterozygous littermates (nu/+) of BALB/c background to different fungi after i.v. challenge.[27] In the chronic state of deep mycoses in humans and laboratory animals, the formation of granulomas is the main pathological finding. However, in the earlier stages, the inflammatory reaction depends on the fungus involved. Towards some fungi, the cellular reaction is mainly made up by the mononuclear cells with assistance from only a negligible number of PMN cells. In other mycoses, the cell infiltration is primarily due to PMN cells in the early stages of infection, whereas in the chronic stages, the killing of the fungus is

Table 1. Susceptibility to mycoses in congenital athymic nude mice (nu/nu) versus their heterozygous littermates (nu/+) of BALB/c background after intravenous challenge; and the dominant type of cells involved in the defense of infection

Fungal infection	Susceptibility of nude mice	Main cellular response
Cryptococcosis		
C. neoformans	Enhanced	Mononuclear
Phaeohyphomycosis		
W. dermatitidis	Enhanced	Mononuclear
Histoplasmosis capsulati		
H. capsulatum. var. capsulatum	Enhanced	Mononuclear
Histoplasmosis duboisii		
H. capsulatum var. duboisii	Enhanced	Mononuclear
Sporotrichosis		
S. schenckii	Enhanced	Mononuclear
Blastomycosis		
B. dermatitidis	Enhanced	Mononuclear/PMN[2]
Paracoccidioidomycosis		
P. brasiliensis	Enhanced	Mononuclear/PMN
Chromoblastomycosis		
F. pedrosoi	Enhanced/lowered[1]	Mononuclear/PMN
Candidosis		
C. albicans	Controversial	PMN/mononuclear
Coccidioidomycosis		
C. immitis	Controversial	PMN/mononuclear
Aspergillosis		
A. fumigatus	None	PMN(mononuclear)
Zygomycosis		
A. corymbifera	None	PMN(mononuclear)

[1]Enhanced at high doses and lowered at low doses.
[2]Polymorphonuclear.

accomplished by the infiltration of macrophages (PMN/mononuclear). Finally, the host defense against aspergillosis and zygomycosis is mainly due to PMN cells, but in the chronic processes of these mycoses granulomas are also formed. In Table 1, the cells playing a main role in the host defense against different fungi are summarized.

EVALUATION OF ANTIFUNGAL AGENTS IN ANIMAL MODELS

Therapeutic choices between microbial agents have traditionally been guided by their activity *in vitro*. However, *in vitro* results for antifungal agents are not necessarily indicative of efficacy *in vivo*. In particular, the azole antifungal agents yield inconsistent sensitivity results and tend to produce higher susceptibility endpoints, depending on components and pH of the medium, inoculum size, incubation temperature, and time of reading.[140] Fluconazole reaches an extreme in terms of the disparity between *in vitro* and *in vivo* activity.[141] Moreover, only by the use of a wide range of animal models was it possible to select and introduce the first broad-spectrum antifungal drug, ketoconazole.[9] For these reasons and the applicability of testing different dispense forms, therapeutic and side effects, etc. the use of animal models of mycoses is of significant importance in the screening for new antifungal agents.

When testing new antifungal agents, as many fungal species as possible should be tested. Moreover, because a number of fungi show strain variation in their virulence, expressed by their median infective dose (ID_{50}) and median lethal dose (LD_{50}) (the dose [colony forming units/kg] which will infect and kill, respectively, 50% of the animals), the number of strains tested should also be high.

Models used in the evaluation of efficacy are classified according to the nature of the infection.[142,143] (1) The basic antimicrobial screening models are commonly used in early evaluation of antifungal agents, and the animals (usually mice) are challenged with a dose that ensures death of all animals. In this model, the ability of agents to prolong survival of infected animals is determined and the estimated median effective dose ED_{50} (mg/kg), the dose that protects 50% of the animals from death, is calculated. Advantages of these models are: infection and treatment are simple; clearly defined endpoints; economical and of a short duration. Disadvantages include: the course of infection is uncharacteristic and fulminant; the antifungal agents are administrated at/or close to the infection; the models are highly sensitive to the size of the infective dose; single or only few doses are given, which may result in pharmacokinetic differences that do not allow comparisons between agents. (2) The *ex vivo* model uses a foreign body containing the organism and is implanted (s.c., i.p., etc.) prior to treatment. During treatment the bodies are removed and the content is analyzed *in vitro*. The bodies may be fibrin clots or dialysis sacks that permit the entry of the agent but restrict the entry of cellular and humoral components of the host defense system. The use of a porous or hollow device permits entry of phagocytes and antibodies, and may be valuable for the determination of these components to penetrate a specific site of infection. This model has thus far not found any practical form in testing antifungal agents, but the "agar implantation" model is an example of its use in mycopathology.[27] (3) In the monoparametric model, a simple indicator of therapeutic effectiveness is measured, as opposed to an ultimative therapeutic cure. In this model the capacity of agents to sterilize infected tissues (e.g., *C. albicans* in murine kidney infections) and concentration of the antifungal agent in tissues is evaluated. In the effort for reducing the use of laboratory animals, monoparametric models should be replaced by discriminative models. (4) The discriminative models are by far the most technically complicated models and are designed to mimic the initiation and progress of infection in humans and higher animals. In these models, multiple parameters are measured and they allow evaluation of drug concentration, adjuvant therapies, etc. In these models, calculated parameters such as the median protective dose (PD_{50}) and median therapeutic dose (TD_{50})(the dose [mg/kg] that protects and cures 50% of the animals, respectively) are determined. In the selection of a discriminative model, the following ideal features should be considered:[143] simple technique for infection; the fungus, route of entry, spread in the body, and tissues involved should be similar to the situation in humans. The severity, course, and duration of the infection should be predictable, reproductive, and amenable to analysis. Furthermore, susceptibility to therapy must be measurable and reproductive. Some models seem to satisfy most of these criteria adequately, e.g., murine pulmonary cryptococcosis, but in most models of mycoses some compromises have to be offered, e.g., in models of dermatophytoses the fungus is usually a zoophilic dermatophyte and the prolonged chronic infections as seen in humans are not produced, and relapse of skin infection may be seen from lesions in internal organs when the infection is established through i.v. inoculation.[9] Another example is that to establish and maintain vaginal candidosis in laboratory animals, they must be oophorectomized and treated with estrogen during the time of infection.[73,77] In Table 2, common animal models of some mycoses used in the testing of antifungal agents are listed.

ANIMAL MODELS AS MYCODIAGNOSTIC TOOLS

A number of fungi are, when only present in a limited amount, grown more regularly *in vivo* than *in vitro*. Therefore, when *in vitro* cultivations of materials under suspicion of content of,

Table 2. Animal models applied in the evaluation of antifungal agents

Fungal infection	Animal	Predisposing factors	Inoculation site	Localization of infection
Dermatophytosis				
T. mentagrophytes and *M. canis*	Guinea pig	Abraded/ none	On skin*	Skin
	Guinea pig	None	I.v.	Skin and dissemination
Pityriasis				
P. ovale and *P. orbiculare*	Guinea pig	Clipped	On skin*	Skin
Sporotrichosis				
S. schenckii	Guinea pig	None	I.v./i.test.	Dissemination
Penicilliosis				
P. marneffei	Guinea pig	Immunosup-pressed/none	I.v.	Dissemination
Blastomycosis				
B. dermatitidis	Mouse	None	I.n.	Lung and dissemination
	Mouse	None	I.n.	Dissemination
Coccidioido-mycosis				
C. immitis	Mouse	None	I.n.	Lung and dissemination
	Mouse	None	I.n.	Dissemination
Histoplasmosis				
H. capsulatum var. *capsulatum*	Mouse	None	I.n.	Lung and dissemination
	Mouse	None	I.v./i.p.	Dissemination
H. capsulatum var. *duboisii*	Guinea pig	None	I. test.	Testicles and dissemination
Paracoccidioido-mycosis				
P. brasiliensis	Mouse	None	I.n.	Lung and dissemination
	Mouse	None	I.n.	Dissemination
Aspergillosis				
A. fumigatus	Mouse	Immunosup-pressed	I.n.	Lung and dissemination
	Chicken	None	Aerosol	Lung and dissemination
	Rabbit	Immunosup-pressed	I. cor.	Cornea
	Rabbit	Intracardial catheter	I.v.	Endocardium and dissemination

190

Table 2. Animal models applied in the evaluation of antifungal agents (continued)

Fungal infection	Animal	Predisposing factors	Inoculation site	Localization of infection
	Guinea pig	Immunosuppressed/none	I.v.	Dissemination
	Mouse	Immunosuppressed/none	I.v.	Dissemination
Cryptococcosis				
C. neoformans	Rabbit	Immunosuppressed	Cisterna magnum	Meninges
	Mouse	None	I. cer.	Meninges and dissemination
	Mouse	Immunosuppressed/none	I.n.	Lung and dissemination
	Mouse	Immunosuppressed/none	I.v./i.p.	Dissemination
	Guinea pig	Immunosuppressed/none	I.v.	Dissemination
Candidosis				
C. albicans	Guinea pig	Clipped and diabetic	On skin	Skin
	Mouse	Immunosuppressed	S.c.	Subcutis
	Mouse	Air s.c.	S.c.	Subcutis
	Rat	Pseudoestrus	I. vag.	Vagina
	Rat	Pseudoestrus and diabetic	I. vag.	Vagina
	Guinea pig	Immunosuppressed and antibiotics	P.o.	Gastrointestinal tract
	Mouse	Immunosuppressed and antibiotics/none	P.o.	Gastrointestinal tract
	Guinea pig	None	I. cor.	Cornea
	Rabbit	Immunosuppressed/none	I. cor.	Cornea
	Rabbit	None	I.v.	Eye and dissemination
	Rabbit	Intracardial catheter	I.v.	Endocardium and dissemination
	Guinea pig	Immunosuppressed/none	I.v.	Dissemination
	Mouse	Immunosuppressed/none	I.v.	Dissemination
	Rat	None	I.v.	Dissemination

*Usually performed under occlusive dressing. Diabetic: alloxan and streptozotocin treated animals. Pseudoestrus: castrated and oestrogen treated animals. Immunosuppressed: X-irradiated, mechlorethamine, prednisolone, hydrocortisone or cyclophosphamide treated animals. Antibiotics: streptomycin and chloramphenicol. Abbreviations, see pg. 170.

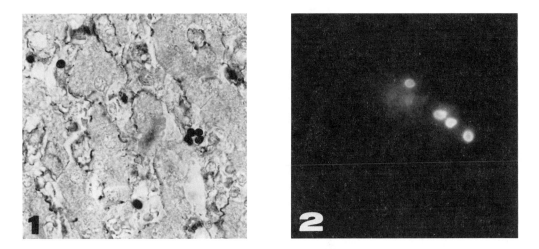

Figure 9. Immunohistochemical identification of *Histoplasma capsulatum* var. *capsulatum*. (1) In the Kupffer's cells, yeast-like organisms are located. (2) Staining of the organisms by specific FITC-labele anti-*H. capsulatum* rabbit globulins confirm the diagnosis of hepatic histoplasmosis. (From H.E. Jensen et al., *APMIS*, 100, 586, 1992. With permission.)

e.g., *B. dermatitidis, H. capsulatum* var. *capsulatum, P. brasiliensis, S. schenckii,* and *C. neoformans,* are negative, animal inoculations (often in mice) are performed with the material.[45] Usually the material is, in combination with antibiotics, given s.c., i.v., i.cran., or i.p., but for *P. brasiliensis* the preferred site for inoculation is the testicles of mountain rats.[45] The specimens are usually of environmental or clinical origin such as soil, pus, granulomas, etc. When growth of the fungus in the animal is suspected at necropsy, its organs are removed and from these *in vitro* cultivation is attempted. Experimental inoculations of mice are also used in the differentiation of some fungi, e.g., *C. carrionii* from *C. bantianum* and the pathogenicity of *C. neoformans* for mice is used in the differentiation of this species from other *Cryptococcus spp.*[26,71] Finally, it should be noted that *in vivo* growth by passage in laboratory animals is presently the only feasible method for the isolation and "cultivation" of *L. loboi*.[26,30]

For the high number of immunological assays used for the diagnosis of different mycoses, the production of specific poly- and/or monoclonal antibodies is essential. Production of polyclonal antibodies is preferably done in rabbits and goats by immunization with different fractions of fungal antigens. Monoclonal antifungal antibodies are produced in mice or rat hybridomas *in vivo* (ascites-production) or *in vitro* (cell cultures). In the evaluation of the sensitivity and specificity of antifungal antibodies controlled experimental infections of laboratory animals are indispensable. For these purposes, animal models have been used extensively in testing, e.g., immunohistochemical assays used in the histopathological differentiation of algae and fungi (Figure 9)[,139,144,145] and in, e.g., enzyme-linked immunosorbent assays (ELISA)[146,147] and agglutination assays[148] developed for the detection of fungal antigen in serum and urine of infected humans and higher animals as an aid in the diagnosis of mycoses. Furthermore, well-characterized antifungal antisera from laboratory animals are often enclosed as references in studies of human antibody reactions, too.[149]

REFERENCES

1. Rippon, J. W., Dermatophytosis and Dermatomycosis, in *Medical Mycology:*3rd ed. W. B. Saunders Company, Philadelphia, 1988, 169.
2. Hironaga, M., Okazaki, N., Saito, K., and Watanabe, S., Trichophyton mentagrophytes granulomas, *Arch. Dermatol., 119, 482, 1983.*

3. Rippon, J. W., Animal models of experimental dermatophyte infections, in *Experimental Models in Antimicrobial Chemotherapy,* vol. 3, Zak, O. and Sande, M. A., Eds., Academic Press, London, 1986, 161.

4. Watanabe, S., Animal models of cutaneous and subcutaneous mycoses, in *Animal Models in Medical Mycology,* Miyaji, M., Ed., CRC Press, Boca Raton, 1987, 53.

5. Takahashi, S., Morphological, biological and physiological studies of Trichophyton rubrum. I. Morphological studies and experimental inoculation of guinea pigs, *Jpn. J. Dermatol., 72, 50, 1962.*

6. Reiss, F., Successful inoculation in animals with Trichophyton parpareum, A*rch. Dermatol. Syph., 54, 242, 1944.*

7. La Touche, C. J., Mouse favus due to Trichophyton quinckeanum (zopf) macleod & muende: a reappraisal in the light of recent investigations, I-III, *Mycopath. et Mycol. Appl., 11, 257, 1959.*

8. Calderon, R. A., Immunoregulation of dermatophytosis, *CRC Crit. Rev. Microbiol., 16, 339, 1989.*

9. Van Cutsem, J., Animal models for dermatomycotic infections, in *Current Topics in Medical Mycology*, Vol. 3, McGinnis, M. R. and Borgers, M., Eds., Springer-Verlag, New York, 1989, 1.

10. Hänel, H., Braun, B. and Löschhorn, K., Experimental dermatophytosis in nude guinea pigs compared with infection in Pirbright White animals, *Mycoses, 33, 179, 1990.*

11. Greenberg, J. H., King, R. H., Kerbs, S., and Field, R., A quantitative dermatophyte infection model in the guinea pig - a parallel to the quantitative human infection model, *J. Invest. Dermatol., 67, 704, 1976.*

12. Kerbs, S. and Allen, A. M., Effect of occlusion on Trichophyton mentagrophytes infection in guinea pigs, *J. Invest, Dermatol., 71, 301, 1978.*

13. Green, F., Lee, K. W. and Balish, E., Chronic Trichophyton mentagrophytes dermatophytosis of guinea pig skin grafts on nude mice, J. *Invest. Dermatol., 79, 125, 1982.*

14. Green, F. and Balish, E., Trichophyton mentagrophytes dermatophytosis in germ free guinea pigs, *J. Invest. Dermatol., 75, 476, 1980.*

15. Van Cutsem, J. and Janssen, P. A. J., Experimental systemic dermatophytosis, J. *Invest. Dermatol., 83, 26, 1984.*

16. Van Cutsem, J., Van Gerven, F. and Janssen, P. A. J., Activity of orally, topically, and parenterally administered itraconazole in the treatment of superficial and deep mycoses: Animal models, *Rev. Infect. Dis., 9, 15, 1987.*

17. Van Cutsem, J., Van Gerven, F. and Janssen, P. A. J., Saperconazole, a new potent antifungal triazol: in vitro activity spectrum and therapeutic efficacy, *Drugs Fut., 14, 1187, 1989.*

18. Van Cutsem, J., Van Gerven, F., Fransen, J. and Janssen, P. A. J., Experimental candidosis in animals and chemotherapy, in: *Candida and Candidamycosis*, Tümbay, E., Ed., Plenum Press, New York, 1991, 107.

19. Van Cutsem, J., Fransen, J. and Janssen, P. A. J., Experimental zygomycosis due to Rhizopus spp. infection by various routes in guinea pigs, rats and mice, *Mycoses, 31, 563, 1988.*

20. Eades, S. M. and Corbel, M. J., Metastatic subcutaneous zygomycosis following intravenous and intracerebral inoculation of Absidia corymbifera spores, *Sabouraudia, 13, 200, 1975.*

21. Fukushiro, R., Maduromycosis, in *Handbook of Dermatology*, Yamamura, Y., Kukita, A., Sano, S. and Seiji, M., Eds., Nakayama Shoten, Tokyo, 1982, 66.

22. Aleksin, R. M., Administration of preparation TF 130, *Veterinariia, 3, 52, 1974.*

23. Dobukovski, E. G., Über Methoden der Trichophytie Bekampfung, *Veterinariia,* 39, 32, 1962.

24. Segal, E., Vaccines for the management of dermatophyte and superficial yeast infections, in *Current Topics in Medical Mycology*, McGinnis, M. R. and Borgers, M., Eds., Springer-Verlag, New York, 1989, 36.

25. Knight, A. G., A review of experimental human infections, *J. Invest. Dermatol., 59, 354, 1972.*

26. Rippon, J. W., The subcutaneous mycoses, in *Medical Mycology*, 3rd ed., W. B. Saunders Company, Philadelphia, 1988, 276.
27. Miyaji, M. and Nishimura, K., Experimental fungal infections, in *Animal Models in Medical Mycology*, Miyaji, M., Ed., CRC Press, Boca Raton, 1987, 1.
28. Reiss, F., Experimental mycotic infections on laboratory animals, in *Medical Mycology*, Simons, R. D. G., Ed., Elsevier, London, 1954, 50.
29. Borelli, D., A method for producing chromomycosis in mice, *Trans. R. Soc. Trop. Med. Hyg., 66, 793, 1972.*
30. Wiersman, J. P. and Niemel, P. L. A., Lobo's disease in Surinam patients, *Trop. Geogr. Med., 17, 89, 1965.*
31. Rippon, J. W., The pathogenic Actinomycetes, in *Medical Mycology*, 3rd ed., W. B. Saunders Company, Philadelphia, 1988, 13.
32. Avram, A., Grains experimentaux maduromycosiques a Cephalosporium falciforme, Monosporium apiospermum, Nadurella mycetomi, et Norcardia asteroides, *Mycopathologia, 32, 319, 1967.*
33. Avram, A., Experimental induction of grains with Cephalosporium falciforme, *Sabouraudia, 5, 89, 1965.*
34. Symmers, D., Experimental reproduction of maduromycotic lesions in rabbits, *Arch. Pathol., 39, 358, 1945.*
35. Fukushiro, R., Kinbara, T., Nagai, T., Ikeda, S. and Kumagai, T., On primary pyoderma-like aspergillosis, *Jpn. J. Med. Mycol., 14, 127, 1973.*
36. Sternberg, T. H., Tarbet, J. E., Newcomer, V. D. and Winter, L. H., Deep infection of mice with Trichophyton rubrum, *J. Invest. Dermatol., 19, 374, 1952.*
37. Satterwhite, T. K., Kageler, W. V., Conkoin, R. H., Portnoy, B. L. and Dupont, H. L., Disseminated sporotrichosis, *J. Am. Med. Assoc., 240, 771, 1978.*
38. Charoenvit, Y. and Taylor, L. R., Experimental sporotrichosis in Syrian hamsters, *Infect. Immun., 23, 366, 1979.*
39. Barbee, W. C., Ewert, A. and Davidson, M., Animal model: sporotrichosis in the domestic cat, *Am. J. Pathol., 86, 281, 1977.*
40. Benham, R. W. and Kesten, B., Sporotrichosis: its transmission to plants and animals, *J. Infect. Dis., 50, 437, 1932.*
41. Hopkins, J. G. and Benham, R. W., Sporotrichosis in New York State, *N. Y. State J. Med., 32, 595, 1932.*
42. Kwon-Chung, K. J., Compararison of isolates of Sporothrix schenckii obtained from fixed cutaneous lesions with isolates from other types of lesions, *J. Infect. Dis., 139, 424, 1979.*
43. Nakahara, T., Studies on the strains of Sporotrichum schenckii isolated from soils, *Jpn. J. Med. Mycol., 12, 30, 1971.*
44. Mackinnon, J. E. and Conti-Diaz, The effect of temperature on sporotrichosis, *Sabouraudia, 2, 56, 1962.*
45. Rippom, J. W., The systemic mycoses, in *Medical Mycology*, 3rd ed., W. B. Saunders Company, Philadelphia, 1988, 373.
46. Brummer, E. and Clemons, K. V., Animal models of systemic mycoses, in *Animal Models in Medical Mycology*, Miyaji, M., Ed, CRC Press, Boca Raton, 1987, 79.
47. Morozumi, P. A., Halpern, J. W. and Stevens, D. A., Susceptibility differences of inbred strains of mice to blastomycosis, *Infect. Immun., 32, 160, 1981.*
48. Brass, C. and Stevens, D. A., Maturity as a critical determinant of resistance to fungal infections: studies in murine blastomycosis, *Infect. Immun., 36, 387, 1982.*
49. Harvey, R. P., Schmid, E. S., Carrington, C. C. and Stevens, D. A., Mouse model of pulmonary blastomycosis: utility, simplicity, and quantitative parameters., *Am. Rev. Resp. Dis., 117, 695, 1978.*
50. Sugar, A. M. and Picard, M., Experimental blastomycosis pneumonia in mice by infection with conidia, *J. Med. Vet. Mycol., 26, 321, 1988.*
51. Landay, M. E., Mitten, J. and Miller, J., Disseminated blastomycosis in hamsters. II. Effect of sex on susceptibility, *Mycopath. Mycol. Appl., 42, 73, 1970.*
52. Conant, N. F., Smith, D. T., Baker, R. D., Calloway, J. L. and Martin, D. S., Eds., *Manual of clinical mycology,* 2nd ed., W. B. Saunders Company, Philadelphia, 1954.

53. Kirkland, T. N. and Fierer, J., Inbred mouse strains differ in resistance to lethal Coccidioides immitis infection, *Infect. Immun., 40, 912, 1983.*

54. Clemons, K. V., Leathers, C. R. and Lee, K. W., Systemic Coccidioides immitis infection in nude and beige mice, *Infect. Immun., 47, 814, 1985.*

55. Huppert, M., Sun, S. H., Gleason-Jordan, I. and Vokovich, K. P., Lung weight parallels disease severity in experimental coccidioidomycosis, *Infect. Immun., 14, 1356, 1976.*

56. Kong, Y. M., Levine, H. B., Madin, S. H., and Smith, C. E., Fungal multiplication and histopathological changes in vaccinated mice infected with Coccidioides immitis, *J. Immunol., 92, 779, 1964.*

57. Schwarz, J., Ed, *Histoplasmosis,* Praeger Publishers, CBS, New York, 1981.

58. Baughman, R. P., Hendricks, D. and Bullock, W. E., Sequential analysis of cellular immune responses in the lung during Histoplasma capsulatum infection, *Clin. Res., 33, 425A, 1984.*

59. Singh, T., Studies on epizootic lymphangitis. Study of clinical cases and experimental transmission, *Indian J. Vet. Sci., 36, 45, 1966.*

60. Singh, T. and Varmani, B. M. L., Studies on epizootic lymphangitis. A note on pathogenicity of Histoplasma farciminosum (Rivolta) for laboratory animals, *Indian J. Vet. Sci., 36, 164, 1966.*

61. Walker, J. and Spooner, E. T. C., Natural infection of the African baboon Papio papio with the large cell form of Histoplasma, J. *Pathol. Bacteriol., 80, 436, 1960.*

62. Butler, T. M., Mystery Case No. 16, *Comp. Pathol. Bull., 21, 1, 1989.*

63. Okudaira, M. and Swartz, J., Infection with Histoplasma duboisii in different experimental animals, *Mycopathologia, 53, 53, 1961.*

64. Lutz, A., Uma mucose pseudo-coccidica localisada no boca e observada no Brazil: contirbuiaco ao conhecimento das hypho-blastomycoses americanas, *Bras. Med., 22, 121, 1908.*

65. Guimeraes, F., Infeccao do hamster (Cricetus auratus Waterhouse) pelo agente da micose de Lutz (blastomicose sul-americana), *Hospital (Rio), 40, 515, 1951.*

66. Brummer, E., Restrepo, A., Stevens, D. A., Azzi, R., Gomez, A., Hoyos, G., McEwen, J., Cano, L. and deBedount, C., Murine model of paracoccidioidomycosis. Production fatal acute pulmonary or chronic pulmonary and disseminated disease: immunological and pathological observations, *J. Exp. Path., 1, 241, 1984.*

67. Pollak, L. and Angulo-Ortega, A., Pathogenesis of paracoccidioidomycosis, Proc. 1st Pan Am. Symp. PAHO and WHO Scientific Publication No. 254, Washington, D.C., 1972, 293.

68. DelNegro, G., Lacaz, C. and Fiorillo, A., Paracoccidioidomycosis: blastomicose Sub-America, Pub. Sarvier-Edusp., Sao Paulo, Brazil, 1982, 78.

69. Iabuki, K. and Montenegro, M. R., Experimental paracoccidioidomycosis in the Syrian hamster: morphology, ultrastructure and correlation of lesions with presence of specific antigen and serum levels of antibodies, *Mycopathologia, 67, 131, 1979.*

70. Restrepo, A. and DeGuzman, E. G., Paracoccidioidomycosis experimental del ration inducida por via aerogena, *Sabouraudia, 4, 299, 1976.*

71. Rippon, J. W., Opportunistic infections, in *Medical Mycology,* 3rd ed., W. B. Saunders Company, Philadelphia, 1988, 532.

72. Van Cutsem, J., Fungal models in immunocompromised animals, in *Mycoses in AIDS Patients,* Vanden Bossche, Ed., Plenum Press, New York, 1990, 207.

73. Yamaguchi, H., Opportunistic fungal infections, in *Animal Models in Medical Mycology,* Miyaji, M., Ed., CRC Press, Boca Raton, FL, 1987, 101.

74. Abe, F., Tateyama, M., Shibuya, H., Azumi, N. and Ommura, Y., Experimental candidiasis in iron overload, *Mycopathologia 89, 59, 1985.*

75. Abe, F., Tateyama, M., Shibuya, H. and Ommura, Y., Experimental candidiasis in iron overload, *Jpn. J. Med. Mycol., 25, 290, 1984.*

76. Odds, F. C., Candidosis of the genitalia, in *Candida and Candidosis,* 2nd ed., Baillière Tindall, London, 1988, 124.

77. Sobel, J. D., Pathogenesis of Candida vulvovaginitis, in *Current Topics in Medical Mycology,* Vol. 3, McGinnis, M. R. and Borgers, M., Eds, Springer-Verlag, 1989, 86.

78. Mardon, D. N. and Robinnette, E. H., Jr., Organ distribution and viability of Candida albicans in noncancerous and tumor-bearing (Lewis lung carcinoma) mice, *Can. J. Microbiol., 24, 1515, 1978.*

79. Johnson, J. A., Lau, B. H. S., Nuater, R. L., Slatar, J. M. and Winter, C. E., Effect of L1210 leukemia on the susceptibility of mice to Candida albicans infections, *Infect. Immun., 19, 146, 1978.*

80. Corbel, M. J. and Eades, S. M., The relative susceptibility of New Zealand Black and CBA mice to infection with opportunistic fungal pathogens, *Sabouraudia, 14, 17, 1976.*

81. Jordan, F. T. W., Diseases of poultry, *Br. Vet. J., 137, 545, 1981.*

82. Jensen, H. E., Basse, A. and Aalbæk, B., Mycosis in the stomach compartments of cattle, *Acta Vet. Scand., 30, 409, 1989.*

83. Jensen, H. E., Krogh, H. V. and Schønheyder, H., Bovine mycotic abortion - a comparative study of diagnostic methods, *J. Vet. Med., B, 38, 33, 1991.*

84. Van Cutsem, J., Antifungal activity of enilconazole on experimental aspergillosis in chickens, *Avian Dis., 27, 36, 1983.*

85. Niki, Y., Bernad, E. M., Edwards, F. F., Schmitt, H. J., Yu, B. and Armstrong, D., Model of recurrent pulmonary aspergillosis in rats, *J. Clin. Microbiol., 29, 1317, 1991.*

86. Bhatia, V. N. and Mohapatra, L. N., Experimental aspergillosis in mice. I. Pathogenic potential of Aspergillus fumigatus, Aspergillus flavus and Aspergillus niger, *Mykosen, 12, 615, 1969.*

87. Bhatia, V. N. and Mohapatra, L. N., Experimental aspergillosis in mice. II. Enhanced susceptibility of the cortisone treated mice to infection with Aspergillus fumigatus, Aspergillus flavus and Aspergillus niger, *Mykosen, 13, 105, 1970.*

88. Sandhu, D., Sandhu, R. S., Damodaran, V. N. and Randhawa, H. S., Effect of cortisone on bronchopulmonary aspergillosis in mice exposed to spores of various Aspergillus species, *Sabouraudia, 8, 32, 1970.*

89. Epstein, S. M., Verney, E., Miale, T. D. and Sideransky, H., Studies on the pathogenesis of experimental pulmonary aspergillosis, *Am. J. Pathol., 51, 769, 1967.*

90. Merkow, L. L., Epstein, S. M., Sideransky, H., Verney, E. and Pardo, M., The pathogenesis of experimental pulmonary aspergillosis, *Am. J. Pathol., 62, 57, 1970.*

91. Sawasaki, H., Horie, K., Naito, Y., Watabe, S., Tajima, G. and Mizutani, Y., Experimental pulmonary aspergilloma, *Mycopathologia, 32, 265, 1967.*

92. Hill, M. W. M., Whiteman, C. E., Benjamin, M. M. and Ball, L., Pathogenesis of experimental bovine mycotic placentitis produced by Aspergillus fumigatus, *Vet. Pathol., 8, 273, 1971.*

93. Cysewski, S. J. and Pier, A. C., Mycotic abortion in ewes produced by Aspergillus fumigatus, Pathologic changes, *Am. J. Vet. Res., 29, 1135, 1968.*

94. Jensen, H. E. and Hau, J., A murine model for the study of the impact of Aspergillus fumigatus inoculation on the foeto-placental unit, *Mycopathologia, 112, 11, 1990.*

95. Jensen, H. E. and Hau, J., Murine mycotic placentitis produced by intravenous inoculation of conidia from Aspergillus fumigatus, *In Vivo, 4, 247, 1990.*

96. Cohrs, P., Jaffe, R. and Meesen, H., Eds., *Pathologie der Laboratoriumstiere,* Vol. 2., Springer-Verlag, Berlin, 1958.

97. Carrizosa, J., Kohn, C. and Levinson, M. E., Experimental aspergillus endocarditis in rabbits, *J. Lab. Clin. Med., 86, 746, 1975.*

98. Golbert, T. M. and Patterson, R., Pulmonary allergic aspergillosis. *Ann. Intern. Med., 72, 395, 1970.*

99. Odds, F. C., Pathogenesis of candidosis, in *Candida and Candidosis,* 2nd ed., Baillière Tindall, London, 1988, 252.

100. Cinander, B., Dubiski, S. and Wardlaw, A. C., Distribution, inheritance, and properties of an antigen, MUB1, and its relation to hemolytic complement, *J. Exp. Med., 120, 897, 1964.*

101. Tarsi, R., Simonetti, N. and Orpianesi, C., Experimental candidiasis in rabbits: protective action of fructose-1,6,-diphosphate, *Mycopathologia, 81, 111, 1983.*

102. Parker, J. C., Jr., Cleary, T. J. and Kogure, K., The effects of transient candidemia on the brain: preliminary observations on a rodent model for experimental deep candidosis, *Surg. Neurol., 11, 44, 1979.*

103. Parker, J. C., Jr., Cleary, T. J., Monji, T., Kogure, K. and Castro, A., Modifying cerebral candidiasis by altering the enfectious entry route, *Arch. Pathol. Lab. Med., 104, 537, 1980.*

104. Louria, D. B., Candida infection in experimental animals, in *Candidiasis*, Bodey, G. P. and Fainstein, V., Eds., Raven Press, New York, 1985, 29.

105. Jensen, H. E., Hau, J., Aalbæk, B. and Schønheyder, H., Experimental candidosis in pregnant mice, *APMIS, 99, 829, 1991.*

106. Thienpont, D., Van Cutsem, J. and Borgers, M., Ketoconazole in experimental candidosis, *Rev. Infect. Dis., 2, 570, 1967.*

107. Balish, E. and Phillips, A. W., Growth, morphogenesis and virulence of Candida albicans after oral inoculation in the germ-free and conventional chick, *J. Bacteriol., 91, 1736, 1966.*

108. Polak, A. and Schaffner, A., A new experimental model of localized candidosis for the study of antifungal chemotherapy, *Mycoses, 32, 398, 1989.*

109. Pope, L. M., Cole, G. T., Guentzel, M. N. and Berry, L. J., Systemic and gastrointestinal candidiasis in infant mice after intragastric challenge, *Infect. Immun., 25, 702, 1979.*

110. Cole, G. T., Lynn, K. T. and Seshan, K. R., Evaluation of a murine model of hepatic candidiasis, *J. Clin. Microbiol., 28, 1828, 1990.*

111. Savage, A. and Tribe, C. R., Experimental murine amyloidosis: experience with Candida albicans as an amyloidogenic agent and liver biopsy as a diagnostic tool, *J. Pathol., 127, 199, 1979.*

112. Miyaji, M. and Nishimura, K., Studies on organ specificity in experimental murine cryptococcosis, *Mycopathologia, 76, 145, 1981.*

113. Watanabe, T., Miyaji, M. and Nishimura, K., Studies on relationship between cysts and granulomas in murine cryptococcosis, *Mycopathologia, 86, 113, 1984.*

114. Karaoui, R. M., Hall, N. K. and Larsh, H. W., Role of macrophages in immunity and pathogenesis of experimental cryptococcosis induced by the airborne route. I. Pathogenesis and acquired immunity of Cryptococcus neoformans, *Mykosen, 20, 380, 1977.*

115. Ritter, R. C. and Larsh, H. W., The infection of white mice following an intranasal instillation of Cryptococcus neoformans, *Am. J. Hyg., 78, 241, 1963.*

116. Graybill, J. R., Ahrens, J., Nealon, T. and Raque, R., Pulmonary cryptococcosis in the rat, *Am. Rev. Resp. Dis., 127, 636, 1983.*

117. Perfect, J. R., Lagn, S. D. R. and Durack, D. T., Chronic cryptococcal meningitis. A new experimental model in rabbits, *Am. J. Pathol., 101, 177, 1980.*

118. Green, J. R. and Bulmer, G. S., Gastrointestinal inoculation of Cryptococcus neoformans in mice, S*abouraudia, 17, 233, 1979.*

119. Dixon, D. M. and Polak, A., In vivo and in vitro studies with an atypical rhinotrophic isolate of Cryptococcus neoformans, *Mycopathologia, 96, 33, 1986.*

120. Dupont, B., Improvisi, L. and Ronin, O., Aspects épidémiologiques et cliniques des infections a Scedosporium et Pseudallescheria, *J. Mycol. Méd., 118, 33, 1991.*

121. Drouhet, E., Dupont, B. and Ravisse, P., Étude expérimentale d'une souche hautement virulente de Scedosporium inflatum isolée d'une arthrite du genou, J. *Mycol. Méd., 118, 16, 1991.*

122. Espinel-Ingroff, A., Oakley, L. A. and Kerkering, T. M., Opportunistic zygomycotic infections — a literature review, *Mycopathologia, 97, 33, 1987.*

123. Ainsworth, G. C. and Austwick, P. K. C., Eds., *Fungal Diseases of Animals*, 2nd. ed., C. A. B., Surrey, 1973.

124. Kitz, J. D., Embree, R. W. and Cazin, J., Comparative virulence of Absidia corymbifera strains in mice, *Infect. Immun., 33, 395, 981.*

125. Waldorf, A. R., Halde, C. and Vedros, N. A., Murine model of pulmonary mucormycosis in cortisone-treated mice, *Sabouraudia, 20, 217, 1982.*

126. Van Cutsem, J. and Boelaert, J. R., Effects of deferoxamine, feroxamine and iron on experimental mucormycosis (zygomycosis), *Kidney Intern., 36, 1061, 1989.*

127. Smith, J. M. B., Experimental mycotic ulceration, *Sabouraudia, 34, 353, 1968.*

128. Jensen, H. E., Hau, J., Aalbæk, B. and Schønheyder, H., Indirect immunofluorescence staining and crossed immunoelectrophoresis for differentiation of Candida albicans and Geotrichum candidum, *Mycoses, 33, 519, 1990.*

129. Spanoghe, L., Devos, A. and Viaene, N., Cutaneous geotrichosis in the red flamingo (Phoenicopterus ruber), *Sabouraudia, 14, 37, 1976.*

130. Segretain, G., Penicillium marneffei N. sp., agent d´une mycose du système réticulo-endothélial, *Mycopath. Mycol. Appl., 11, 327, 1959.*

131. Deng, Z., Yun, M. and Ajello, L., Human penicilliosis marneffei and its relation to the baboo rat (Rhizomys pruinosus), *J. Med. Vet. Mycol., 24, 383, 1986.*

132. Faergemann, J., Experimental tinea versicolor in rabbits and humans with Pityrosporum orbiculare, *J. Invest. Dermatol., 72, 26, 1979.*

133. Faergemann, J., Tinea versicolor and Pityrosporum orbiculare: mycological investigations, experimental infections and epidemiological surveys, *Acta. Dermatol. Venereol., 86, 1, 1979.*

134. Connor, D. H. and Neafie, R. C., Protothecosis, in Pathology of Tropical and Extraordinary Diseases, Vol. 2, Bindford, C. H. and Connor, D. H., Eds., Armed Forces Institute of Pathology, Washington, D. C., 1976, 684.

135. Frank, N., Ferguson, L. C., Cross, R. F. and Redman, D. R., Prototheca, a cause of bovine mastitis, *Am. J. Vet. Res., 30, 1785, 1969.*

136. Migaki, G., Garner, F. M. and Imes, G. D., Bovine protothricosis - a report of three cases, *Pathol. Vet., 6, 444, 1969.*

137. Imes, G. D., Lloyd, J. C. and Brightman, M. P., Disseminated protothecosis in a dog, *Onderstepoort J. Vet Res., 44, 1, 1977.*

138. Rogers, R. J., Connole, M. D., Norton, J., Thomas, A., Ladds, P. W. and Dickson, J., Lymphadenitis of cattle due to infection with green algae, *J. Comp. Pathol., 90, 1, 1980.*

139. Sudman, M. S. and Kaplan, W., Identification of the Prototheca species by immunofluorescence, *Appl. Microbiol., 25, 981, 1973.*

140. Bennett, G. and Grant, S., Eds., Antifungal activity, in *Fluconazole an Overview*, Fortune Printing Co., Hong Kong, 1990, 7.

141. Odds, F. C., Cheesman, S. L. and Abbott, A. B., Antifungal effect of fluconazole (UK-49858), a new triazole antifungal, *in vitro, J. Antimicrob. Chemother., 18, 473, 1986.*

142. Zak, O. and O'Reilly, T., Minireview — animal models in the evaluation of antimicrobial agents, *Antimicrob. Agents Chemother., 35, 1527, 1991.*

143. Zak, O. and Sande, M. A., Eds., Introduction: the role of animal models in the evaluation of new antibiotics, in *Experimental Models in Antimicrobial Chemotherapy*, Vol. 1, Academic Press, Orlando, 1986, 1.

144. Jensen, H. E. and Schønheyder, H., Immunofluorescence staining of hyphae in the histopathological diagnosis of mycoses in cattle, *J. Med. Vet. Mycol., 27, 33, 1989.*

145. Jensen, H. E., Bloch, B., Henriksen, P., Dietz, H. H., Schønheyder, H. and Kaufman, L., Disseminated histoplasmosis in a badger (Meles meles) in Denmark, *APMIS, 100, 586, 1992.*

146. Dupont, B., Huber, M., Kim, S. J. and Bennett, J. E., Galactomannan antigenemia and antigenuria in aspergillosis: studies in patients and experimentally infected rabbits, *J. Infect. Diseas., 155, 1, 1987.*

147. Jensen, H. E., Latgé, J. P., Frandsen, P. L. and Schønheyder, H., Application of ELISA and immunoblotting for the diagnosis of systemic bovine aspergillosis and zygomycosis, *Proc. VIth Int. Symp. World Assoc. Vet. Lab. Diag., 1992, 39.*

148. Van Cutsem, J., Meulemans, L., Van Gerven, F. and Stynen, D., Detection of circulating galactomannan by Pastorex Aspergillus in experimental invasive aspergillosis, *Mycoses, 33, 61, 1990.*

149. Latgè, J. P., Moutaouakil, M., Debeaupuis, J. P., Bouchara, J. P., Haynes, K. and Prévost, M. C., The 18-killodalton antigen secreted by Aspergillus fumigatus, *Infect. Immun., 59, 2586, 1991.*

Chapter 16

Animal Models in Cancer Research

Jørgen Rygaard

CONTENTS

INTRODUCTION

Cancer is a common term for all malignant tumors. Cancers can be divided into main groups depending on their origin. Tumors originating from the mesenchyme are called sarcomas. They comprise malignancies arising from connective tissue, muscle, endothelial and related tissues, and blood. Carcinomas are derived from epithelial cells. They contribute the main part of malignancies in humans, such as tumors of the skin, breast, lungs, and the gastrointestinal and urinary tract. Also, malignant melanomas are usually included in this group, which poses the most serious problems in the clinic and therefore is given special emphasis in the experimental laboratory.

Basic characteristics of cancers in humans and in other vertebrates are the same. They show autonomous growth, disregarding the social order of the multicellular organism from which

0-8493-4390-9/94/$0.00+$.50

they arise. They invade locally, destroying neighbor cells and tissues, and most seriously they can spread in the organism and form metastases. If left untreated, cancers will almost inevitably lead to the death of the individual. Humans and animals alike fall victim to this. Therefore, animal models of cancer can be considered relevant tools in biomedical research. They can help us understand what causes cancers, how cancers develop, and — hopefully — how they can be treated. It should be stressed that much of our present-day knowledge has been achieved in the test tube or tissue culture flask, thanks to the fact that cell lines can be propagated in such circumstances and will respond to cancer-provoking stimuli, carcinogens, and to therapeutic agents in much the same way as they do in the intact organism. One important aspect is lost, however, namely the interaction between the tumor and the host organism. This can be remedied by working with transplantable animal tumors in animals. But still, laboratory animals *are* animals and extrapolations have to be made from the model to the human situation.

This dilemma can be solved midway by using human tumor material heterotransplanted into and maintained in animals with spontaneous or induced immunodeficiencies, primarily the athymic nude mouse and rat, and the SCID mouse.

After giving a brief outline of the roots of experimental cancer research, this presentation will focus on the laboratory mouse, thereby omitting the mention of some animal models such as rat, hamster, rabbit, and dog often used in long term carcinogenesis studies, since these applications may be of more interest in toxicology.

As pointed out by Sivak[1] "...the single most cogent reason for the use of mice is the availability of a wide variety of inbred strains of markedly different properties. The use of these inbred strains with their wide range of properties relevant to the induction of cancer, and the ability to obtain genetically known hybrid strains of mice to examine the hereditary basis for these properties make available a unique animal resource among the small rodents that are used in carcinogenesis research." The same arguments can be expressed in relation to tumor biology studies and experimental cancer therapy. Since the statement was made, the mouse-based models have been supplemented with transgenic mice, some of which are of major interest in cancer research.

Also, successful research is strongly dependent on ready access to relevant chemicals, which today mean well-defined monoclonal antibodies and reagents to demonstrate mediators such as, e.g., cytokines, probes for *in situ* hybridization, etc. The range of such reagents directed against mouse cells and molecules by far outdoes what is available against the cells and molecules of other animal species, which is another pragmatic argument for focusing on the mouse in cancer research.

ORIGIN OF EXPERIMENTAL CANCER RESEARCH
CHEMICAL CARCINOGENESIS

Experimental cancer research using laboratory animal models started in 1914 with the observation by Yamagiwa and Ichakawa[2] that repeated painting of rabbits' ears with tar would lead to the formation of carcinomas of the skin, similar to squamous cell carcinomas in humans. They may have gotten their inspiration from the finding by Pott[3] 140 years earlier that former chimney-sweeper boys who had been exposed to tar and soot during infancy would in many cases develop cancers of the scrotum, again squamous cell carcinomas. The knowledge of chemical carcinogens increased over the next few years, leading to the identification of various carcinogens, e.g., the polycyclic hydrocarbon compound DMBA (7,12-dimethylbenz(a)anthracene) which is still one of the most used chemical carcinogens, and showing also that mice would develop skin tumors after exposure to tar products.[4] This initiated the leading role of the laboratory mouse in cancer research. Further experiments demonstrated that the efficiency of chemical carcinogens could be increased if the exposed skin was pretreated with a substance that could induce hyperplasia, but which was not necessarily carcinogenic in itself.[5] One such promoter which is still widely used is croton oil, which contains 12-o-tetradecanoylphorbol-13-acetate, TPA. This finding led to the establishment of the so-called two-stage or initiation-promotion model.[6]

VIRAL AND OTHER CARCINOGENS

Today we know a range of viruses that can cause cancer *in vitro* and *in vivo*.[1,7] They comprise both DNA and RNA viruses in many species, ranging from frog to chicken, mouse, rabbit, dog, cow, and humans. Although the evidence for viral carcinogenesis in humans is weak, Burkitt's lymphoma is associated with the presence of Epstein-Barr virus, and some types of human papilloma virus are suspected of causing cancer of the uterine cervix.

Other well-known techniques for inducing cancers in laboratory animals include irradiation and hormone treatment.

SPONTANEOUS TUMORS

A wide range of spontaneous tumors are known to arise in laboratory animals, with the highest frequency in some inbred strains of mice,[8] but also in the laboratory rat, again showing some strain difference.[9] Spontaneous animal tumors metastasize with a species and strain dependent frequency that is generally lower than that of tumors in humans. A large number of well-defined cultured cell lines have been established from spontaneous animal tumors and form an important tool in experimental cancer research.

Readers who are particularly interested in these aspects will find ample general information in textbooks on pathology and cancer. The scope of this chapter does not allow detailed information on spontaneous and induced tumors in mouse and rat, which must be sought elsewhere.[8,9]

The latest addition to the field of cancer research is the demonstration of oncogenes and techniques for producing transgenic animal models with defined genetic changes that may enhance or inhibit the development of cancer.

ONCOGENES

In the late 1970s, a prominent group of cancer related genes, the proto-oncogenes, was discovered, and during the next decade several members of this group were identified. Today, probably one hundred such proto-oncogenes have been described. Most oncogenes were discovered in one of the following two ways: they were the transforming genes of certain viruses able to cause cancer in laboratory animal models,[10,11] or they were genes identified in DNA extracts from cancer cells which could be shown to transform mouse fibroblasts *in vitro* into cells with certain malignant characteristics.[12,13] The oncogenes were later shown to have a normal counterpart, called a proto-oncogene, present in all nucleated normal cells. They appear over a wide span of evolution, indicating that their functions are essential for the survival of cells.

The next step was the discovery in the early 1980s that many of the proto-oncogenes are in fact identical with genes coding for growth factors such as PDG (platelet derived growth factor), and EGFR (epidermal growth factor receptor); other proto-oncogene products have been identified as membrane-bound kinases, signal transducers, or regulators of transcription. Also, genes with a growth restriction function, which may indirectly promote growth when inactivated, have been foreseen and later described. The first member of this group, the retinoblastoma gene, *Rb*, was molecularly cloned in 1986.[14] Genes belonging to this group are also termed anti-oncogenes and tumor-suppressor genes, a somewhat misleading designation as it implies that the main role of such genes is to prevent tumors from arising. For a review, see Reference 15.

The genetic mutations most frequently described in human cancers occur in the p53 tumor-suppressor gene. This mutation has been constructed in transgenic mice, which may become of great importance in cancer research.

HETEROTRANSPLANTATION MODELS

In early attempts to transplant human malignant tumors into animal hosts, the anterior eye chamber of the rabbit or the brain of heterologous species,[16] and the hamster cheek pouch[17] were used for implantation. The success was reasonable as regards take, but growth time was limited, and observation of the implant was difficult. Whole-body irradiated animals[18] or corticosteroid treated hosts[19] rendered better possibilities for implantation in places where the fate of the implant could be monitored, but both irradiated and hormone treated animals were affected by the treatment, which could also influence the growth of the implants. The introduction of the athymic nude mouse in the late 1960s, of the athymic nude rat, and not least the SCID mouse in the early 1980s, followed by the development of the SCID-hu model, has provided important animal model possibilities for cancer research.

In the following, immunomodulated and spontaneously immunodeficient models will be described, and their applicability in cancer research will be commented on.

IMMUNOMODULATION

Immunomodulation is an urgent issue in experimental cancer research, in part as a tool in tumor immunologic intervention, but also for the establishment of heterotransplantation models.

X-ray and Cytostatic Treatment

Agents that have a general inhibitory effect in the multicellular organism will also possess immunosuppressive characteristics. X-ray irradiation is a potent proliferation inhibitor and was — and to some extent still is — widely used as an immunosuppressant. In laboratory animal models, lethal or sublethal irradiation can be combined with transplantation of bone marrow or selected lymphocyte subpopulations. In this respect, irradiated animals are similar to animals with some congenital immunodeficiencies. Side effects may occur due to irradiation of other tissues/organs than the immune system.

Drugs with a wide spectrum of action, such as cytostatic drugs and corticosteroids, will affect immune responsiveness. Their action is dose dependent within certain limits. They may, however, as is the case of X-irradiation, have undesirable side effects. Therefore, more specific approaches depending on the part of the system one wishes to influence, can be recommended. Such procedures will be described in relation to the cellular components of the immune system.

T-cell Modulation

T cells are responsible for cell-mediated immune responses and are necessary to initiate B-cell responses to thymus-dependent antigens. Since T cells mature in neonatal life in the thymus (although some extrathymic development may take place), neonatal thymectomy can delete T-cell responses as demonstrated by Miller;[20] foreign grafts are accepted, and immune responses to many antigens are poor, resulting in wasting and death at a young age. In the adult mouse (or other laboratory animal), T cells have spread to the whole organism. Adult thymectomy must therefore be combined with X-irradiation in order to remove mature T cells. Since the irradiation, as mentioned above, will damage not only T cells, but also other cells, including B cells, irradiation must be followed by the transfer of B-cell containing bone marrow in order to establish B competence.

A more specific removal of T cells can be achieved by treatment with anti-lymphocyte serum (ALS) or better anti-thymocyte serum (ATS) — polyclonal sera from rabbits or other species. Also drug treatment can be used to abort T-cell responses. The most promising example of this category is Cyclosporin A, which has a pronounced anti-T cell activity and fewer side effects on other components of the immune system, although not totally free of side effects in other organs, e.g., the kidneys. The introduction of monoclonal antibodies in experimental and clinical work may offer an improved treatment. Using monoclonal antibodies, highly specific subsets of lymphocytes can be defined (the CD system) and isolated.

Since thymus is the organ responsible for T-cell maturation, thymic hormonal factors have been introduced under various names. Results from experimental and clinical investigations are discordant. More steady results can be obtained with lymphokines (e.g. interleukines, interferons), which can now be produced in large amounts using recombinant techniques.

Specific T-cell potentiation in the experimental setup can be obtained with transfer of specific T cells, educated and sorted, or selected by cloning procedures. Priming with tumor cells can be used to specifically boost T-cell responses.

B-cell Modulation

B-cell responses in the neonatal mouse can be suppressed totally or to a wide extent by treatment with anti-μ immunoglobulin, directed against heavy chains of IgM immunoglobulin. Potentiation of B cells follows the same general line as that of T cells: priming and lymphokine treatment.

SPONTANEOUS IMMUNODEFICIENCY MODELS

Immunodeficient laboratory animal mutants have been known for more than 25 years. Their genetically determined deficiency does not include the side effects seen in irradiated or heavily drug-treated models. They are highly susceptible to microorganisms from the environment and therefore call for optimal housing conditions (for review of murine immunodeficiencies, see: Langdon and Smyth[21]). In the following, some immunodeficient mutants are described with main emphasis on the athymic nude mouse and the SCID mouse.

The Athymic (Nude) Mouse

The athymic (nude) mouse has been used in biomedical research since 1968.[22-24] The athymic condition is due to a recessive autosomal mutation, *nude*, the symbol for which is *nu*. Based on the genetics of the mutation, various breeding schemes can be set up. In proper microbiological conditions, nude females are fertile, but they have difficulty in weaning their young. Nude males are generally fertile although infections in the genital tract may cause infertility.

Breeding of nude mice can be based on the mating of heterozygous males and females, or — preferably — on the mating of homozygous males with heterozygous haired females, which will give a 50% nude offspring in contrast to heterozygous/heterozygous matings, where only an average of 25% are athymic.

Due to its lack of T-cell responses, the nude mouse accepts grafts of allogeneic and xenogeneic tissue, including malignant tumors. Full immunocompetence can be established with a thymus graft, and partial immunocompetence with spleen cells or selected T-cell subpopulations.

The Natural Killer (NK) Cell — Immunological Surveillance

The natural killer (NK) cell was first described in the nude mouse. In 1975, Kiessling et al.[25] and Herberman et al.[26] gave simultaneous descriptions of this cell type, which appears in various percentages in nude mice, depending on their genetic background. Much interest has focused on NK cells and their suggested anti-cancer potential. The hypothesis of Immunological Surveillance[27] predicted that thymus-dependent cell-mediated immune responses were responsible for the constant removal of malignant cells, which were postulated to be generated continuously in the organism, in mice as well as in humans. Observations in athymic nude mice, which do not develop malignant tumors with a higher frequency than do normal mice of the same genetic background,[28] strongly advocated against the Immune Surveillance hypothesis. Today — in spite of much conflicting experimental evidence, and although by definition not belonging to the immune system *sensu stricte* — the NK-cell seems to have taken over the role of Immune Surveillance from the T lymphocyte.

The Athymic (Nude) Rat
The athymic (*nude*) rat[29,30] has characteristics similar to those of the *nude* mouse, including the ability to host human malignant tumors. Immunocompetence can be established in part or totally with thymus grafts or selected T-cell subpopulations.

The Beige Mouse
The beige mouse[31] has no NK-cell activity. Double mutants of *nude* and *beige* mice can be bred, lacking both NK- and T-cell functions.

The Xid Mouse
The xid mouse[32] has an x-linked immunodeficiency with a partly impaired B-cell function.

The SCID Mouse (Severe Combined Immunodeficiency)
The SCID mutation[33] has a severe combined immunodeficiency, involving both T and B cells. A low percentage of SCID mice are leaky, i.e., they have polyclonal B-cell activation, leading to the production of high levels of (nonsense) immunoglobulin. The SCID mouse accepts grafts of human malignant tumors, and — most important — also grafts of normal human lymphoid cells so that a human immune system can be constructed in it (SCID-hu).[34] This combination of mouse and humans offers highly interesting possibilities for immunomodulatory studies and not least for the study of specific cell-mediated immune responses against (even) autologous tumor tissue.

HETEROTRANSPLANTATION

Human malignant tumors transplanted into nude mice and later into SCID mice have been widely used in many areas of cancer research. For a review, see Reference 35. Tumors retain their human characteristics: histological and cytological morphology, karyotype, molecular structures including oncogenes,[36] and the ability to express clonal evolution.

TRANSPLANTATION TECHNIQUES
Since the first human malignant tumor was implanted subcutaneously in nude mice in 1969, the subcutaneous tissue seems to have been the most popular site for implantation,[23] as based on a survey of the literature, and this seems to hold also for the limited experience in SCID mice. Tumors can be implanted s.c. as solid blocks, as needle biopsies by use of a trochar, or as cell suspensions. In all instances, a space is easily prepared either by surgical procedures or by the pressure of the throcar or the inoculated cell suspension. The area is richly vascularized so that blood supply and lymph drainage can be easily established. The free mobility of the skin allows an expansion over the growing tumor.

Mode of Growth
In the nude mouse, tumors implanted s.c. will in nearly all cases grow locally, encapsulated in a connective tissue capsule, thus mimicking the growth mode of benign tumors in humans. Only in rare instances have metastases been observed. In the SCID mouse, tumors will be locally invasive and a few weeks after implantation metastases can be demonstrated in the

peritoneum, spleen, lymph nodes, and lungs.[37] This difference in growth pattern between nude and SCID mouse is a striking feature that must be taken into consideration when choosing a heterotransplantation model. A recently identified nude mutant substrain on a partly BALB/c background allows a range of human malignant tumors to metastasize with a frequency close to that of SCID mice. This mutant is presently under study in our laboratory.

Regional Growth Differences

Tumors implanted into nude mice show pronounced regional growth rate differences. This fact was noticed also in murine tumors grown in their syngeneic hosts by Auerbach.[38] There seems to be a significant predeliction for tumor growth in the anterior (occipital) region of the mouse trunk as opposed to the posterior (caudal) region. Anterior tumors may grow 3 to 4 times as rapidly as posterior tumors. Also, there is a growth difference between tumors transplanted in the dorsal and ventral region, ventral tumors developing more rapidly than dorsal tumors. There are no differences between the right side and the left side of the mouse trunk. The reason for the difference in growth in the various regions is not known. Obviously, immunological factors cannot account for the difference. It is important to be aware of this phenomenon, particularly when comparing tumor sizes.

Age Dependent Differences in Tumor Take

Tumor grafts are more readily accepted in young animals than in older animals. It has been shown that cancer cell lines were accepted significantly more often in young compared to adult animals, and the maximum tumor size in young mice was found to be twice that in adult mice. In nude mice, lymphoid cells with T-cell markers are found with increasing frequency with age, but it is not clear whether this phenomenon accounts for the difference in take rate between young and old. The difference should be kept in mind when working with tumor transplantation in this model.

Tumorigenicity

Based on observations of extensive materials, it is obvious that some tumor types are extremely difficult to establish in nude mice, and also that several factors such as background strain of the mice, age of host, site of inoculation, addition of feeder cells with the implant, etc. may influence the outcome. This is of importance because tumorigenicity in nude mice is used as a characteristic of tumor cell lines, for instance in the American Tissue Culture Collection Catalogue, and also in oncogene studies. From what has been mentioned, it will be obvious that tumorigenicity in the unadulterated nude mouse is not an absolute value. A more well-defined model for tumorigenicity may be needed. The SCID mouse may actually represent a better tumorigenesis model, but at the present time evidence is still too scarce to allow final conclusions.

Monitoring Tumor Growth

Traditionally, the size of subcutaneously implanted tumors have been described by measurement with a slide caliper in two or in some instances three dimensions. There can be several objections to this. The measurement in only two dimensions (length x width) does not of course mathematically describe the volume of the tumor, but only the two measured dimensions. By using suitable formulas the two measurements can be transformed into an approximation of tumor volume. For discussion of this, see Reference 35.

TRANSGENIC ANIMAL MODELS

As mentioned above, mutations in the p53 tumor-suppressor gene are the most frequently observed genetic lesions in human cancers. The normal physiological role of the gene seems to be in the regulation of the cell cycle. Donehower et al.[39] introduced a null mutation into the

206

gene by homologous recombination in murine embryonic cells. Mice that are homozygous for the mutation appear normal, but they will develop a variety of neoplasms by 6 months of age. The authors conclude that the absence of the p53 gene predisposes to neoplastic disease, and further that an oncogenic mutant form of the p53 gene is not obligatory for the genesis of many types of tumors.

Tumors have been observed from the age of 8 weeks in these transgenic mice, and the spectrum is very wide, most tumors observed thus far being sarcomas. These mice, GenPharm® TSG-p53 transgenic mice, are now commercially available and may be of great interest in both toxicology and cancer research.

Heterozygous TSG-p53 are also available. They have a low spontaneous level of tumorigenesis, but a shorter latency period in carcinogenesis experiments compared to nontransgenic mice. It can be expected that several types of transgenic mice of interest to cancer research will appear in the years to come, probably supplying cancer research with more refined tools "than dreamt of in our philosophy".

DISCUSSION AND COMMENTS

Is it reasonable in a presentation of animal models in cancer research to focus so relatively narrow-mindedly on heterotransplantation models? In the author's opinion, they represent the closest approximation to the human situation when used with due consideration. Advantages and disadvantages are discussed extensively elsewhere.[40] After nearly 25 years in laboratory use, they have not given definitive clues to an overall understanding of cancer or to a miracle cure, nor has any other model or test system during the same period.

Just before this volume went to press, a paper appeared reporting a cure of xenografted human carcinomas by an immunoconjugate (BR96-DOX) between chimeric monoclonal antibody BR96, directed against Le^y antigen expressed on the surface of many human carcinomas, and the anticancer drug doxorubicin®. Complete regression was induced in xenografted human lung, breast, and colon carcinomas growing s.c. in athymic nude mice, and 70% of mice bearing extensive metastases of a human lung carcinoma were cured. Given to athymic rats with s.c. growth of human lung carcinoma, it cured 94%. This is remarkable since the rats, in contrast to mice, express the BR96 target antigen in their normal tissues.

ACKNOWLEDGMENTS

The experimental work in our laboratory underlying this presentation was supported by the Danish Medical Research Council, the Danish Cancer Society, Ejnar Willumsens Mindelegat, Meta & Håkon Baggers Legat, and Simon Spies Fonden. My son, Kåre Rygaard, cand. med., has been a helpful sparring partner during the preparation of the manuscript.

REFERENCES

1. Sivak, A., Chemical carcinogenesis, in *The Mouse in Medical Research, Vol. 4: Experimental Biology and Oncology,* Foster, H. L., Small, J. D. and Fox, J. G., Eds., Academic Press, New York, 1982, chp. 19.
2. Yamagiwa, K. and Ichikawa, K., Über die atypische Epithelwucherung, *Gann,* 11, 1914.
3. Pott, P., Chirurgical observations relative to the cataract, the polypus of the nose, the cancer of the scrotum, the different kinds of ruptures, and mortification of the toes and feet. Hawes, Clarke and Collins, London, 1775. Reprinted in: *Natl. Cancer Inst. Monograph,* 10, 7, 1963.
4. Kennaway, E. L., On the cancer-producing factor in tar. *Int. Med. J.,* 1, 564, 1924.
5. Berenblum, I., The cocarcinogenic action of croton resin. *Cancer Res.,* 1, 44, 1941.

6. Berenblum, I. and Shubik, P., A new, quantitative approach to the study of chemical carcinogenesis in mouse's skin. *Br. J. Cancer*, 1, 383, 1947.

7. Medina, D., Mammary tumors, in *The Mouse in Medical Research, Vol. 4: Experimental Biology and Oncology,* Foster, H. L., Small, J. D. and Fox, J. G., Eds., Academic Press, New York, 1982, chap. 21.

8. Murphy, E. D., Characteristic tumors, in *The Biology of the Laboratory Mouse*, Green, E. L., Ed., McGraw-Hill, New York, 1966, chap. 27.

9. Peckham, J. C., Experimental oncology, in *The Laboratory Rat, vol. II, Research Applications*. Baker, H. J., Lindsey, J. R. and Weisbroth, S. H., Eds., Academic Press, 1980, chap. 6.

10. Stehelin, D., Varmus, H. E., Bishop, J. M. and Vogt, P. K., DNA related to the transforming gene(s) of avian sarcoma viruses is present in normal avian DNA. *Nature*, 260, 170, 1976.

11. Levinson, A. D., Oppermann, H., Levintow, L., Varmus, H. E. and Bishop, J. M., Evidence that the transforming gene of avian sarcoma virus encodes a protein kinase associated with phosphorylation. *Cell*, 15, 561, 1978.

12. Shih, C., Padhy, L. C., Murray, M. and Weinberg, R. A., Transforming genes of carcinomas and neuroblastomas introduced into mouse fibroblasts. *Nature*, 290, 261, 1981.

13. Blair, D. G., Cooper, C. S., Oskarsson, M. K., Eader, L. A. and Vande Woude, G. F., New method for detecting cellular transforming genes. *Science*, 218, 1122, 1982.

14. Friend, S. H., Bernards, R., Rogelj, S., Weinberg, R. A., Rapaport, J. M., Albert, D. M. and Dryja, T. P., A human DNA segment with properties of the gene that predisposes to retinoblastoma and osteosarcoma. *Nature*, 323, 643, 1986.

15. Bishop. J. M., The molecular genetics of cancer, *Science*, 235, 305, 1987.

16. Greene, H. S. N. and Lund, P. K., The heterologous transplantation of human cancers, *Cancer Res.,* 4, 24, 1944.

17. Lutz, B. R., Fulton, G. P., Patt, D. I. and Handler, A. H., The growth rate of tumor transplants in the cheek pouch of the hamster (Mesocricetus auratus), *Cancer. Res.*, 10, 321, 1950.

18. Clemmesen, J., On transplantation of tumor cells to normal and pre-irradiated heterologous organisms, *Am. J. Cancer*, 29, 313, 1937.

19. Toolan, H. W., Growth of human tumors in cortisone-treated laboratory animals: The possibility of obtaining permanently transplantable human tumors. *Cancer Res.*, 13, 389, 1953.

20. Miller, J. F. A. P., Immunological function of the thymus. *Lancet,* 2, 748, 1961.

21. Langdon, S. P, and Smyth, J. F., Types of immunodeficiency in mice, in Boven, E. and Winograd, B. Eds. *The Nude Mouse in Oncology Research*. CRC Press, Boca Raton, Ann Arbor, Boston, London, 1991, chap. 2.

22. Pantelouris, E. M., Absence of thymus in a mouse mutant. *Nature,* 217, 370, 1968.

23. Rygaard, J. and Povlsen, C. O., Heterotransplantation of a a human malignant tumour to "nude" mice. *Acta Pathol. Microbiol. Scand.*, Sect. A, 77, 758, 1969.

24. Rygaard, J. Thymus and Self. *Immunobiology of the Mouse Mutant nude*. FADL, Copenhagen, 1973; John Wiley and Sons, London, 1975; Japanese ed. Tuttle-Mori, Tokyo, 1979.

25. Kiessling, R., Klein, E. and Wigzell, H., 'Natural' killer cells in the mouse. I. Cytotoxic cells with specificity for mouse Moloney leukemia cells. Specificity and distribution according to genotype. *Eur. J. Immunol.*, 5,112, 1975.

26. Herberman, R. B., Nunn, M. E. and Lavrin, D. H., Natural cytotoxic reactivity of mouse lymphoid cells against syngeneic an allogeneic tumors. Distribution of reactivity and specificity. *Int. J. Cancer*, 16, 216, 1975.

27. Burnet, F. M., *Immunological Surveillance*, Pergamon Press, Sydney, 1970.

28. Rygaard, J. and Povlsen, C. O., The nude mouse vs. the hypothesis of immunological surveillance. *Transplantat. Rev.,* 28, 43, 1976.

29. Schuurman, H.-J., Rozing, J., van Loveren, H., Vaessen, L. M, B, and Kampinga, J. The athymic nude rat. In Wu, B.-Q, and Zheng, J. Eds., *Immune-Deficient Animals in Experimental Medicine*. Karger, Basel, 54, 1989.

30. Hougen, H. P., *The athymic nude rat*. Thesis, Copenhagen. APMIS 99, Suppl. 21, 1991.
31. Roder, J. C., The *beige* mutation in the mouse. I. A stem cell predetermined impairment in natural killer cell function. *J. Immunol.*, 123, 2168, 1979.
32. Amsbaugh, D. F., Hansen, C. T., Prescott, B., Stashak, P. W., Barthold, D. R. and Baker, P. J., Genetic control of the antibody response to type III pneumococcal polysaccharide in mice. *J. Exp. Med.*, 136, 931, 1972.
33. Bosma, G. C., Custer, R. P. and Bosma, M. J., A severe combined immunodeficiency mutation in the mouse. *Nature*, 301, 527, 1983.
34. Mosier, D. E., Immunodeficient mice xenografted with human lymphoid cells: new models for in vivo studies of human immunobiology and infectious diseases. *J. Clin. Immunol.*, 10, 185, 1990.
35. Boven, E. and Winograd, B., Eds., *The Nude Mouse in Oncology Research*. CRC, Boca Raton, FL, 1991.
36. Rygaard, K., Sorenson, G. D., Pettengill, O. S., Cate, C. C. and Spang-Thomsen, M., Abnormalities in structure and expression of the retinoblastoma gene in small cell lung cancer cell lines and xenografts in nude mice. *Cancer Res.*, 50, 5312, 1990.
37. Xie, X., Brünner, N., Jensen, G., Albrectsen, J., Gotthardsen, B. and Rygaard, J., Comparative studies between nude and scid mice on the growth and metastatic behavior of xenografted human tumors. *Clin. Exp. Metastasis*, 10, 201, 1992.
38. Aurbach, R., Morrissey, L. W. and Sidky, Y. A., Regional differences in the incidence and growth of mouse tumors following intradermal or subcutaneous inoculation. *Cancer Res.*, 38, 1739, 1978.
39. Donehower, L. A., Harvey, M., Slagle, B. L., McArthur, M. J., Montgomery, C. A. Jr., Butel, J. S. and Bradley, A., Mice deficient for p53 are developmentally normal but susceptible to spontaneous tumours. *Nature*, 356, 215, 1992.
40. Trail, P. A., Willner, D., Lasch, S. J., Henderson, A. J., Hofstead, S., Casazza, A. M., Firestone, R. A., Hellström, I. and Hellström, K. E., Cure of xenografted human carcinomas by BR96-doxorubicin immunoconjugates, *Science*, 261, 212, 1993.

INDEX